Hairdressing for NVQ 1 and 2

BOB WOODHOUSE

In association with
City & Guilds

Hodder & Stoughton
A MEMBER OF THE HODDER HEADLINE GROUP

Orders: please contact Bookpoint Ltd, 130 Milton Park, Abingdon, Oxon OX14 4SB. Telephone: (44) 012354 827720, Fax: (44) 01235 400454. Lines are open from 9.00–6.00, Monday to Saturday, with a 24 hour message answering service.

British Library Cataloguing in Publication Data
A catalogue record for this title is available from The British Library

ISBN 0 340 773014

First published 2000
Impression number 10 9 8 7 6 5 4 3
Year 2005 2004 2003 2002

Typeset by Wearset, Boldon, Tyne & Wear
Printed in Italy for Hodder & Stoughton Educational, a division of Hodder Headline Plc, 338 Euston Road, London NW1 3BH by Printer Trento.

Contents

Acknowledgements

Hairdressing And Beauty Industry Authority

The publishers would like to acknowledge the Hairdressing and Beauty Industry Authority (HABIA) for the development of the NVQ and SVQ at levels 1, 2 and 3.

The authors and publishers would like to acknowledge the following photographic sources.

The author and publishers would like to acknowledge the assistance of West Kent College, Tonbridge, Kent in providing facilities for the following photographs.

Photographer: David Guy Technical Director: Bob Woodhouse Figures 2.2, 2.3, 2.4, 2.5, 2.6, 2.7, 2.8, 2.9, 2.10, 2.11, 2.12, 2.15, 3.2, 3.3, 3.4, 3.5, 3.6, 3.7, 3.8, 3.9, 3.10, 3.11, 3.12, 3.13e, 4.1a, 4.3a, 4,31, 4.32, 4.33, 5A.7, 5A.13, 5A.17, 5A.18, 5A.19, 5A.20, 5A.21, 5A.22, 5A.23, 5A.24, 5A.25, 5A.26, 5A.27, 5A.31, 5A.32, 5A.33, 5A.34, 5A.35, 5A.36, 5A.37, 5A.38, 5A.39, 5A.40, 5A.43, 5A.46, 6.39, 6.40, 6.41, 6.42, 6.43, 6.44, 6.45, 6.46, 6.47, 6.48, 9.1, 11.1, 11.2, 11.4, 11.6, 11.7, 11.8, 11.13, 11.38, 11.47, 11.52, 11.54, 11.58, 12.1, 12.2, 12.3, 12.4, 12.5, 12.6, 12.9, 12.10, 12.13, 12.14, 12.15, 12.22, 12.24, 12.31, 13.3, 13.4, 13.5, 13.6, 13.7, 13.8, 13.9, 13.10, 13.12, 13.13, 13.15, 13.17, 13.18, 13.19, 13.20, 13.21, 13.22, 13.23, 13.24, 13.25, 13.26, 13.29, 13.30, 13.31, 13.32, 13.34 and 13.36.

The following photographs originally appeared in *Milady's Standard Textbook of Cosmetology*, © 1994 Milady Publishing Company (A Division of Delmar Publishers Inc.) Photographers: Michael A. Gallitelli, Steven Landis, Eric Von Lockhart, Gillette Research Institute, New Image's Salon System.

Figures on page 14 and page 15, and Figures 3.13a, 3.13b, 3.13c, 4.2, 4.3, 4.4, 4.5, 4.6, 4.7, 4.8, 4.9, 4.12, 5A.1, 5A.9, 5A.10a, 5A.10b, 5A.10c, 5A.10d, 5A.41, 5A.44, 5A.45, 5B.2, 5B.10, 5B.3, 5B.6, 5B.7, 5B.9, 5B.10, 5B.11, 6.1a, 6.1b, 6.2, 6.3, 6.4, 6.9, 6.11, 6.13, 6.14, 6.15, 6.16, 6.19, 6.26, 6.28, 6.29, 6.30, 6.33, 6.34, 6.35, 6.49, 7.1, 7.2, 8.1, 9.2, 11.28, 11.29, 11.30, 11.31, 11.32, 14.8, 14.11, 14.12, 14.13 and 14.28.

Additional photographs as follows: Price Associates: Figures 5B.12, 5B.13, 5B.14, 13.27 and 13.28 David Sparrow: Figure 4.1b West Kent College: Figure 3.13c The National Medical Slide Bank/The Wellcome Trust: Figures 14.16, 14.17, 14.18, 14.19, 14.20, 14.27 and 14.29.

If any acknowledgement has been inadvertently omitted, the omission will be rectified at the earliest possible oportunity.

About this book

To the student

This book will provide you with the essential knowledge required to help you acquire the skills necessary for professional ladies' and men's hair-dressing. Within this is the underpinning knowledge needed to help you achieve the current National Vocational Qualification or Scottish Vocational Qualification (NVQ or SVQ) at Levels 1 and 2. Within each chapter you will be provided with information and instructions on how to acquire practical skills. Colour illustrations will help you to understand the practical tasks. Each chapter also includes questions that you may use to test yourself (with model answers in chapter 15) and check your learning, together with suggestions for tasks to further your learning and help you to demonstrate competence.

You may use the whole of this book, or you may follow those sections that apply to your current needs, at the appropriate level. On pages 307–312 is a 'skill check' you may use this to identify your existing skills and direct you to those areas that require development. The skill check may be copied for your personal use to chart your progress, and will provide evidence of your personal professional development in your job role.

To the trainer/lecturer

This book is designed to support the emerging hairdresser and may be used as a support to a structured programme of delivery, both as a course textbook and as a reference text. It will facilitate the flexible candidate-centred ethos of Vocational Qualifications by enabling those whose preferred style of learning is self-supported study to work at their own pace, providing the necessary underpinning knowledge together with instruction in how to exercise hairdressing skills. This book will enable the student to achieve a basic grasp of these skills. For those candidates who follow a more formalised style of directed learning, this book provides reference points as well as both visual and text direction in how to carry out hairdressing tasks.

The Personal Skill Check (see page 307) may be used by the candidate to identify any previously acquired learning and to chart and review progress towards developing skills and understanding. This chart may be photocopied for multiple use by the owner of this book.

THE WORLD OF HAIRDRESSING

Welcome to the profession of hairdressing. Hairdressing offers you a career of variety which can reflect your own particular personality and creative ability. This profession is dynamic: it is fashion-related and, as innovative concepts and techniques are continually being introduced, you will never stop learning and developing your skills to fit your job role. Hairdressing is a profession in which you can move from one focus to another and in which one experience can open new doors to another. There are opportunities which make use of:

- creative artistic skills – hairstylist, artistic director, platform artist, photographic session hairdresser, theatrical/television/film hairstylist

- social caring skills – hairstylist, hospital-based hairstylist, wig fitter
- technical/scientific skills – trichologist, technical demonstrator/representative, product tester, researcher
- commercial skills – business manager, personnel manager, retailer, merchandiser, sales representative, hairstylist, wig fitter
- educational skills – hairdressing teacher/trainer, hairdressing skills assessor, product demonstrator, training/assessment coordinator
- ancillary skills – wigmaker, wig fitter/dresser, hair implanter, manicurist, beautician, receptionist.

Many of those opportunities listed above require a foundation of basic hairdressing skills, and these skills must be learned and practised often enough to become automatic responses to particular situations. This dedication to learning is essential in becoming a professional with professional skill levels (remember: the learning process never ends).

The National/Scottish Vocational Qualification provides the opportunity to develop and extend your skills and to gain recognition for these.

The skills recognised may be those directly related to the technical skills of hairdressing. They may also include supportive skills of management and/or customer service.

As a hairdresser you will be responsible for the way people look and feel. You must enjoy working with people, both as a member of a team and as an individual with your client. The skills of hairdressing are used throughout the world and therefore as a qualified professional you may enjoy the opportunity to work world-wide.

Hairstylist

The hairstylist may find employment in a variety of commercial situations. There are many opportunities within hairdressing salons of differing types, often catering for differing customer bases.

- There are high street salons within most cities, towns and villages. In-store salons are often found within larger department stores. Some are single salons, but there are groups of salons owned by one company, and there are groups of salons which, while individually owned, work together as groups for mutual business benefits. Franchise salons trade individually through the guidance of the named franchise service.
- A freelance hairstylist may operate as a home visiting service, styling his or her clients' hair in their own homes, or may offer professional services within a salon.
- Large businesses often employ residential hairstylists for their staff.
- The leisure industry often incorporates hairdressing within hotels, airports and airlines and fitness/leisure centres.
- The care sector frequently incorporates hairdressing services – appreciating the benefits of hairdressing to the well-being of its patients and those for which they care.

Hairstylists may specialise in a particular style of work or cover a wide range in either or both ladies' and men's hairstyling. There are opportunities as a hairstylist to travel:

- As a technical demonstrator for a product manufacturer, demonstrating to and training either the public or other professionals.
- As a hairstylist on board cruise ships, which have hairdressing and beauty facilities for their guests.
- As a resident hairstylist for a theatrical/show company.

Colour/perm specialist

The technology linked with chemical processes, including hair colouring and perming, is wide ranging. In many larger salons or salon groups there are often specialists performing these chemical procedures. These specialists have a high degree of knowledge and skill in the service offered. They would not usually have their own client base, but would offer their skills to all of the salon's clients.

Most hairdressing product manufacturing houses employ specialists to demonstrate and teach the use of their products.

Receptionist

The smooth running of the day-to-day business of the hairdressing salon depends largely on the correct control and direction of the client base. Correct reception procedures include the phasing of appointments to maximise use of the salon's staff team and avoid delays in clients' time. The receptionist is often the first point of contact with the salon for the client, either via the telephone or face to face, therefore giving that 'first impression' to the potential client. Receptionists may be asked about the services and products used and sold by the salon, and asked for guidance on their suitability. Should there be a problem or a delay for the client it is often the receptionist who will handle this or will be responsible for directing the client to someone who can help and advise. At the end of the visit it is usually the receptionist who deals with payment by the client and arranges for follow-up appointments.

Retail/merchandising specialist

Retail sales of hair care and ancillary products require specialist skills. Product wholesalers often employ specialists to maintain retail merchandising stands. Knowledge of the features and benefits of products is required, as well as skill in sales techniques and display. Usually sales skills are more important than skills and knowledge of hairdressing, as the features and benefits of a product may be learned by a sales person.

Beautician

The beautician complements the work of the hairstylist in enhancing the appearance of the client, and beauty treatment is often included as a service offered in the hairdressing context. Beauty services include facial treatments, cleansing, massage and make-up as well as manicure and pedicure. This role does not necessarily require a knowledge of or skill in hairdressing, but the ability to offer both hairdressing and beautician skills can be an employment advantage.

Trainer/educator

Passing your skill and knowledge on to others can be very rewarding. This can take the form of teaching those who are new to the profession and are learning basic skills, or working with experienced hairdressers who wish to update their skills or to learn how to perform a specific task.

Trainer/educators are employed in colleges and hairdressing schools and in manufacturers' training centres, where they work with groups of people learning hairdressing techniques. Some salon chains have their own trainers who undertake the training of their staff either by visiting the individual salons, or by the staff attending a school.

Technical representatives, working for product manufacturers, may visit individual salons to undertake training in the use of their company's products. In addition to hairdressing experience and qualifications, a teaching or training qualification is desirable.

Salon owner/manager/director

While owning a hairdressing business does not require hairdressing skills, it will be a considerable advantage to have a knowledge of hairdressing, and for an owner/stylist this will be essential. As well as hairdressing skills, skills of business management including planning, budgeting, personnel management and knowledge of relevant legislation are all desirable when taking on this role. As a salon owner you would have a high level of control over the direction of the business, and as a manager you might be responsible for the running of the business within the framework of the requirements of the business owner. As a director of a company you would have a say in the direction of the business, in consultation with other directors.

Qualifications

There is a raft of currently applicable qualifications for the hairdresser. National Vocational Qualifications and Scottish Vocational Qualifications focus upon a person's ability to perform a task or range of tasks to a competent standard and their relevant knowledge and understanding. They are achieved by demonstrating the ability to perform tasks competently in a range of situations.

Level 1 Hairdressing

For those undertaking hairdressing activity supporting others. For example shampooing, contributing to reception, perming, colouring and relaxing hair.

Level 2 Hairdressing

For those undertaking a range of basic hairdressing skills to a competent level. These skills may be either ladies or mens hairdressing or both. These skills include haircutting, styling, colouring, perming and relaxing. For men's hairdressing it can include shaping facial hair and shaving.

Level 3 Hairdressing

For those undertaking a range of advances hairdressing skills as well as training, assessing hairdressing skills, promotional work and/or supervisory aspects.

Level 4 Management

For practising managers with responsibility for: allocating work, achieving specific results, carrying out policy, controlling limited financial budgets and contributing to recruitment and guiding change.

Level 4 Business Management and Development

For owner managers who undertake business planning, manage finance, renew business performance, develop marketing plans for their business.

National Standards

A government report 'Education and training working together' (1985) resulted in the introduction of National Vocational Qualifications and Scottish Vocational Qualifications. These qualifications are based on National Standards of competence that are relevant to a particular industry or sector.

National Standards for Hairdressing indicate the standard of competent performance, knowledge and understanding that is expected of someone working within hairdressing. To ensure that these National Standards remain relevant to the industry that they serve, they are reviewed regularly.

National Training Organisations

As the Industry Training Organisation for Hairdressing – the Hairdressing Training Board (HTB) has the responsibility for developing training for hairdressing. The Hairdressing Training Board is part of the National Training Organisation (NTO) Hairdressing and Beauty Industry Authority (HABIA), NTO's have a strategic role in identifying current and future skill needs and assuring that arrangements are in place for meeting those skill needs. The authors acknowledge the role and contribution that the NTO has played in these standards.

Achieving NVQ or SVQ

NVQs and SVQs are achieved by demonstrating that you are competent within your job role and that you have the knowledge and understanding of the principles and practices which underpin these skills. The National Standards define what the job role is; they determine which tasks are normally undertaken by a person within that role (units) and then separate each task into its component stages (elements). Each element describes an activity that is judged against performance criteria; that is, how someone should carry out that activity. It may be necessary to prove competence within the activity in a range of situations or variables.

Competence is the ability to undertake a task to the standards which are expected of that industry.

To prove competence, knowledge and understanding against these National Standards you must produce evidence; that is, something that proves you can do what you claim. The most effective way of providing such proof is to undertake the activity within a real client–hairdresser situation and this can be observed by a qualified assessor who is also a competent hairdresser. This is by far the most effective method of proving competence. For limited areas it may be possible to simulate a real event, in place of an actual client–hairdresser activity. This can be done when demonstrating competence in areas which rarely occur or in which when they do occur there is an element of risk. This is not usually acceptable for hairdressing styling skills.

It is not always possible for an assessor to observe every task within all the variables required and in those cases it may be necessary for you to provide alternative evidence of your performance for assessment by the assessor. These alternatives may include your personal statement or description of the process undertaken, actual forms/record cards completed by you, testimony by others (possibly your client, a colleague, an employer or supervisor), or projects or assignments which are a collection of various forms of evidence. If you have existing hairdressing or other relevant qualifications, or have undertaken previous training or have previous relevant experience it may be possible to present this as evidence. Any evidence must prove competence that is current and must be relevant to the National Standards being proven.

In some cases, when it has not been appropriate to demonstrate competence through your own performance, whether it is observed by an assessor or not, competence may be proven by producing evidence of potential capability subject to agreement with your assessment centre.

Records of assessment and other evidence being used to prove competence, knowledge and understanding are presented, for certification, in the form of a portfolio. This is the collection of evidence, indexed and cross-referenced to the National Standards.

Note. Those who wish to pursue an NVQ or SVQ are recommended to discuss and plan their evidence collection and presentation with their assessor, each awarding body and assessment centre will have their own specific requirements, though all will work within the same National Standards framework.

As a candidate working towards the achievement of a National/Scottish Vocational Qualification it is your responsibility to present evidence assessment. When you consider yourself ready for assessment you should discuss this with your allocated assessor. Your assessor will support you in determing if you are ready for a formative or summative assessment.

You will be guided towards the suitability of forms of evidence and/or tasks undertaken in relation to the Units/Elements that you wish to achieve. With your assessor you will agree a plan for assessment that will confirm: the evidence to be presented; the task to be undertaken which the evidence will confirm; the elements of the NVQ\SVQ against which the evidence will be judged; the timescale for the assessment; agreed review dates.

During this planning process you should feel free to contribute your thoughts regarding how you will prove your competence. Each assessment centre will have procedures to follow if agreement cannot be made.

Remember – it is your role to present evidence of competence – your assessor will provide you with support, guidance and encouragement to undertake this in a manner that is acceptable to the Awarding Body.

HOW TO USE THIS BOOK

You may read this textbook starting from the beginning or you may use it as a source of essential knowledge and a training manual by locating the particular skill that you require, either through the index or by using the cross-referencing grid that is included in this section.

The main topics of each chapter of the book are listed in the centre column of the grid, and by reading the columns to either side you will find the location of the supporting information. Each chapter is cross referenced to aid access. The column to the left will guide you to the location of Level 1 material, the column to the right to Level 2. Level 1 material is indicated throughout by a

■ in the margin and by the tinted yellow text alongside (blue in boxed text). All material in the book is useful to those of you following Level 2.

The review questions and further study sections at the end of each chapter will help you to produce evidence of competence in essential knowledge and understanding. Discuss them with your assessor.

Chapter 14, 'The Hair and Scalp' will provide you with essential knowledge about the hair and skin. The model answers contained in chapter 15 are there for you to confirm correct responses to the review questions. Use them wisely, and remember that you only fool yourself if you claim to be more knowledgeable than you really are. Model answers are best used to confirm correct responses, not as a means to quick learning, as they cover only a limited range of the essential knowledge.

Your own Personal Skill Check, on pages 307–312, will enable you to review your progress from the beginning of your programme of study through to the achievement of your chosen award. You may make a single photocopy of pages 307–312 for your own use, so that you may review your progress regularly. This will help you to identify your existing competence and to identify when you are ready for assessment, where you still need practice and where you need training. This Skill Check will also prompt you to identify how you can prove your competence in any particular skill.

Level 1	Topic	Level 2	
	Introduction, ⇓ The world of hairdressing, ⇓ Career opportunities.		
	Level 1 ⇔ Level 2 Common information ⇓		
Unit 104	Client care procedures ⇓	Unit 201 Unit 203	Unit 207 Unit 208
Unit 101 Unit 104	Shampooing & conditioning ⇓	Unit 201 Unit 202 Unit 205A	Unit 205B Unit 206 Unit 209
Unit 101 Unit 104 Unit 105	Drying hair into shape ⇓	Unit 201 Unit 203	Unit 209 Unit 213
	Hair cutting ⇓	Unit 201 Unit 204	Unit 209 Unit 210
Unit 101 Unit 102A/B Unit 104 Unit 105	Permanent waving ⇓	Unit 201 Unit 202 Unit 205A/B	Unit 208 Unit 209
Unit 101 Unit 102B Unit 104 Unit 105	Relaxing hair ⇓	Unit 201 Unit 202 Unit 205B	Unit 208 Unit 209
Unit 101 Unit 102A/B Unit 104 Unit 105	Hair colouring ⇓	Unit 201 Unit 202 Unit 206	Unit 208 Unit 209
Unit 103 Unit 104	Customer reception ⇓	Unit 201 Unit 207	Unit 208 Unit 209
Unit 103 Unit 104 Unit 105	Working with others ⇓	Unit 201 Unit 208 Unit 209	
Unit 104 Unit 105	Effective use of resources ⇓	Unit 209	
Unit 105	Health & Safety ⇓	Unit 209	
	Setting & Dressing Hair ⇓	Unit 201 Unit 203 Unit 209	
	Barbering skills ⇓	Unit 201 Unit 203 Unit 204 Unit 208 Unit 209	Unit 210 Unit 211 Unit 212 Unit 213
	Shaving & massage ⇓	Unit 201 Unit 209	Unit 211 Unit 212
Unit 105	Hair & scalp ⇓	Unit 201 Unit 202	
	Your personal skill check		

CHAPTER 1

Client care procedures

This section will provide the essential knowledge to help you understand the skills used in client care, and will help you to be aware of the need for consultation and negotiation in satisfying your clients' requirements.

Level 1	
Element 104.1	Develop effective working relationships with clients
Element 104.2	Develop effective working relationships with colleagues
Element 104.3	Develop self within job role
Level 2	
Element 201.1	Consult with and maintain effective working relationships with clients
Element 201.2	Advise clients on salon products and services
Element 201.3	Advise clients on after-care procedures
Element 203.2	Dry and finish hair to style
Element 205.3	Set and dress hair to style
Element 207.1	Attend to clients and enquiries
Element 208.1	Develop and maintain effective team work and relationships with colleagues

Contents

INTRODUCTION

The quality of service and care provided throughout the entire hairdressing experience is a major factor in satisfying a client. Compare your own reaction, when you visit a business where you receive an attentive, courteous service and are kept aware of what the process is that you will experience, to your feelings when you visit a similar category of business where you are treated without courtesy, and are not kept informed about what the process is or how long it should take.

All members of the hairdressing team should be responsible for customer care, no matter what level they are at within the business.

COMMUNICATION

You will not be able to satisfy your client's needs if you do not, in the first place, establish what those needs are. Without understanding them you will be unable to establish a personal action plan to achieve in the most efficient manner.

1 Your style of communication with the client should establish a professional and caring relationship with them. The exact style you use will differ according to the individual client, the hairdresser/stylist and the salon procedures. At all times you must be courteous, friendly and professional towards your client. The novice hairdresser must take care to maintain this approach to the client at all times, no matter what their own personal feelings. Do not air your stresses or personal grievances with or in front of the client. If you have any problems with your work in the salon discuss this with your trainer/tutor/manager at a mutually agreed time, where confidential guidance and rational discussion may take place.

Salon procedures may determine how your client is addressed; if you use clients' first names, you need to decide how to greet a client whose name you do not know (a new client). Ensure that you are fully aware of any of your salon's guidelines for client approach. Ask your trainer/tutor/manager for guidance if you are unsure. You should ensure that your clients can understand your style of speech (pace, vocabulary or accent). If you have a communication disadvantage make arrangements to ensure effective communication with your clients. Discuss this with your trainer/tutor/manager.

Never assume that the client understands your communication. Check for signs indicating a lack of comprehension; these will typically include a vague or quizzical expression on the client's face, and a lack of response. If you feel that the client has not understood what you are trying to say be prepared to spend a little time to discuss it with them. Remember some clients may have communication difficulties: these may include hearing, language and sight limitations and lack of attention.

> ***TIP*** Unless you are aware of your client's wishes you will not be able to work towards satisfying them. Communication is the key.

You must inform your client about any delay or disruption in the hairdressing process. The reason for the delay or disruption and the implications for your client's treatment should be explained to them, in understandable terms. Give your client a realistic view of how long a delay is likely to be; discuss options with your client, such as alternative appointments, alternative hairstylists or alternatives to sitting waiting. Should the delay or disruption be known about in advance your client may be contacted and alternatives suggested, therefore preventing confrontation within the salon. Remember that your client may have a tight time schedule and disruption, if notified far enough in advance, can often be accommodated, provided that it is not a regular occurrence.

CLIENT CONSULTATION

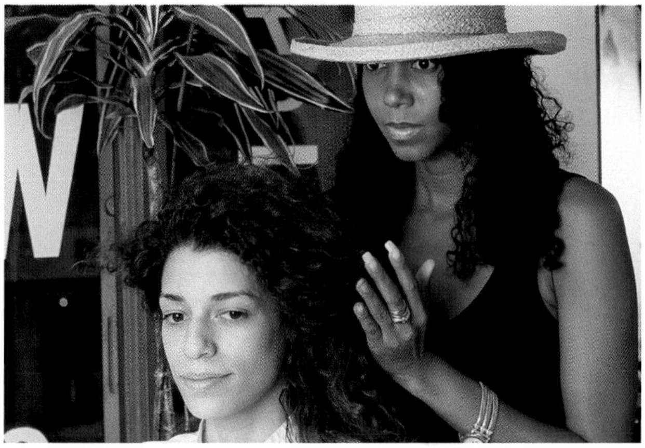

Consultation with your client will enable you to identify any factors that may limit or affect the services and products that you use. This is the opportunity to determine the most suitable techniques, products and equipment to enable you to create the agreed effect, and that both hair and scalp are suitable for these intended treatments.

Effective communication between you and your client is essential before beginning the hairdressing process, to ensure that your client's wishes are met. The use of style books, photographs, fashion magazines, computerised style viewers and wigs can help as aids to understanding proposed outcomes. Your consultation will normally take place when both you and your client are seated, facing each other, discussing their wishes with regard to their chosen hairstyle.

You as the hairstylist will consider the suitability of the requested treatment and hairstyle for the client. Here is a list of critical influencing factors and questions to ask yourself:

- your client's life style
- does the hair style fit the client's employment requirements?
- does the client's face and head shape suit the requested hairstyle?
- does the client's haircut suit the requested hairstyle?
- does the texture and length of the hair suit the requested hairstyle?
- are there any hair growth patterns that may adversely affect the required hairstyle?
- are there any previous chemical treatments remaining in the hair?

> ***TIP*** Failure to consult effectively with your client may result in loss of business to your salon, damage to your client's hair and scalp, and failure to fulfil your client's wishes.

There may be occasions when the style/treatment requested by your client is not, in your opinion, achievable on, or suitable for the client. Your negotiation skills will be required to counsel and guide your client towards a more suitable choice. You will need to be honest and sincere, and objective enough to justify your statements to your clients.

Records of previous consultations and services given to your client should be viewed, enabling you to check on previous products used and outcomes. Many salons maintain a written record of clients and their consultations/treatments. This will usually take the form of alphabetically indexed cards containing information about previous findings and the products used on the client, the dates of use and the outcomes of these services. There are computerised customer information systems available, offering the same facility as the written record, but often making retrieval of the information much easier and more rapid. Maintaining these client records will provide a reference should a customer complain at a later stage. It will also help to ensure continuity when a previous treatment is to be repeated. The information contained in client records should be considered confidential (refer to Data Protection Act 1998 page 185). Many salons have a policy that your client may not have access to this information. Check with your trainer/tutor/manager for advice on this before giving out information.

> ***TIP*** Remember, your client must feel that they can trust your judgement and guidance. Honest recommendations and advice on additional services will produce repeat business from clients who want you to guide them in their purchase. Your clients will buy their hair care products from the salon with your guidance rather than from retail outlets who are unable to offer professional advice.

Always consider additional services that will enhance the finished look and make maintenance of that look easier and more realistic for your client. Your client will look to you, as their hairstylist, for advice and guidance about their look and about which additional services, such as colour or permanent wave, may enhance this look. Hair colour may be used to improve the overall look of the hair, or to accentuate features of a particular hairstyle. The use of permanent waves or straighteners may help in the style retention and enable certain fashion effects to be achieved. Your client may not fully appreciate the effect that these additions to the service may have, so suggestions from hairstylists are an important part of their responsibility towards clients. While these additional services may cost the client more, they will be justified provided they add to client satisfaction and their appearance.

Your professional ability will be reflected in the finished look and its ease of maintenance.

> ***TIP*** Remember, if your client has confidence in your professional ability they will more readily accept your advice in these matters. This confidence will be developed by a professional approach to your work, your apparent knowledge and confidence in decision making and in the hairstyles produced on previous clients. All discussions and information given to you by your client should be considered confidential to your salon and not discussed with other clients or those outside the salon.

After-care products for home use, may be suggested at this stage. You should explain their features and benefits to your client and give guidance about particular products and how they should be used. These products will include haircare with shampoos and conditioners. Styling and finishing products, hair ornamentation and personal haircare tools, including heated tongs, brushes etc. should be included. As a professional you will be able to guide your client towards the appropriate items for their particular needs. To be able to do this you must be fully conversant with all retail products available from your salon, their features and benefits.

Having completed your pre-service consultation confirm the decisions with your client, explain to them what the process will be, in understandable terms, give an indication of the time that this will take and the actual cost to your client of this treatment.

Keep a record of products used on your clients and those that your clients purchase for after-care. This will provide you with guidance on future visits. Some salons record these details on 'treatment plans' a copy of which is given to your client and a copy retained by the salon.

Consultation is a continuous process while working with the client. Throughout the hairdressing process you, the stylist, will consult with the client about their wishes. Watch the client for signs of discomfort or agitation, which may indicate dissatisfaction with the process so far, if this becomes apparent discuss this with the client. In order for you to deal with a problem you
must first of all be fully aware of what the problem is. Should your client express a concern that is 1
beyond your responsibility, excuse yourself from the client, and discretely inform your supervisor of the situation. The client may require confirmation of the progress towards completion, they may require reassurance that the requested result can be achieved, they may have changed their mind about the required outcome or they may be experiencing physical discomfort. It is important to solve these problems as soon as possible to prevent them becoming barriers in communication. For complex problems, deal with each aspect of the problem individually rather than attempting to deal with it all in one.

> ***TIP*** Your salon may provide each client with a written record of their consultation, treatment plan and after-care regime. This can be an effective communication tool and support your client in maintaining their look.

HAIR ANALYSIS

Much of your time, as a hairdresser, is taken up with servicing and styling clients' hair. For this reason, you should be able to recognise the condition and types of hair and be able to analyse them.

Condition of the hair

Knowledge of hair and skill in determining its condition can be acquired by constant observation using the senses available to you: sight, touch, hearing and smell.

- **Sight.** Observing the hair will immediately give you some knowledge about its condition. Being able to look at hair is a major factor in its analysis, and touching the hair is the final determining factor.
- **Touch.** Hairdressers are guided by the touch or feel of the hair in making a professional hair analysis. When the senses of touch is fully developed, fewer mistakes will be made, by you, in judging the hair.
- **Hearing.** Listen to what your clients tell you about their hair, health problems, reactions to cosmetics and medications they might be taking. You will be in a better position to analyse the condition more accurately.
- **Smell.** Unclean hair and certain scalp disorders create an odour. If your client generally is healthy, you might suggest regular shampooing and proper rinsing.

Qualities of the hair

Qualities by which human hair is analysed are *texture, porosity* and *elasticity.*

> ***TIP*** Be aware of hair skin and scalp conditions that may preclude hairdressing treatments. Refer to Chapter 14 for further information.

Texture

Hair texture refers to the degree of coarseness or fineness of the hair (thick or thin), which may vary on different parts of the head. Variations in hair texture are due to:

- *Diameter of the hair,* whether coarse, medium, fine or very fine. Coarse hair has the greatest diameter; very fine hair has the smallest.
- *Feel of the hair,* whether harsh, soft or wiry: usually determined by the condition of its outer layer.

Medium hair is the normal type most commonly seen in the salon. This type of hair does not present any special problem. *Fine* or *very fine hair* requires special care. Its microscopic structure usually reveals that only two layers, the cortex and cuticle, are present. *Wiry hair,* whether coarse, medium, or fine, has a hard, glassy finish caused by the cuticle scales lying flat against the hair shaft. It takes longer for chemicals such as permanent wave solutions, tints, or lighteners to penetrate this type of hair.

Porosity

Hair porosity is the ability of all types of hair to absorb moisture (*hygroscopic quality*). Hair has *high porosity* when the cuticle layer is raised from the hair shaft and easily absorbs moisture and chemicals. *Medium porosity* (normal hair) is most often seen in the salon. Usually hair with moderate porosity presents no problem when receiving hair services, whether permanent waving, hair tinting or lightening. *Low porosity* (resistant hair) exists when the cuticle layer is lying close to the hair shaft and absorbs the least amount of moisture. *Uneven porosity* is when there are areas of uneven porosity along the hair's length or on differing areas of the head. This can result in an uneven absorption of chemicals into the hair and may produce an uneven result. A range of pre-chemical treatments are available that will aid in evening the hair's porosity along its length. Hair with other than moderate porosity requires thorough analysis and strand tests before the application of hair cosmetics.

Elasticity

Hair elasticity is the ability of hair to stretch and return to its original form without breaking. Hair can be classified as having high levels of elasticity, normal levels of elasticity and low levels of elasticity. (Refer to the section on permanent waving for more information.) Hair with normal elasticity is springy and has a lively lustrous appearance. Normal hair, when dry, is capable of being stretched by about 20% of its length; it springs back when released. Wet hair can be stretched 40% to 50% of its length. Porous hair stretches more easily than resistant hair, though it may have a low level of elasticity, as once stretched it often does not return to its original form.

HAIR GROWTH PATTERNS

The direction of hair growth will have an effect upon the hairstyle recommended to the client. As a general rule hairstyles will remain in place longer if they follow or go with the direction of hair growth. There are times when additional height can be achieved by styling the hair against this direction.

Strong directions of hair growth, including *nape whorls* and *double crowns* will require special consideration to reduce the adverse effect that they can have on the finished hairstyle. Often additional hair length is required to reduce this effect.

Direction of hair growth, page 282

HEAD AND FACE SHAPES

The best results are obtained when each of your clients facial features are properly analysed for strengths and shortcomings. Your job is to accentuate a client's best features and play down features that do not add to the person's attractiveness.

You must develop the ability to recommend hairstyles for your clients. Each client deserves a hairstyle that is properly proportioned to their body type, is correctly balanced to their head and facial features, and frames their face to its best advantage. The essentials of artistic and suitable hairstyles are based on the following general characteristics:

- Shape of the head: front view (face shape), profile, and back view.
- Characteristics of features: perfect as well as imperfect features, defects, or blemishes.
- Body structure, posture, and poise.

Hair structures, page 279

Facial types

Each client's facial shape is determined by the position and the prominence of the facial bones. There are seven facial shapes: oval, round, square, oblong, pear-shaped, heart-shaped, and diamond-shaped. To recognise each facial shape and to be able to give correct advice, you should be acquainted with the outstanding characteristics of each.

The face is divided into three areas: forehead to eyebrows, eyebrows to end of nose, and end of nose to bottom of chin. When creating a style for a client, you will be trying to create the illusion that each client has the ideal face shape (see Figure 1.1).

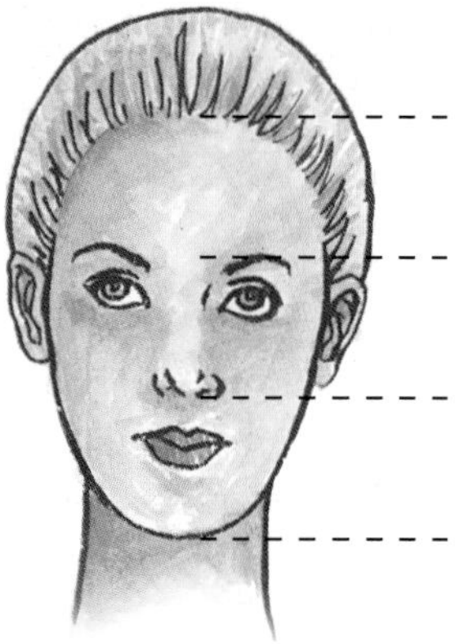

Figure 1.1 Ideal face proportions

Oval facial type

The oval-shaped face is generally recognised as the ideal shape. The contour and proportions of the face form the basis for modifying all other facial shapes.
Facial contour: The oval face is about 1.5 times longer than its width across the brow. The forehead is slightly wider than the chin.

Special considerations, page 13

A person with an oval-shaped face can wear any hairstyle unless there are other considerations, such as spectacles, length and shape of nose, or profile (see Figure 1.2).

Round facial type

Facial contour: Round hairline and round chin line; wide face.

Aim: To create the illusion of length to the face.

Create a hairstyle with height by arranging the hair on top of the head. You can place some over the ears and cheeks, but it is also appropriate to keep the hair up on one side, leaving the ears exposed. Style the fringe to one side (see Figure 1.3).

Square facial type

Facial contour: Straight hairline and square jawline; wide face.

Aim: To create the illusion of length; offset the square features. The problems of the square facial type are similar to the round facial type. The style should lift off the forehead and come forward at the temples and jaw, creating the illusion of narrowness and softness in the face. Asymmetrical hairstyles work well (see Figure 1.4).

Pear-shaped facial type

Facial contour: Narrow forehead, wide jaw and chin line.

Aim: To create the illusion of width in the forehead.

Build a hairstyle that is fairly full and high. Cover the forehead partially with a fringe of soft

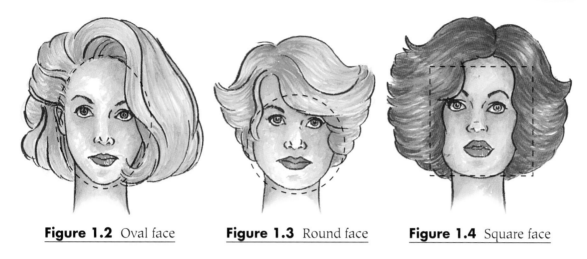

Figure 1.2 Oval face

Figure 1.3 Round face

Figure 1.4 Square face

hair. The hair should be worn with a soft curl or wave effect dressed over the ears. This arrangement adds apparent width to the forehead (see Figure 1.5).

Diamond facial type

Facial contour: Narrow forehead, extreme width through the cheekbones, and narrow chin.

Aim: To reduce the width across the cheekbone line.

Increasing the fullness across the jawline and forehead while keeping the hair close to the head at the cheekbone line helps create an oval appearance. Avoid hairstyles that lift away from the cheeks or move back from the hairline (see Figure 1.6).

Heart-shaped facial type

Facial contour: Wide forehead and narrow chin line.

Aim: To decrease the width of the forehead and increase the width in the lower part of the face.

To reduce the width of the forehead, a centre parting with the fringe flipped up or a style slanted to one side is recommended. Add width and softness at the jawline (see Figure 1.7).

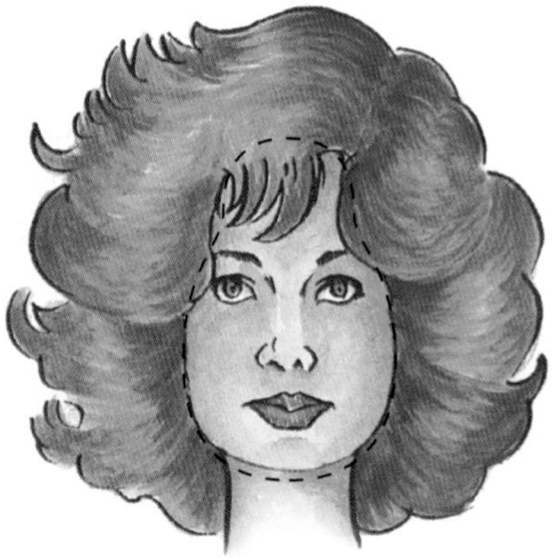

Figure 1.5 Pear-shaped face

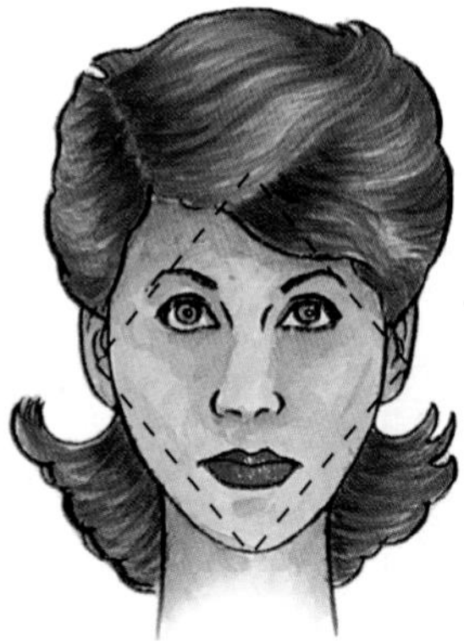

Figure 1.6 Diamond face

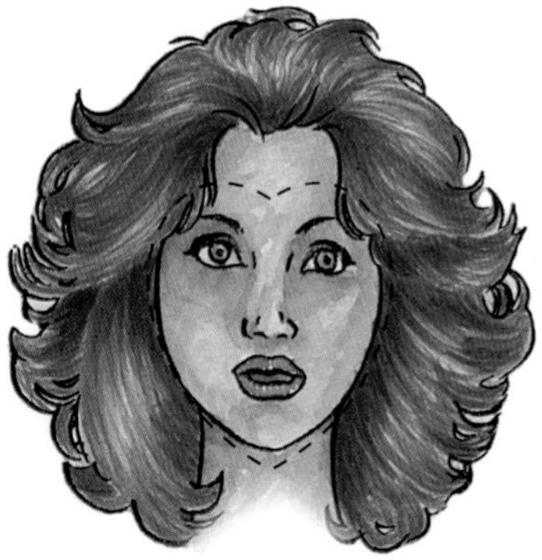

Figure 1.7 Heart-shaped face

Profiles

Always look at your client's profile. When creating a hairstyle, the profile (side view) can be a good indicator as to the correct shape of hairstyle to choose.

Straight profile

This is considered the ideal. It is neither concave nor convex, with no unusual facial features. Usually, all hairstyles are becoming to the straight or normal profile (see Figure 1.8).

Concave (prominent chin)

The hair at the nape should be styled softly with a movement upward. Do not build hair onto the forehead (see Figure 1.9).

Convex (receding forehead, prominent nose, and receding chin)

Place curls or a fringe over the forehead. Keep the styles close to the head at the nape (see Figure 1.10).

Low forehead, protruding chin

Create an illusion of fullness to the forehead by building a fluffy fringe with height. An upswept temple movement will add length to the face. Soft curls in the nape area soften the chin. Do not end the style line at the nape – this draws attention to the chin line. Rather, create a line that is either higher or lower than the chin line (see Figure 1.11).

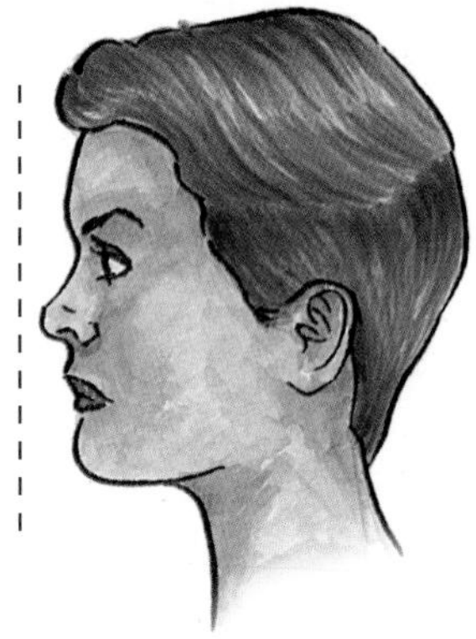

Figure 1.8 Straight profile

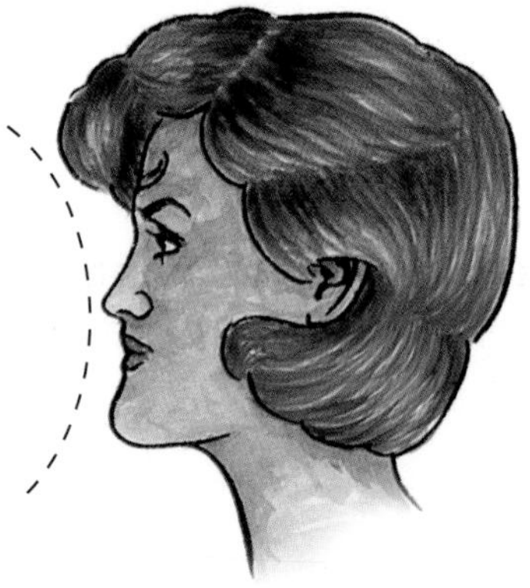

Figure 1.9 Concave profile

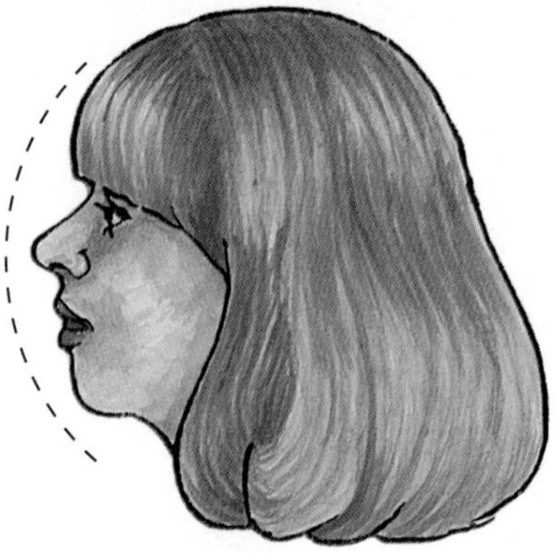

Figure 1.10 Convex profile

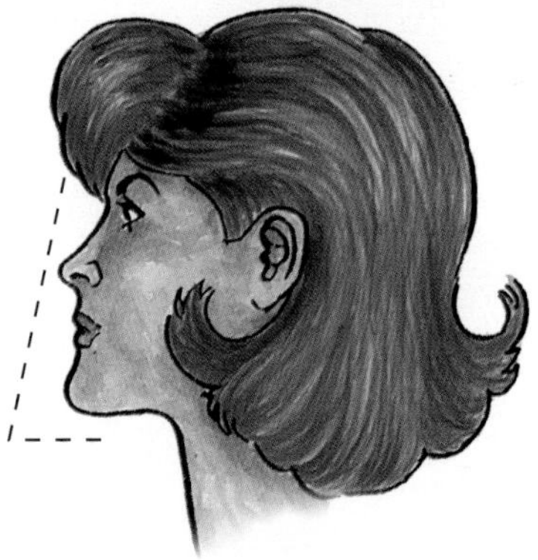

Figure 1.11 Low forehead, protruding chin

Nose shapes

Nose shapes are closely related to profile. When studying your client's face, the nose must be considered both in profile and in full face.

Turned-up nose

This type of nose is usually small and accompanied by a straight profile. The small nose is considered to be a childlike quality; therefore it is best to design a hairstyle that is not associated with children. The hair should be swept off the face creating a line from the nose to the ear. This will add length to the short nose. The top hair should move off the forehead to give the illusion of length to the nose (see Figures 1.12 and 1.13).

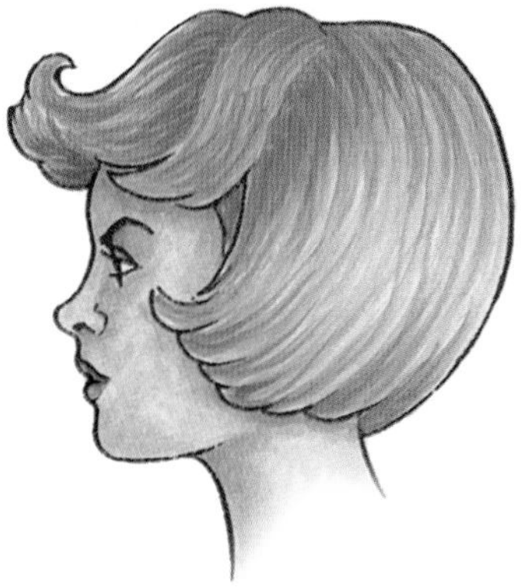

Figure 1.12 Wrong

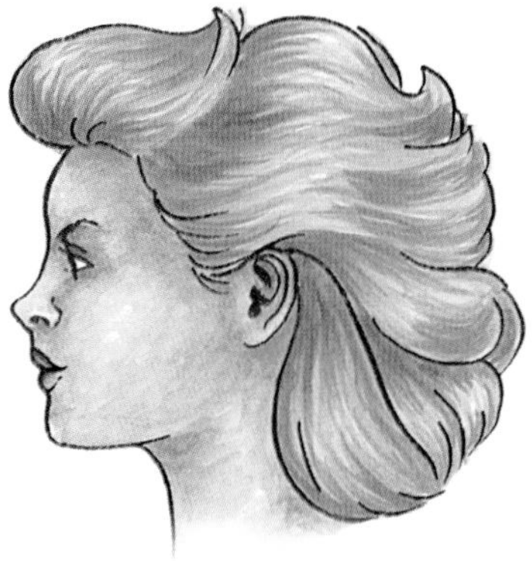

Figure 1.13 Right

Prominent nose (hooked, large, or pointed)

In order to draw attention away from the nose, bring the hair forward at the forehead with softness around the face (see Figures 1.14 and 1.15).

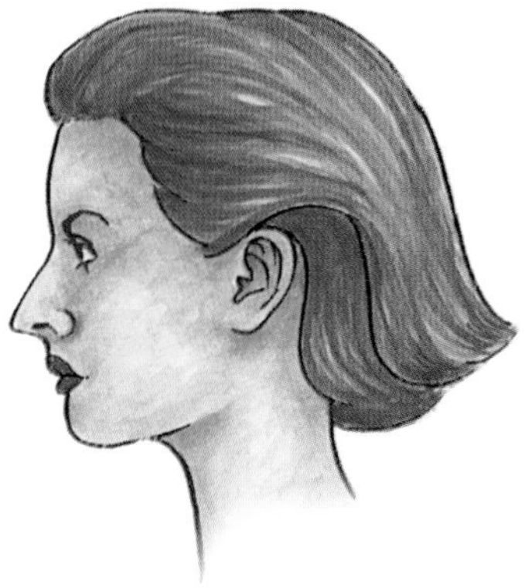

Figure 1.14 Wrong

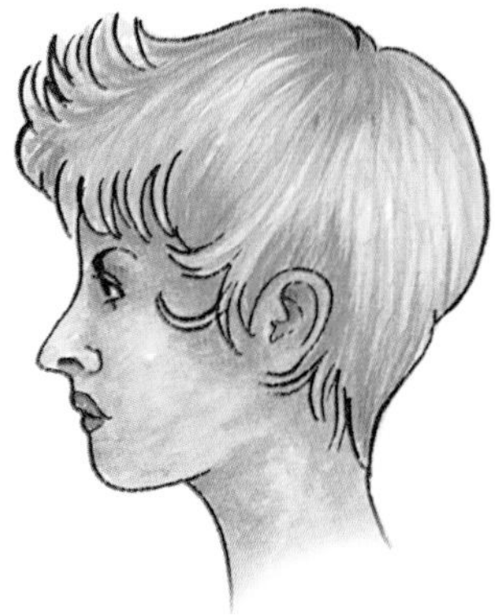

Figure 1.15 Right

> ***TIP*** Symmetrical hairstyles are evenly balanced styles. Asymmetrical hairstyles are unevenly balanced but still aesthetically pleasing.

Crooked nose

To minimise the conspicuous crooked nose, style the hair in an off-centre manner that will attract the eye away from the nose. Asymmetrical styles are best. Any well-balanced hairstyle will accentuate the fact that the face is not even (see Figures 1.16 and 1.17).

Wide, flat nose

A wide, flat nose tends to broaden the face. In order to minimise this effect, the hair should be drawn away from the face. In addition, a centre parting tends to narrow the nose, as well as draw attention away from it (see Figures 1.18 and 1.19).

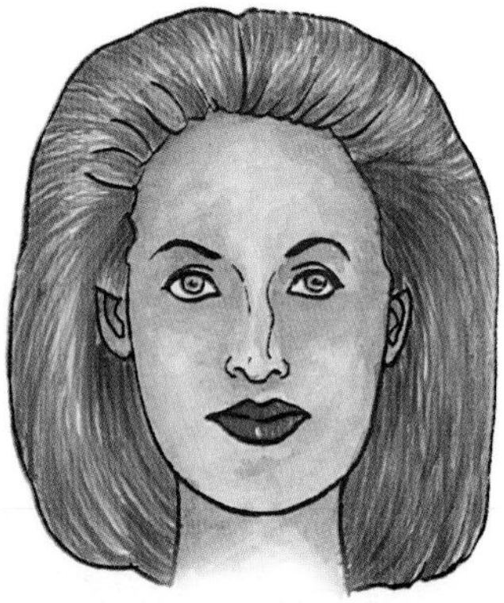

Figure 1.16 Wrong

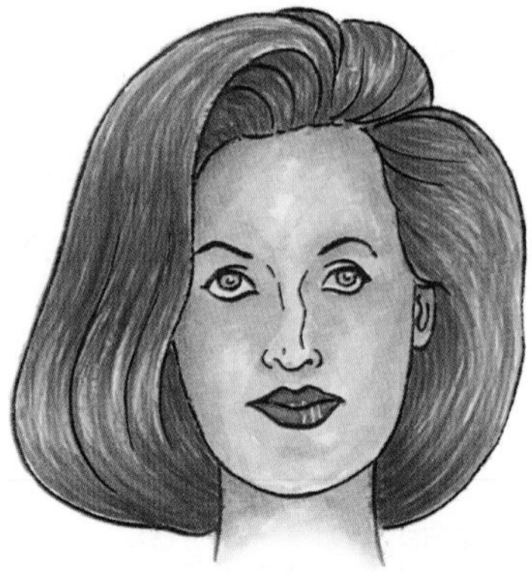

Figure 1.17 Right

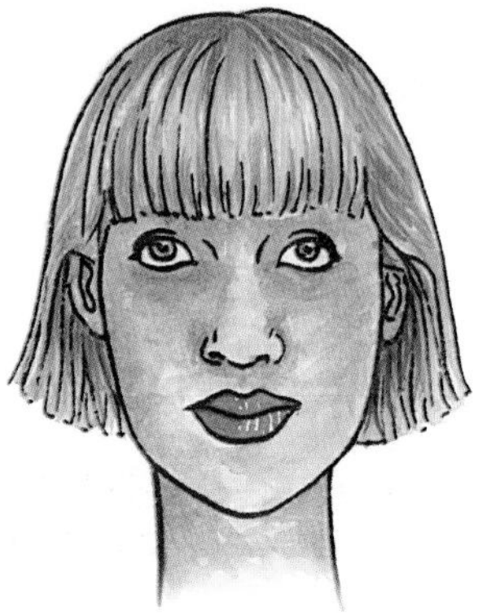

Figure 1.18 Wrong

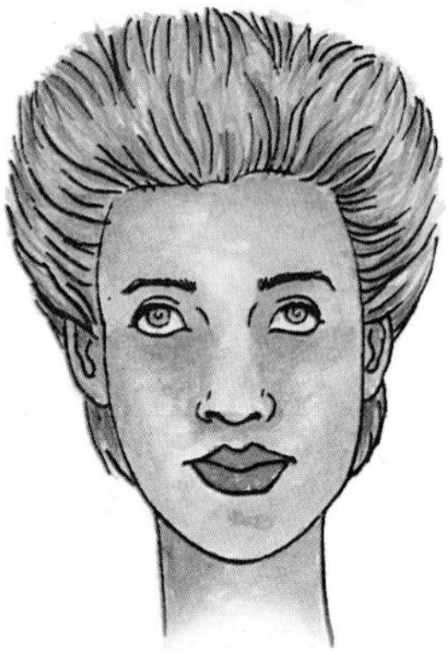

Figure 1.19 Right

Eyes

The eyes are the focal point of a face. Be prepared to create hairstyles that bring out the best in a client's eyes.

Wide-set eyes

Usually found on a round or square face. You can minimise the effect by lifting and fluffing the top of the hair and fringe area. A side fringe helps to draw attention away from the space between the eyes (see Figures 1.20 and 1.21).

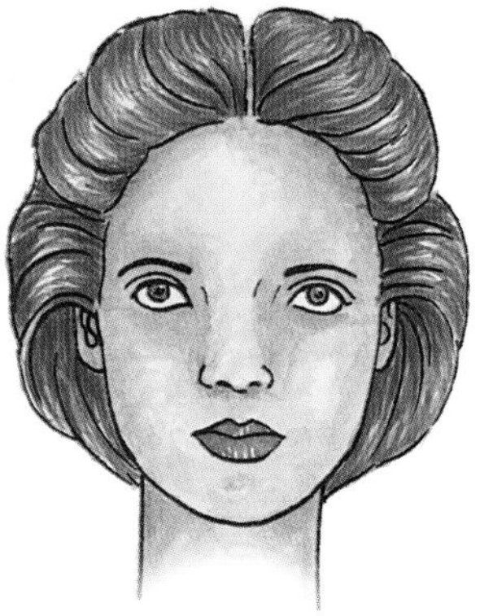

Figure 1.20 Wrong

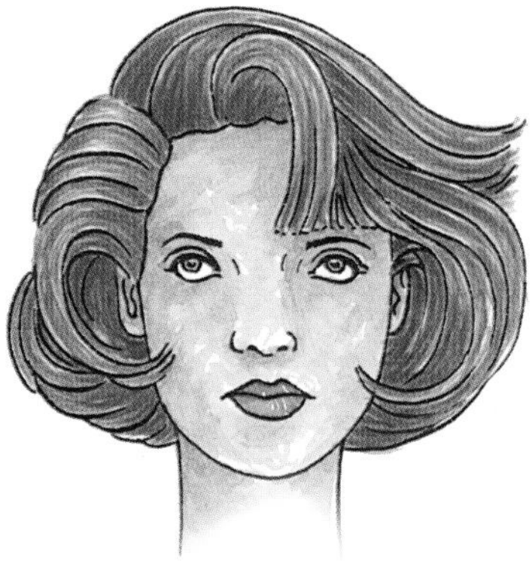

Figure 1.21 Right

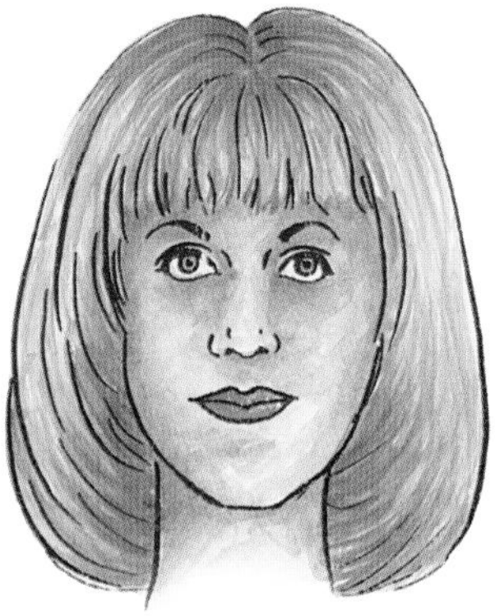

Figure 1.22 Wrong

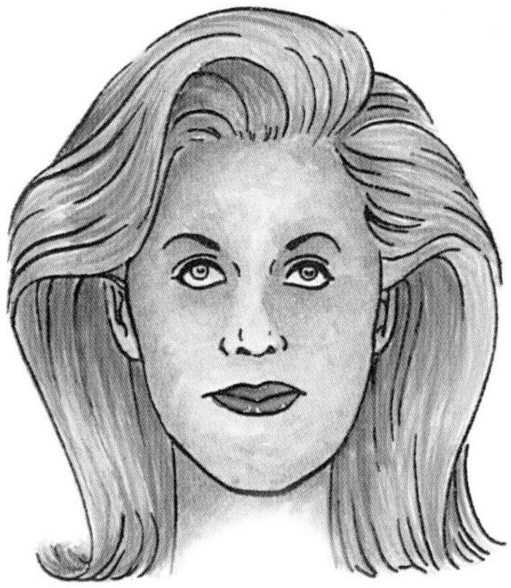

Figure 1.23 Right

Close-set eyes

Usually found on long, narrow faces, try to open the face with the illusion of more space between the eyes. Style the hair fairly high with a side movement. The hair ends should turn outward and up (see Figures 1.22 and 1.23).

Head shapes

The shape of your client's head is just as individual as other physical features. As with the face, the oval is considered the ideal shape. Your goal when designing hairstyles should be to give them the illusion of an oval. As you evaluate your client's head shape, mentally impose an oval picture over it. Where there is flatness, plan to build volume (see Figures 1.24 to 1.29).

Special considerations

Very few, if any, of your clients will have a perfect set of features. Your goal is to analyse their features and accentuate the best ones. In addition you will need to consider the particular features of various ethnic groups.

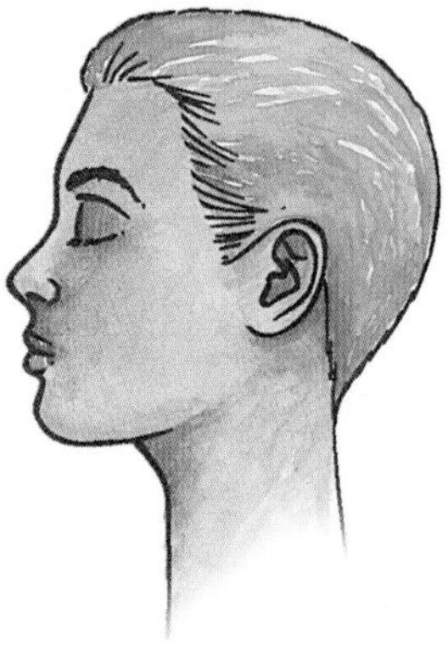

Figure 1.24 Perfect oval

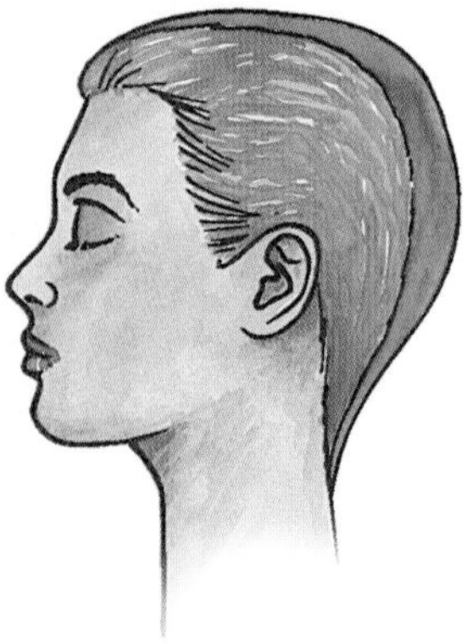

Figure 1.25 Narrow head, flat back

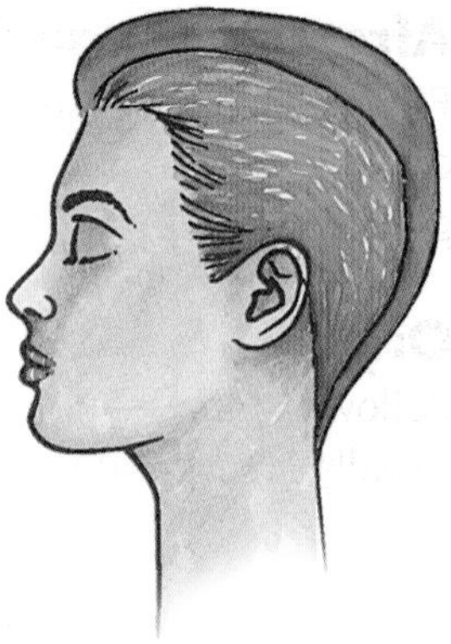

Figure 1.26 Flat crown

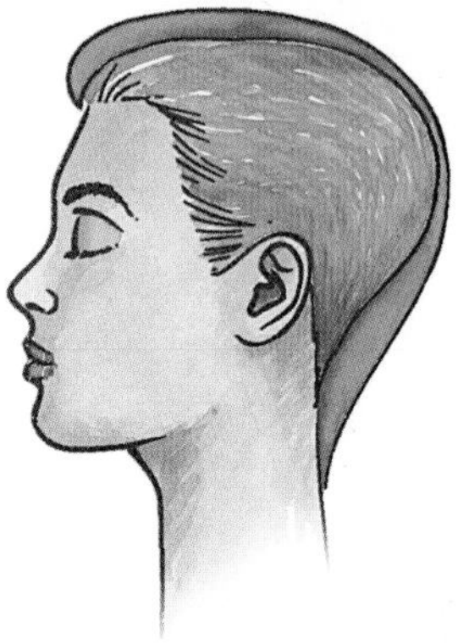

Figure 1.27 Pointed head, hollow nape

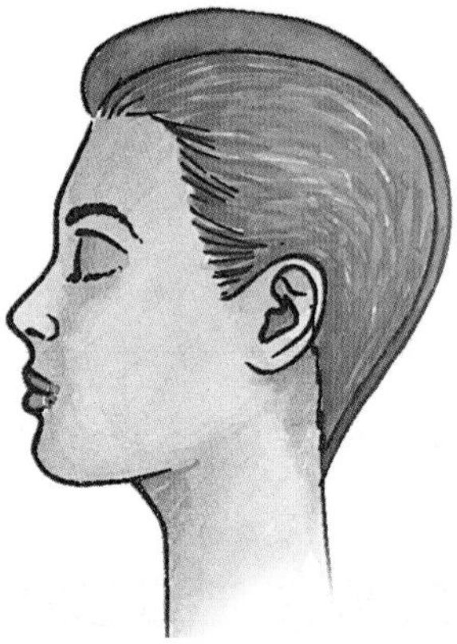

Figure 1.28 Flat top

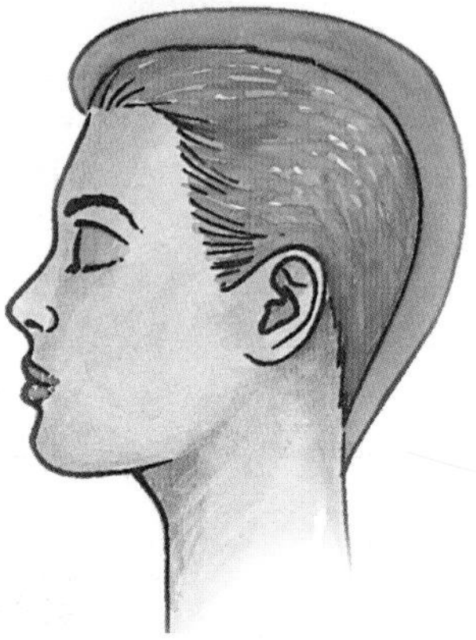

Figure 1.29 Small head

Plump with short neck

Aim: To create the illusion of length.

Corrective hairstyle: Sweep the hair up to give length to the neck. Build height on top. Avoid hairstyles that give fullness to the back of the neck and hairstyles with horizontal lines (see Figure 1.30).

Long, thin neck

Aim: To minimise the appearance of the long neck.

Corrective hairstyle: Cover the neck with soft waves. Avoid short or sculptured necklines. Keep the hair long and full at the nape (see Figure 1.31).

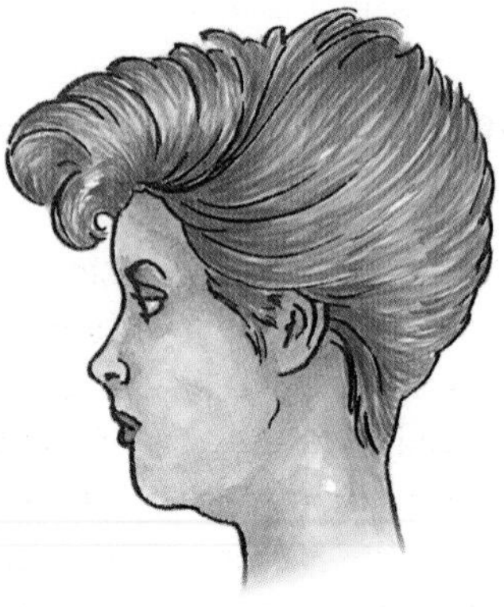

Figure 1.30 Plump with short neck

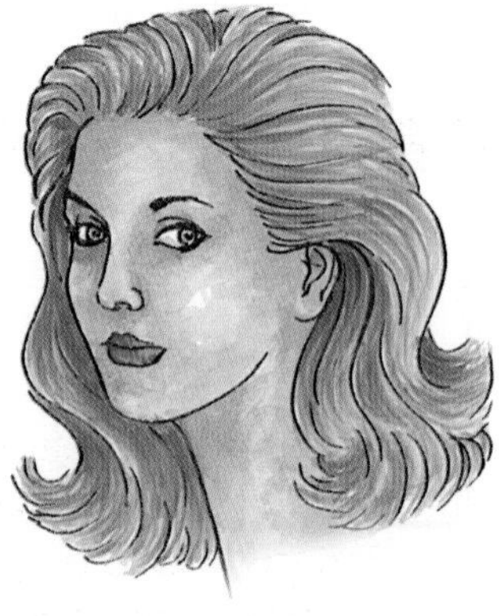

Figure 1.31 Long, thin neck

Afro-Caribbean features

Follow styling rules that relate to the particular face shape. If the hair has been straightened, set it on large rollers. If not, press it thermally with a large barrel iron. Either method will allow you to gain more control in order to style the hair according to design principles (see Figure 1.32).

Oriental features

Follow styling rules that relate to the particular face shape. Keep in mind that oriental hair is usually strong and may require more precise handling (see Figure 1.33).

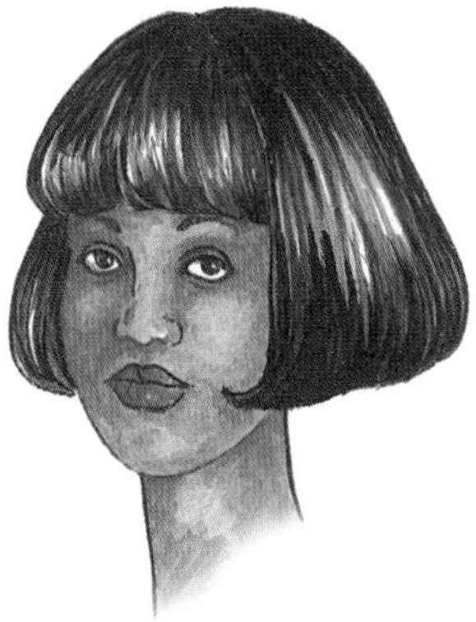

Figure 1.32 Afro-Caribbean client

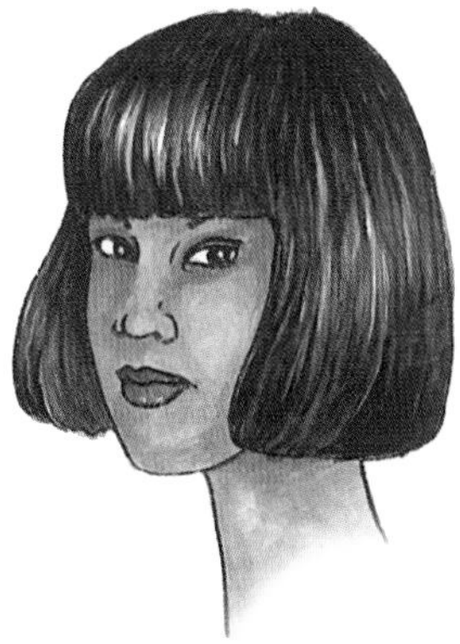

Figure 1.33 Oriental client

EDUCATING YOUR CLIENT

Your client will require educating in how to maintain their hair and the style that you have created. This will include correct choice and use of products on their hair. Clients will need guidance in how frequently they should visit you in the salon to maintain their hair. Follow up services for clients with new looks may be offered as a salon policy. All clients should be encouraged to make return appointment reservations before leaving the salon. This will enable you, the hairstylist, to plan your work as well as helping to ensure an ongoing client relationship.

> ***TIP*** Remember, your client will become a mobile advertisement for your work. It is important that your client is able to maintain their look to the best advantage. You will improve your efficiency if you educate your client in the care of their hair between visits.

RETAIL AND HOMECARE PRODUCT SALES

As more products are added to salon operations, selling is becoming an increasingly important responsibility of the hairdresser. The hairdresser who is equally proficient as a hairstylist and a salesperson is most likely to be the one to succeed in business. Advising clients about the appropriate products to use in their hair care programme will not only add to your income, but will better enable your clients to maintain the look you worked so hard to achieve. The sale of suitable homecare products should be considered an integral part of the hairdressing process and all part of the need to satisfy the client's expectations, the one service supporting the good work of the other.

> ***TIP*** Do not ignore the buying signals that your client gives. Clients who display interest in a product will often respond positively if provided with honest, professional guidance in their suitability. Part of your role, as a hairdresser, is to support your client in effectively caring for their hair.

The largest percentage of home hair care products are sold in the high street retail shops, where advice in appropriate selection and correct use is given usually by non-hairdressers. You are at an advantage for these reasons:

- You are a well informed professional.
- Your client will be able to purchase products that complement the products which you have used on their hair.
- Your client will have indicated their willingness to purchase, by coming to you for advice and a professional service.
- The ambience of hair care and beauty will set the mood for considering the purchase of products related to this.

To be successful in sales you need ambition, determination, and a good personality. The first step in selling is to sell yourself. Clients must like and trust you before they will purchase hair care services, products, or other merchandise. Every client who enters the salon is a prospective purchaser of additional services and merchandise. The manner in which you treat that person lays the foundation for suggestive selling. Recognising the needs and preferences of clients makes the intelligent use of suggestive selling possible.

Selling principles

To become a proficient salesperson you must understand and be able to apply the following selling principles:

- Be familiar with the features and benefits of each service and product.
- Adapt your approach and technique to meet the needs of each client.
- Be self-confident.
- Generate interest and desire, which may lead to a sale.
- Look for indications of interest in products and services. Clients may be nervous about declaring interest, but they may look at the product or linger by the merchandising stand, asking questions about the product or service.
- Never misrepresent your service or product.
- Use tact when selling to a client.
- Don't underestimate the client or the client's intelligence.
- To sell a product or service, deliver a sales talk in a relaxed, friendly manner and, if possible, demonstrate its use.
- If selling a product, allow your client to handle the item.
- Recognise the right psychological moment to close (complete) any sale. Once the client has offered to buy, stop selling – don't oversell, except to praise the client for the purchase and assure them that they will be happy with it.
- Do not be embarrassed when informing the client of the cost of the purchase; the product does have a value.

Types of clients

The hairdresser who is most likely to be successful in selling additional services or merchandise to clients is one who can recognise the many different types of people and knows how to deal with each type.

The following are four of the most usual types you are likely to meet. Each people type might be treated in the way suggested.

- *Shy, timid type.* Make the client feel at ease. Lead the conversation. Don't force the conversation. Be cheerful.
- *Talkative type.* Be a good listener. Tactfully switch the conversation to hair care product need.
- *Nervous, irritable type.* Does not want much conversation. Wants simple, practical hairstyle and a fast worker. Get started and finished as quickly as possible.
- *Inquisitive, over-cautious type.* Explain everything in detail. Show him or her facts – information leaflets, brand names. Ask for the client's opinion.

The psychology of selling

Each person who enters a salon is an individual with specific needs. No matter how good a hairdressing service or product may be, you will find it difficult to make a sale if the client has no need for it. Thus, your first task is to determine whether the client needs or is interested in a service or product.

FURTHER STUDY

- Find out what services are available within your salon, how long they take and what they cost. 1
- Ensure that you are fully aware of the products that are available for retail sale in your salon and their particular features and benefits.
- Create a style guide, a portfolio of current hairdressing fashion that you may use as a communication aid when discussing styles with clients.
- Attending manufacturers' product use demonstrations will help you to learn about their use and their features and benefits.
- Develop your skills of negotiation with clients, particularly how to guide a client towards the correct choice of hairstyles.
- Produce a fact sheet about the retail products available in your salon. List the features, benefits and costs. This may become a useful reference for yourself, your colleagues and your clients. Discuss the use of the fact sheet with your supervisor or manager.

REVIEW QUESTIONS

1. List the information required for the customer records retained in your salon. 1
2. To whom, within your salon, do you refer if the client expresses concern with service in the salon?
3. Suggest two indicators that a client does not understand your com-munication.
4. Describe how a new client is addressed when visiting your salon.
5. Which hair or scalp conditions may preclude hairdressing processes? What advice would you give the client with one of these conditions?
6. Which term is used to describe the coarseness or fineness of the hair?
7. Which term is used to describe the ability of hair to absorb moisture?
8. Does hair stretch more easily when wet or when dry?
9. Describe two strong hair growth patterns.

CHAPTER 2

Shampooing and conditioning the hair and scalp

This section will give you the essential knowledge you need to understand and carry out shampooing and conditioning of the hair and scalp.

Level 1	
Unit 101	
Element 101.1	Maintain effective and safe methods of working when shampooing, conditioning and drying hair.
Element 101.2	Shampoo and surface condition hair
Unit 104	
Element 104.1	Develop effective working relationships with clients
Element 104.2	Develop effective working relationships with colleagues
Element 104.3	Develop self within the job role
Level 2	
Element 201.1	Consult with and maintain effective working relationships with clients
201.2	Advise clients on salon products and services
202.1	Maintain effective and safe methods of working when shampooing and conditioning hair
202.2	Shampoo hair and scalp
202.3	Condition hair and scalp
205A.2	Perm hair using basic techniques
205B.2	Perm hair using basic techniques
206.3	Permanently change hair colour
206.4	Create highlight and lowlight effects in hair
209.2	Support health, safety and security at work

Contents

INTRODUCTION

Following consultation, shampooing is usually the first of a great many salon services, preparing the hair for the following hairdressing processes. In salons where the stylist undertakes the shampoo, the client may use this initial experience to evaluate the professional expertise of the stylist. Clients are likely to assume that a stylist who shampoos professionally will perform all additional services with that same level of competency and concern. In salons where a trainee or other member of staff undertakes the shampoo, the client may use the experience to judge the professionalism of the salon as a whole. Therefore, the client who enjoys the shampoo service is more likely to request additional services and to recommend the stylist and the salon to potential clients.

Shampooing is an important preparatory step for a variety of hair services and is performed primarily to cleanse the hair and scalp. However, the psychological effects of a pleasurable and relaxing experience at the shampoo bay will help to ensure that the client visits the salon on a regular basis.

To be effective, a shampoo must remove all dirt, oils, cosmetics and skin debris without adversely affecting either the scalp or hair. It is important to analyse the condition of the client's hair and scalp and to check for contagious diseases and disorders. A client with an infectious disease of the scalp should not be treated in the salon and should be referred to a medical practitioner.

Unless the scalp and hair are cleansed regularly, the accumulations of oil and perspiration, which mix with the natural scales and dirt, offer a breeding place for disease-producing bacteria. This can lead to scalp disorders. See Chapter 14.

Hair should be shampooed as often as necessary, depending on how quickly the scalp and hair become soiled. As a general rule, oily hair should be shampooed more often than normal or dry hair.

> ***TIP*** Your employer will arrange for you to be instructed in the safe use of chemicals and products. For more information refer to the Control of Substances Hazardous to Health (COSHH) Regulations 1992.

WATER

Chemically, water is composed of hydrogen and oxygen (H_2O). Depending on the kinds and qualities of other minerals present, it can be classified as either hard or soft water. You will be able to make a more professional shampoo selection if you know whether the salon water is hard or soft.

Soft water is rain water or water that has been distilled or chemically softened (deionised). It contains relatively small amounts of minerals and, therefore, allows shampoos to lather freely. For this reason, it may be preferred for shampooing.

Hard water contains minerals that reduce the ability of shampoo to lather. However, hard water can be softened by a chemical process. Calcium deposits from the hard water can build up limescale, blocking the jets of the shower head (also called the rose).

SHAMPOOING

Required materials and implements

Before giving a shampoo, gather all the necessary materials and implements. Don't forget that the client should be properly gowned to protect their clothing. The relaxing mood and the professional quality of the shampoo is destroyed if you dash off to get a forgotten item, leaving the client wet and dripping at the basin. The materials and implements required are:

- towels
- gown
- wide-toothed comb
- hair brush
- appropriate shampoo and conditioner.

> ***TIP*** Take time to discover what types of shampoo are available for use in your salon. Find out their suitability for differing hair and scalp types and conditions.

> ***TIP*** If personal protective equipment is provided use when handling certain products you have a responsibility to use these. For more information refer to the Control of Substances Hazardous to Health (COSHH) Regulations 1992.

Selecting the correct shampoo

Many types of shampoos are available. As a professional hairdresser, you should learn the properties and actions of a shampoo to determine whether or not it will serve your intended purpose. Read the product label and the accompanying literature carefully so that you can make an informed decision.

A pre-shampoo consultation with the client will enable you to decide on the appropriate shampoo to use. Question your client about their hair and scalp: ask when the hair was last shampooed, how often the hair is shampooed and why the hair is shampooed at that frequency (whether it is for cleanliness or for styling). Ask about previous hair treatments. Shampoo manufacturers give guidance for shampoo selection. You will probably need to handle the hair to confirm your findings.

Select the shampoo according to the condition of the hair and scalp, bearing in mind any previous treatments. Also consider treatments that are likely to be used after the shampoo. Hair is not considered normal if it has been:

- lightened
- abused by the use of harsh shampoos
- toned or tinted
- damaged by improper care
- permanently waved
- damaged by exposure to sun, cold, heat or wind
- chemically relaxed
- affected by client ill-health.

If uncertain about the choice of shampoo, consult with your trainer/tutor/manager for advice.

Dry shampoos

If your client is unable to get their hair wet, whether due to illness, a lack of water or when there is insufficient time, a dry shampoo may be used. These shampoos are not suitable for preparing the hair for any subsequent chemical service on your client, nor do they enable the 'wetting' of the hair necessary to produce a set or blow-dry.

Dry spirit shampoo is a foaming spirit, that, while it wets the hair, evaporates very quickly. The spirit is applied to the hair and massaged through the hair to produce a foam. This foam suspends the dirt from the hair. The foam is wiped from the hair using a cupped hand or a towel, and the hair dries very quickly.

Dry powder shampoo is a powder consisting of a mixture of talc and chalk. It is applied to the hair and brushed through. The powder absorbs any grease and attracts the dirt from the hair.

Neither of the dry shampoos is as effective a cleanser as wet shampoos.

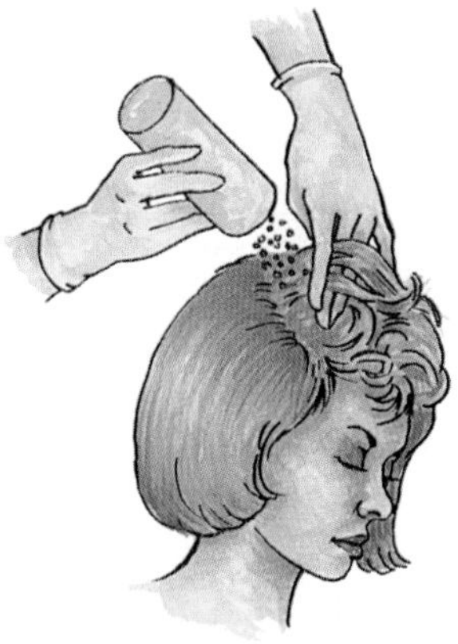

Figure 2.1 Applying dry shampoo

1 Brushing

Hairbrushes made of natural bristles are recommended for hair brushing. Natural bristles have many tiny overlapping layers, or scales, which clean and add lustre to the hair, while nylon bristles are shiny and smooth and recommended for hairstyling.

You should include a thorough brushing as part of every shampoo and scalp treatment, with the following exceptions:

- Do not brush before giving a chemical treatment.
- Do not brush if the scalp is irritated.

Brushing stimulates the blood circulation to the scalp and helps remove dust, dirt, tangles and hairspray build-up from the hair (see Figure 2.2). Therefore, you should brush the hair whether the scalp and hair are in a dry or an oily condition. Do not use the comb to loosen scales from the scalp.

To brush the hair, first part it through the centre from front to nape. Then part a section about 1.25cm ($\frac{1}{2}$") off the centre parting starting at the nape. Holding this strand of hair in the left hand between the thumb and fingers, lay the brush (held in the right hand) with the bristles well down on the hair close to the scalp; rotate the brush by turning the wrist slightly, and sweep the bristles the full length of the hair. Repeat three times. Then part the hair again 1.25cm ($\frac{1}{2}$") above the first parting and continue until the entire head has been brushed (see Figure 2.3).

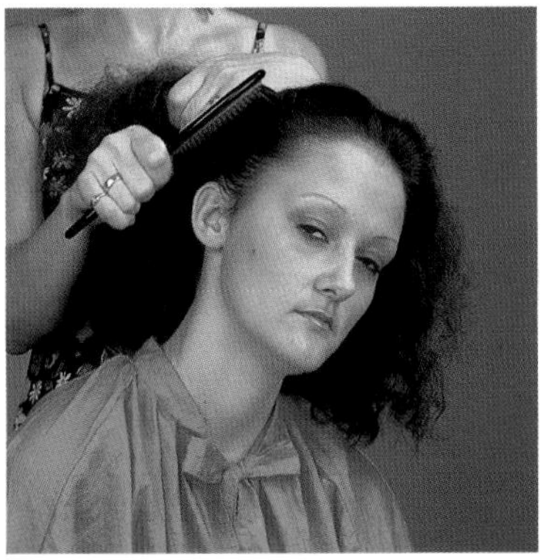

Figure 2.2 Brushing the hair

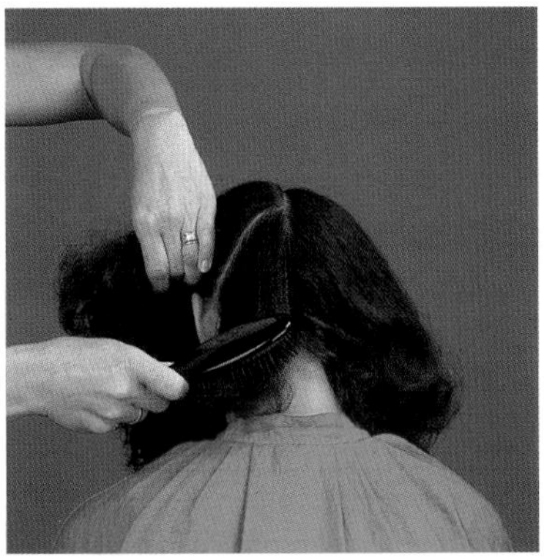

Figure 2.3 Hair sectioned and brushing started

Avoid placing the hair under undue tension. If the hair is tangled, commence by removing tangles at the points, then work steadily back towards the root area.

Shampoo procedure

Preparation

1. Seat your client comfortably at your work station.
2. Select and arrange the required materials.
3. Wash/cleanse your hands.
4. Place the shampoo cape around your client's neck (be sure that the client's clothing lies smoothly under the gown and cape). See Figure 2.4.
5. Remove any hairpins and combs from the hair.
6. Ask your client to remove earrings and glasses and put them in a safe place. Your salon may have a policy and procedures for this.
7. Examine the condition of your client's hair and scalp to determine the correct shampoo choice, check for any contra-indications to shampooing: open cuts or sores on the scalp, contagious disorders.
8. Brush the hair thoroughly.
9. Seat your client comfortably at the shampoo basin, ensuring that your client is seated in such a position that their neck makes an efficient water seal between it and the basin (assuming that it is a back wash style basin. See Figure 2.5).

> ***TIP*** Check with your supervisor on the salon procedure for looking after clients' valuables.

10. Ensure that towels are correctly located to protect the client. Two towels will be required. Some salons place a towel around the neck at the front of the client and then the second around the neck at the back. Other salons place one towel around the back of the neck, keeping the second in reserve for use when the shampoo is completed.
11. Adjust the volume and temperature of the water spray.

To avoid scalding yourself and the client turn on the cold water flow first and then gradually introduce the hot water until a temperature which is com-fortable to the client is established. Test the temperature of the water by spraying it on the back of your hand or the inside of your

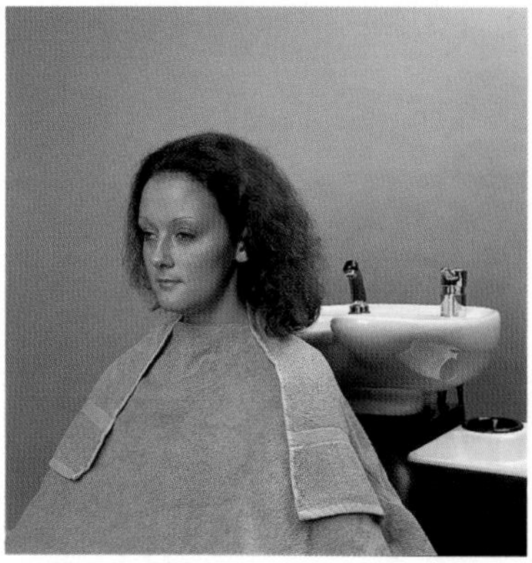

Figure 2.4 Completed shampoo gowning

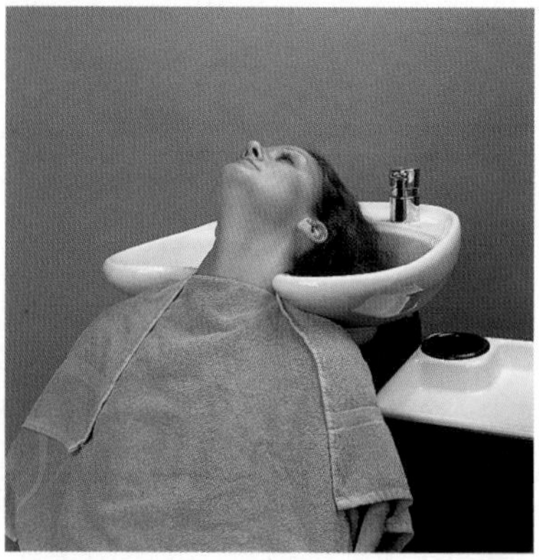

Figure 2.5 Client at back wash basin

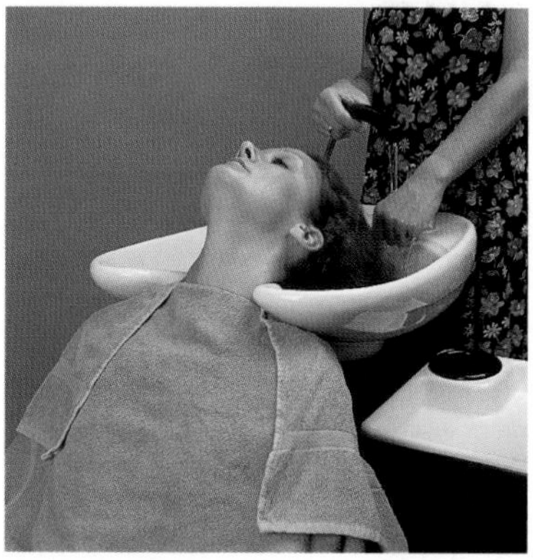

Figure 2.6 Testing water temperature

wrist, as these areas are more sensitive to temperature than the palm of the hand. The temperature of the water must be constantly monitored by keeping one finger over the edge of the spray nozzle (rose) and in contact with the water (see Figure 2.6).

REMINDER In massaging the scalp, do not use firm pressure if:

- You will be giving your client a chemical service after the shampoo.
- Your client's scalp is tender or sensitive.
- Your client requests less pressure.

When you are shampooing excessively greasy hair, the shampooing may be more effective if the shampoo is added to the hair before water is added. This will aid the emulsification of the oil.

Procedure

1. Wet hair thoroughly with warm water spray. Lift the hair and work it with your free hand to saturate the scalp. Shift your hand to protect the client's face, ears and neck from the spray when working around the hairline (see Figure 2.7).

2. Apply small quantities of shampoo to the hair. First emulsify the shampoo on the palms of the hands. This will aid distribution and remove any chill. Beginning at the hairline and working back apply the shampoo with the effleurage massage technique. Work into a lather using the pads or cushions of the fingers (the rotary massage technique).
3. Manipulate the scalp using rotary massage.
   a) Use pads of the fingers and thumbs working them in small rotary movements on the scalp.
   b) Begin at the front hairline and work in a back-and-forth movement until the top of the head is reached (see Figure 2.8).

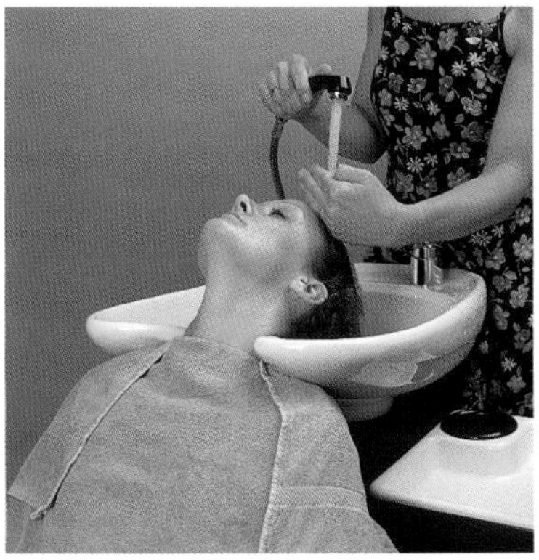

Figure 2.7 Shielding client's face during shampooing

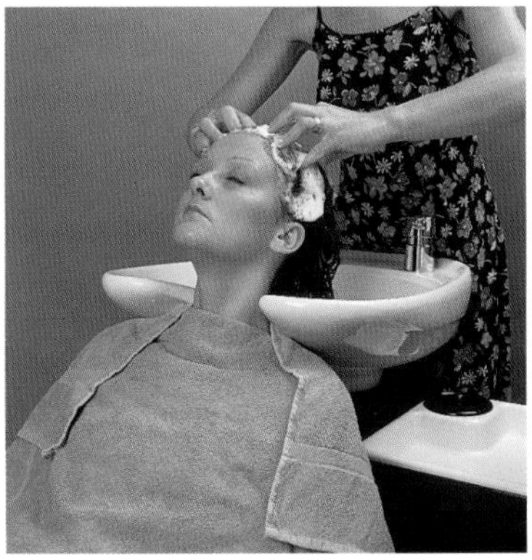

Figure 2.8 Rotary massage technique

   c) Continue in this manner to the back of the head, shifting your fingers back 2.5 cm (1") at a time.
   d) Lift the client's head, with your left hand controlling the movement of the head. With your right hand, start at the top of the right ear and, using the same movement, work to the back of the head.
   e) Drop your fingers down 2.5 cm (1") and repeat the process until the right side of the head is covered.
   f) Beginning at the left ear, repeat the previous two steps.
   g) Allow the client's head to relax and work around the hairline with your thumbs in a rotary movement.
   h) Repeat these movements until the scalp has been thoroughly massaged.
   i) Remove excess shampoo and lather by gently squeezing the hair.
4. Rinse the hair thoroughly.
   a) Lift the hair at the crown and back with the fingers of your left hand to allow the spray to rinse the hair thoroughly.
   b) Cup your hand along the napeline and pat the hair, forcing the spray of water against the base scalp area.

REMINDER When you are shampooing very long hair take care not to tangle the hair by your massage technique. Drawing your fingers from the root area to the hair points will help to untangle the hair.

5. Repeat the process.
   a) If necessary, repeat the procedure using the steps 2, 3 and 4 as outlined above. You will need less shampoo because partially clean hair lathers more easily.

   b) It may not be necessary to repeat this process when shampooing recently shampooed hair or when the hair is excessively fine.
6. Surface hair conditioning.
   a) If required, a surface conditioner may be applied at this time.
   b) Remove excess moisture from the hair by squeezing the hair in the hands.
   c) Using your hands or a specialised applicator, apply the conditioner to the hair and distribute throughout the hair, using an effleurage massage movement, (see pages 36–37).
   d) Rinse the excess conditioner from the hair, following the manufacturer's instructions.
   e) If you are in doubt about whether a surface-active conditioner is required, consult with the hair stylist.
7. Partially towel dry.
   a) Remove excess moisture from the hair at the shampoo basin.
   b) Wipe excess moisture from around the client's face and ears with the towel, take care not to allow the corners of the towel to contact the client's eyes. Folding the ends of the towel back on themselves will help to prevent this (see Figure 2.10).
   c) Lift the towel over the back of the client's head and wrap the head with the towel.
   d) Place your hands on top of the towel and massage until the hair is partially dry (see Figure 2.10). Use the effleurage technique.

Surface-active conditioners, page 30

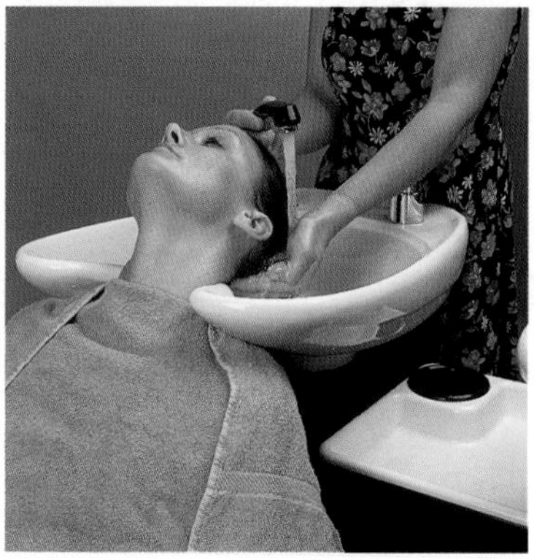

Figure 2.9 Rinsing shampoo from the nape area

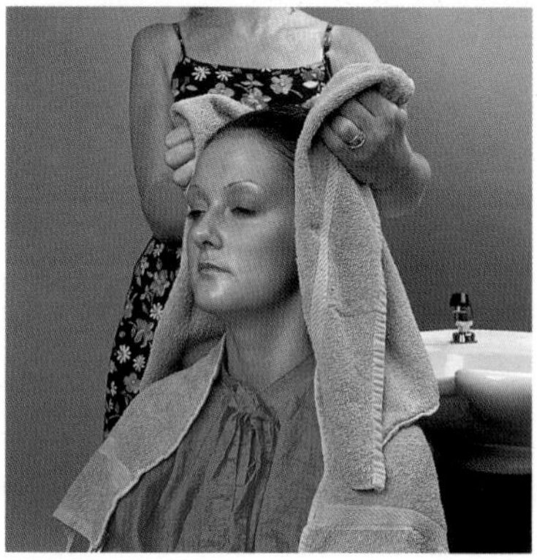

Figure 2.10 Towel drying the hair

Completion

1. Comb the hair, using a wide-toothed comb, beginning with the ends at the nape of the client's neck. This will help to prevent unnecessary tension on the hair.
2. Change the towel around the client's neck, if necessary.
3. Style the hair as desired.

Clean-up

1. Dispose of used materials, and place unused supplies in their proper places.
2. Wipe the basin area clear of hair and water.
3. Place used towels in the towel bin.
4. Remove hair from combs and brushes and wash them with hot, soapy water; rinse and place in wet disinfectant for the required time.
5. Wash your hands.

TIP Remember – do not leave a client sat, following a shampoo, with water dripping onto their face, neck or clothes. Your salon may have policies and procedures for clients to remain with their head wrapped in a towel or combed back off the face, while waiting for styling.

WHAT THE EXPERT SAYS Shampooing is one of the first skills that you learn as a novice hairdresser. It should not be regarded as an unimportant task to be carried out by an unskilled person. One of the first procedures that your client will experience within the salon, shampooing prepares the hair for most hairdressing processes and success in these subsequent processes may often depend on effective preparation of the surface on which the hairstylist creates.

The shampooist is an important member of the hairdressing salon team. When carrying out a shampoo, remember that you have the opportunity to create a rapport with your client. The shampoo should relax your client, so carry it out in a style that is likely to do this. While speed of work is important for business efficiency, this speed should be achieved without making your client feel rushed. A prepared and methodical approach to the process will enable you to achieve the speed but at the same time to relax and reassure your client that they are in the hands of a knowledgeable professional. By being adequately prepared, you will have all the tools you need at hand. This will help to ensure that your client receives a process that flows and is not interrupted by frantic periods when you are searching for the correct product or leaving the client to fetch tools that should have already been at hand.

There are opportunities for you to show your professional skill during the shampoo. Remember that you are the professional, who in most cases has a greater knowledge of the procedures and products being used. Advise your client in the correct choice of product, this may include the choice of shampoo or cleanser. Advise your client about appropriate conditioning for their hair. You will have a greater knowledge about the range of products used within your salon, your client has come to you for a service and your advice is part of that service.

Home-use hair care products may be suggested during the shampoo process, particularly suitable shampoos and conditioners. Watch out for signs of interest shown by your client in the products you are using. Retail lines which complement the products used within your salon should be available.

Salon cleanliness

Occasionally try to see the salon in the way that your client does. At the shampoo area consider what view of the salon they have. From the shampoo chair does your client see areas that require cleaning? Often from the seated position your client will see under shelves, basins and other fixtures that from a standing position appear perfect. However, when seated a client may get a different view.

TIP Rotary massage – a surface massage where the pads of the fingers move in rotary movement on the scalp with light pressure. The fingers may be regularly lifted and drawn along the lengths of the hair to remove tangles when shampooing long hair.

TIP Effleurage massage – a stroking movement often used to distribute shampoo across the scalp and along the hairs length.

TIP Avoid using extremes of water temperature when shampooing greasy hair as both very warm and very cold water can stimulate the sebaceous glands that produce the grease (sebum).

THE CHEMISTRY OF SHAMPOO

To determine which shampoo will leave your client's hair in the best condition for the intended service you must understand the chemical ingredients of shampoos. Most shampoos have many common ingredients. It is often small differences in formulation that makes one shampoo better for a particular hair texture or condition.

The ingredient that most shampoos have in common, and it usually is number one on the list to show that there is more of it than any other ingredient, is water. Generally, it is not just plain water, but purified or deionised water. From there, ingredients are listed in descending order according to the percentage of each ingredient in the shampoo.

Classification of shampoos

The second ingredient that most shampoos have in common is the base surfactant or base detergent. These two terms, surfactant and detergent, mean the same thing, cleansing or 'surface-active' agent. The term surfactant describes organic compounds brought together by chemical synthesis (combining chemical elements to form a whole) to create wetting, dispersing, emulsifying, solubilising, foaming or washing agents (detergents).

TIP It is useful to know the basic properties of the main classifications of surfactants.

Anionic	lowers the surface tension of water.
Cationic	attracted to the hair, has a positive charge.
Non-ionic	acts as a foam stabiliser.
Ampholytic	acts as a foam stabiliser, makes shampoo less irritating to the eyes.

The base surfactant or combination of surfactants determines into which class a shampoo will fall. The base surfactants used in shampoos fall into four broad classifications: anionic, cationic, non-ionic and ampholytic.

Most manufacturers use detergents from more than one classification. It is customary to use a secondary surfactant to complement or offset the negative qualities of the base surfactant. For example, an ampholytic that is non-irritating to the eyes can be added to a harsh anionic to create a product that is more comfortable to use.

TYPES OF SHAMPOO

The choice of shampoo is determined by:

- the condition of the scalp (dry, greasy or dandruff-affected)
- the texture and condition of the hair (damaged, porous, fine or chemically treated)
- subsequent hairdressing treatments (permanent wave and permanent hair colouring).

> ***TIP*** Some shampoos can affect the pH of the hair (see Chapter 5A). This can affect subsequent hairdressing treatments. Read manufacturer guidance with care.

Shampoo manufacturers' guidelines should be followed in determining the appropriate choice for your client.

Those shampoos available today include those intended for use on:

Normal hair – these shampoos are designed to cleanse the average head of hair, leaving it in good condition for subsequent styling,

Dry hair – these shampoos will help nourish the hair, add moisture to the hair and make the hair easier to comb.

Greasy hair – these shampoos will be effective in the removal of sebum from the hair and scalp and may contain additives which will help to reduce the activity of the sebaceous glands.

Dandruff-affected – these shampoos will help to combat the causes of dandruff and to remove dandruff scales from the hair and scalp. Additives including selenium sulphide and zinc pyrethione are often included within these shampoos.

Fine hair – these shampoos are designed to reduce the softening effect of shampooing.

Artificially coloured hair – these shampoos are designed to reduce the colour fade caused by shampooing the hair.

Pre-perm – these shampoos are designed to cleanse the hair and to prepare the hair for subsequent permanent curling.

> ***HEALTH AND SAFETY*** Ensure that you thoroughly rinse and dry your hands after carrying out a shampoo. Failure to do this may result in dry, chapped skin (dermatitis).
>
> If shampoo is allowed into the eye, the eye should be rinsed with copious supplies of sterile water.
>
> Should your client indicate that the shampoo is causing scalp irritation, this may indicate a possible allergic reaction. Alternative shampoos should then be used. In severe cases you should recommend that your client seek medical advice.

Conditioning hair and scalp

There are a number of hair and scalp conditions that may be treated by the professional hairdresser. It is essential that, in offering this service, the hairdresser is able to identify those conditions that may be safely treated and those that require referral to a medical practitioner.

Modern technology has enabled manufacturers to produce a wide range of professional treatments that may be offered by the hairdresser. In some cases these treatments take the form of 'one-off' products that may be applied to either the hair and/or scalp, independently of any other product used with your client. There are also treatment systems available that offer a range of products which may be used in conjunction with each other. These usually take the form of a range of shampoos (cleansers), treatment lotions or creams, styling aids and a range of 'take home' products which complement those used in the salon. These treatment ranges usually have a regime of use, which leads the hairdresser through the process of analysis of the hair and scalp, selection of the appropriate products and their correct method of application.

➤The hair and scalp, pages 278–300

> ***TIP*** A full awareness of the procedures for using these products is an essential part of offering them as treatments. Always follow the manufacturer's directions.

Hair conditioning

Treatment conditioning

Hair cannot care for itself, and once damaged is unable to repair itself.

Hair that is out of condition is usually rather dry, brittle and rough to the touch. This may be caused by the use of chemical processes on the hair (permanent waving, bleaching and tinting), the use of poor quality tools (rough combs or brushes with sharp bristles), excessive heat on the hair (too frequent or incorrect use of heated styling tools), your client's ill health or even the weather (excessive sun).

The result of this may be a roughening of the outside layer of the hair, the cuticle, or, in its worst state, the breakdown of the hair's structure, causing the hair to break.

Surface-active conditioning

Following a shampoo, the client's hair is often conditioned to compensate for the drying effect of these processes. A surface-active conditioner would be used. The action of a surface conditioner is to coat the hair. This fills the gaps on the roughened surface of the cuticle, making it easier to comb and less liable to tangle. It also helps to soften the hair. The action of the surface conditioner will usually last until the next shampoo, the effect gradually disappearing as the hair is brushed, combed and subjected to treatment.

To apply a surface conditioner following the shampoo, remove excess moisture from your client's hair by pressing it between your hands. Place a small amount of the conditioner on your hands and then distribute this throughout the hair, paying particular attention to those areas worst affected by any dryness. Gently work the conditioner through the hair using your fingers and then rinse thoroughly from the hair. Note that some conditioners are not rinsed from the hair: check the manufacturer's guidelines. A coating of conditioner will be left on the hair until it is next shampooed – during this time it gradually breaks down.

> ***TIP*** Always follow the manufacturer's guidelines when using a product.

Penetrating conditioners

These conditioners penetrate the surface of the hair. Their actions are varied but in the main their effect is to build artificial bonds that form in the cortex layer of the hair, replacing those natural bonds which have been lost due to the causes listed earlier. Many of these conditioners also neutralise the effect of chemical treatments on the hair, returning the hair to its normal pH of between 4.5 and 5.5. This helps to prevent any further action by the chemical treatment.

Penetrating conditioners are available in liquid, cream and oil forms. The liquid form is the most suitable where softening the hair is not desirable. The cream format often has the benefit of both the surface-active and the penetrating conditioner in one product. Oil-based products usually consist of vegetable oils. Sulphonated vegetable oils are more easily shampooed from the hair following the treatment as they act both as an oil, conditioning, and a detergent, cleansing. When using a plain vegetable oil, apply to hair before it has been made wet, add shampoo and emulsify this with the oil before adding any water.

> ***TIP*** Always follow the manufacturer's directions when using these products. The manufacturer's advice on Health and Safety should be followed.

Protective conditioning

Some conditioners may be used to protect the hair during chemical processes. Liquid conditioners, called **pre-treatment conditioners**, may be applied before a permanent wave to even the porosity of the hair. This will produce a more even absorption, by the hair, of the perming solution. Those parts of the hair that are more porous and therefore require more protection absorb more of the pre-perm conditioner, therefore being self selective. Follow the manufacturer's directions at all times when using these products.

Certain cream-based conditioners may be used as protective barriers when perming hair. Those areas of the hair coated with the conditioner will not easily absorb the perming lotion. This technique may be used when root perming or when protecting highly delicate hair during a perming process.

A sunscreen surface-active conditioner may be applied to the hair, either as a cream or as a liquid spray. This lies on the surface of the hair and acts as a screen against harmful rays from the sun, which dry and lighten the hair.

Scalp treatments

> ***TIP*** The Electricity at Work Regulations 1989, requires that all electrical equipment used in your salon must be electrical safety checked. Check with the person responsible before using unchecked equipment that you or other may have brought into the salon.

Mild scalp conditions may often be treated by specialist treatment systems. There is a variety of product ranges available, including treatments to combat dandruff (*Pityriasis simplex*), greasy scalp (*Seborrhea*) and even forms of hair loss (*Alopecia*). As the cause of a scalp condition must normally be established before a successful treatment can be determined, and as this often requires the specialist knowledge of a trichologist, these products may not always be able to offer the remedy required. Therefore when offering a treatment to a client it is advisable to indicate that success is not guaranteed. When using specialist scalp treatments, always follow the manufacturer's guidelines on the method and frequency of application.

Following these treatments always update the client records. Remember, if you are unsure which treatment is most appropriate for your client, or how the treatment should be applied, consult with your trainer.

> ***TIP*** Take care always to wear protective gloves, if recommended by the product manufacturer.

SCALP MASSAGE

1 This will help to stimulate capillary blood flow, which feeds the hair root and follicle. It will also help to stimulate the production of sebum (the hair and skin's natural oil) from the sebaceous glands that open into the hair follicle. Scalp massage will also relax and soothe your client.

Scalp massage may be given by hand or mechanically, and is usually given when the hair and scalp have been treated with a conditioning cream. This lubricates the surface of the hair and scalp, enabling the massage to take place without the client suffering discomfort.

Do not carry out any form of scalp massage if there are open sores or cuts on the scalp, if there is any contagious scalp disorder or if your client complains of pain or discomfort during the massage.

Hand applied scalp massage

Petrissage is a massage movement using the pads of the fingers, in a gripping, kneading movement (see Figure 2.11), co-ordinated together. Often when you start the scalp massage, the scalp

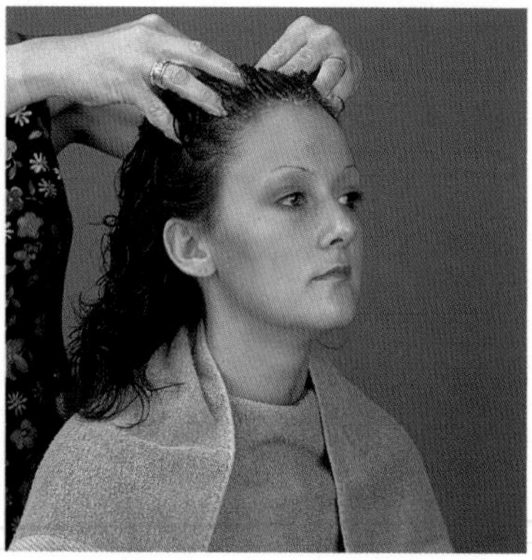

Figure 2.11 Petrissage massage movement

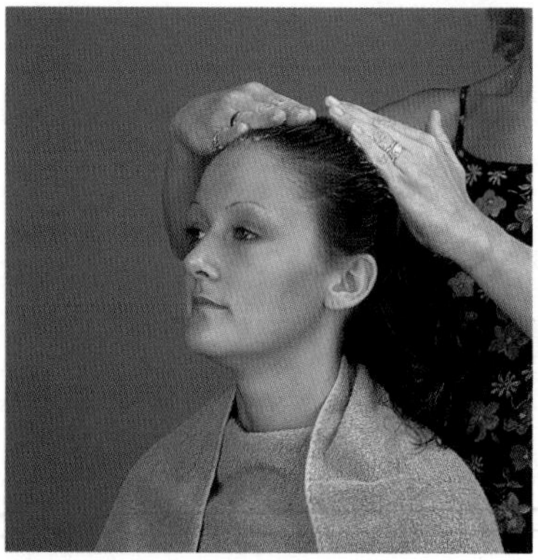

Figure 2.12 Effleurage massage movement

is tight and therefore this massage should be started gently on the scalp and as the scalp manipulation loosens the scalp, the massage may become more intense, though never rough. The massage movement should follow an organised pattern over the scalp with both hands using an even pressure. Take care not to exert too much pressure on the sensitive areas of the scalp, the temporal and mastoid areas.

Effleurage is a stroking movement using the fingers and palms of the hands (Figure 2.12) and has a soothing effect, helping to distribute the increased blood flow.

> ***TIP*** The Electricity at Work Regulations 1989 requires that portable electrical tools should be regularly tested (PAT) for electrical safety

Mechanically applied scalp massage

Direct massage

You may provide scalp massage by using the vibro massager, which is a gun-like apparatus with a 1
spiked applicator. Ensure that the applicator is attached firmly to the vibro massager. Gently press the applicator onto the scalp and move in an organised pattern over the scalp in small circular movements (see Figure 2.13). Lift the applicator away from the hair and scalp occasionally to prevent tangling the hair. This must be done more frequently if you are massaging the scalp of a client with long hair.

> ***TIP*** Your salon may have procedures for visual checking of electrical appliances and reporting faults. Find out what your salon's procedures are for this.

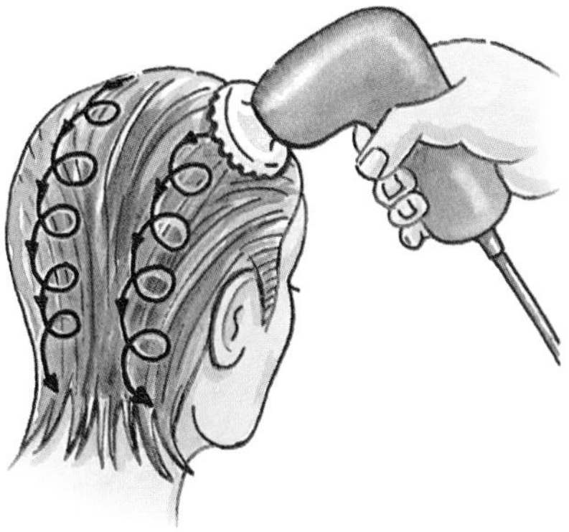

Figure 2.13 Using a vibro massager on the scalp

When using the vibro massager on your client for the first time, allow the client to become accustomed to its sensation by applying it for a few moments to the back of their hand. The duration of the treatment may be extended gradually, at each application, to a maximum of ten minutes.

Other applicators are designed for use on specific areas of the body:

- sponge – on the face
- suction bell – for deep skin toning
- flat applicator – for surface muscles
- hard vulcanite applicator – for large flat muscles.

Remember to ensure that all applicators are washed, dried and sterilised after each use.

Indirect massage

In indirect massage your hands become the applicators that make contact with your client's scalp. A style of vibro massager is strapped to the back of each hand, causing your hand to vibrate. You may then use your hands to make both petrissage and effleurage massage movements on the client's scalp.

THE USE OF HEAT

During the application of a cream conditioner heat may be used to aid penetration of the hair by the product, as well as speeding up any chemical processes. Moist heat swells the hair shaft, making this action easier. Heat may be provided in several ways including:

- the scalp steamer
- the thermal cap
- radiated heat
- scalp heat.

The scalp steamer

The scalp steamer is an apparatus with a hood that may be adjusted to fit over the scalp area of your client. It has a reservoir which holds a supply of distilled or deionised water. This water feeds into a small boiler that produces steam. This steam is fed to a series of jets that distribute it within the hood (Figure 2.14).

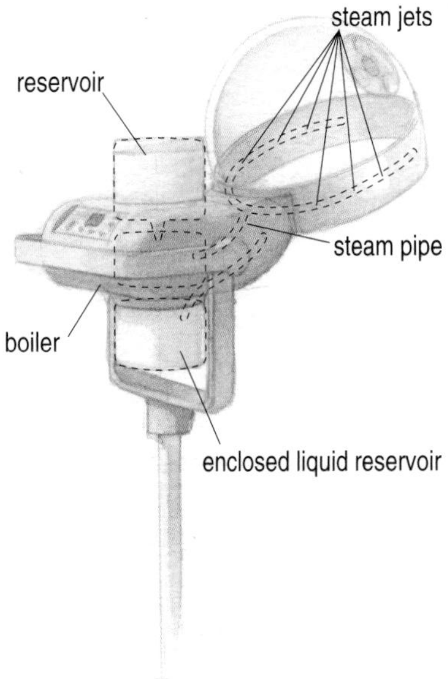

Figure 2.14 How a scalp steamer works

Before use ensure that the machine is clean. Check the inside of the hood for traces of previously used products and ensure that the reservoir has a sufficient supply of water. Pre-heat the steamer and, once steaming, adjust any temperature settings and locate the hood carefully over the scalp area, ensuring that the hood and vents are adjusted so as to avoid steam escaping onto your client's neck. Ensure client comfort at all times, and ensure that your client is able to inform someone should they experience any discomfort.

The thermal cap

A thermal cap is a close-fitting hood with an electrically heated element, similar to that in an electric blanket, built into the fabric. Once connected to an electrical supply the interior of the cap becomes warm. This heat is conducted to the hair and any products lying on the hair. As the surface is water proof the moisture is retained. Care must be taken to ensure client comfort at all times.

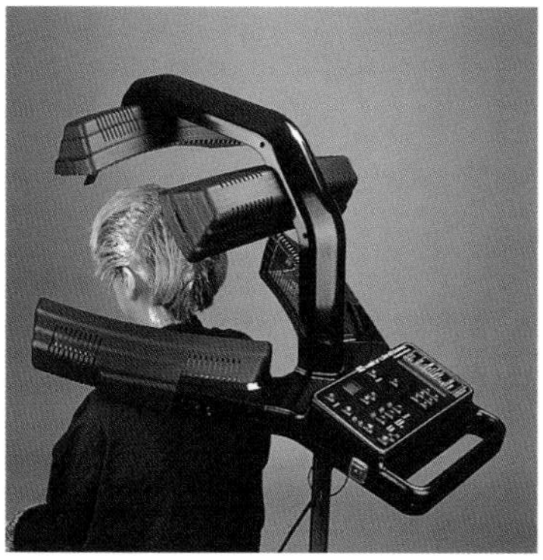

Figure 2.15 Accelerator in use on client

Radiated heat

There are a number of appliances that may be used to radiate heat onto the hair and scalp. Some use specialised light bulbs to generate this heat; others use heating elements (Figure 2.15). Care must be taken to locate elements correctly around the head, to ensure even heating and to prevent 'hot spots' on the head. As the product's moisture is not trapped within any hood, check to ensure that the hair does not dry out during the process. If this happens moisten the hair.

> ***TIP*** Never use electrical equipment if you do not know how to. Always read the manufacturer's directions or ask your trainer for guidance in correct use.

Scalp heat

Scalp heat, if retained, may be used to aid penetration by conditioning products. The scalp area is enclosed within a polythene cap that, in turn, is enclosed within a towel. The polythene cap prevents moisture loss and the towels insulates reducing heat loss.

FURTHER STUDY

- Find out the features and benefits of the shampoos used in your salon, so that you can advise upon and select appropriate products for use on your client both in the salon and for home care.
- Many manufacturers produce treatment ranges that have cleansers (shampoos), which are complemented with hair and scalp conditioners and styling products. You should make yourself aware of these and how they are selected for the client.
- The hairdresser should be aware of what retail hair care products are available from non-hairdresser retail outlets so that comparisons may be discussed with your client.
- Develop your selling skills, look for signs, from your clients, of interest in retail products.
- Produce a fact sheet about the shampoos and conditioning products available in your salon. Include details of specific safety aspects when using these.

> ***TIP*** Some products, particularly oils, may become more liquid and run when heat is applied, so your client must be adequately protected by gowns and towels.

HEALTH AND SAFETY Before using any electrical appliance make a visual check of all outer casings, cables and plugs. Should any loose connections or other damage be apparent, report this to your line manager. Do not use equipment which appears to be unsafe. Do not handle electrical appliances with wet hands. If you are not fully aware of how to use an item of equipment read the manufacturer's instructions or seek instruction from your trainer.

REVIEW QUESTIONS

1. List the range of shampoos used within your salon and indicate the hair and scalp types for which they are designed.
2. What effect can hard water have on the shower head at the basin?
3. On what occasions would you use 'dry' shampoos?
4. When shampooing, how is the water temperature tested?
5. Describe 'rotary' massage.
6. List two ingredients often found in 'anti-dandruff' shampoos.
7. What is the pH of normal hair?
8. Describe the action of a surface conditioner.
9. Give two occasions when protective conditioning may be appropriate.
10. Give two benefits to be gained by the client from scalp massage.
11. Describe Petrissage massage movement.
12. Give two contra-indications to the use of vibro scalp massage.
13. What benefits are obtained from using heat in conjunction with a reconditioning cream?
14. What fluid is used in the scalp steamer?

CHAPTER 3

Drying hair into shape

This section gives you the essential knowledge to help you understand the processes of drying hair to create a finished look. This includes a variety of fashion styling techniques.

Level 1	
Unit 101	
Element 101.3	Blow dry one length hair which is below shoulder length
Unit 104	
Element 104.1	Develop effective working relationships with clients
Element 104.2	Develop effective working relationships with colleagues
Element 104.3	Develop yourself within the job role
Unit 105	
Element 105.2	Support health and safety at work
Level 2	
Unit 201	
Element 201.1	Consult with and maintain effective relationships with clients
Element 201.2	Advise clients on salon products and services
Element 201.3	Advise clients on after-care procedures
Unit 203	
Element 203.1	Maintain effective and safe methods of working when drying and setting hair
Element 203.2	Dry and finish hair to style
Unit 209	
Element 209.2	Support health, safety and security at work
Unit 213	
Element 213.1	Maintain effective and safe methods of working when drying hair
Element 213.2	Dry and finish hair

Contents

INTRODUCTION

The client leaves the hair stylist wishing to look their best. Fulfilling this wish ensures the client's satisfaction and helps to establish good customer relations. The way that the client looks when they leave the hair stylist indicates, both to the client and other potential clients, the professional ability and character of the hairstylist. This finished hairstyle becomes an advertisement for the stylist's work and the salon's standard of hairdressing.

CLIENT CONSULTATION

The choice of drying and dressing technique used will depend upon the finished outcome required (this will be agreed with the client by consultation), the hair type being dressed and the preferences of the client. This selection and choice of hairstyle and technique will be made by advice given to and negotiation with your client during consultation, which would normally take place between the hairstylist and client before the hairdressing process begins and may be reviewed throughout the treatment.

As you are a trainee, your stylist will guide you towards the most suitable style for the 1
client and one that will satisfy their requirements. Ensure that you fully understand the stylists instructions before starting the dry. If you experience any problems during the dry, the stylist should be asked for guidance, this should be done discreetly, according to the salon's policy. Failure to request help when problems have been identified may lead to wastage of both the client's and salon's time, as well as incorrect results.

> ***TIP*** Remember, ensure that the client is fully aware of the intended finished result before starting to dry the hair.

As your client will become an advertisement of your hairdressing skills it is important that they are able to maintain their hair at its best between visits. Educate your client in how to maintain the style, particularly following the introduction of a new look to the client. Home use products that complement the products used in your salon and will enable the style to be maintained should be recommended and offered for sale. Always ensure that the client is aware of how to correctly use these products.

The styling process includes:

- Client consultation – establishing what the required hairstyle is
- Shampooing – this cleanses and wets the hair allowing it to be 'stretched' and formed into a new shape. Hydrogen and sulphur bonds within the cortex of the hair are temporarily broken down by the water, allowing the hair to be stretched (see Figure 3.1). Hair stretches more easily when wet, and shampooing the hair wets it more effectively than just damping with a trigger spray.
- Drying – during this stage the hair is stretched into a new shape and dried into that shape. The hydrogen and sulphur bonds in the hair reform and hold the hair in the shape in which it was dried.
- Reforming – when the hair is wetted again it returns to its natural shape and may be restyled again. Hair absorbs moisture from the atmosphere (it is hygroscopic) and therefore the hairstyle gradually falls, falling more rapidly in moist damp conditions

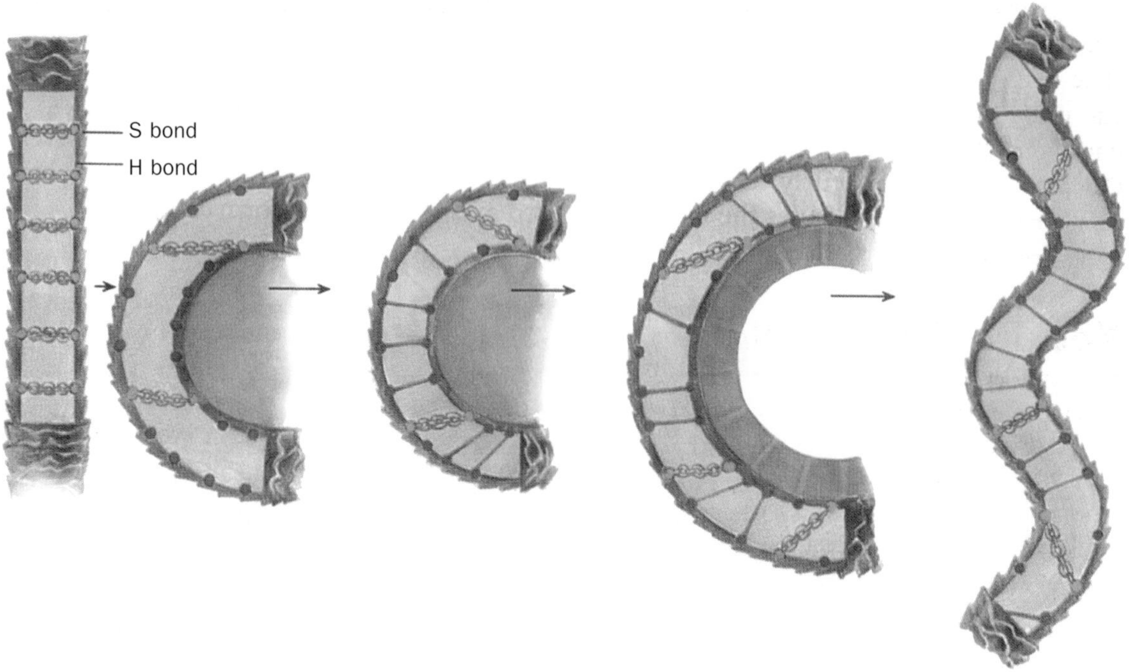

Figure 3.1 Chemical bonds within hair

(high humidity). Styling aids often place a coating on the hair to slow down this absorption of moisture, delaying elastic recoil, and therefore extending the life of the style.

Gowning your client

1 The purpose of gowning your client is to protect them and their clothing from damage or contamination during the hairdressing process (see Figure 3.2). The exact method of gowning used will depend upon your salon's policy and the nature of the hairdressing processes you are about to carry out and may be varied during your client's visit to the salon.

Gowning for your client when carrying out treatments where the hair is wet will require you to prevent moisture from causing discomfort to the client or damage to clothing. However, gowning when using styling irons has different requirements, as there will not be any moisture present.

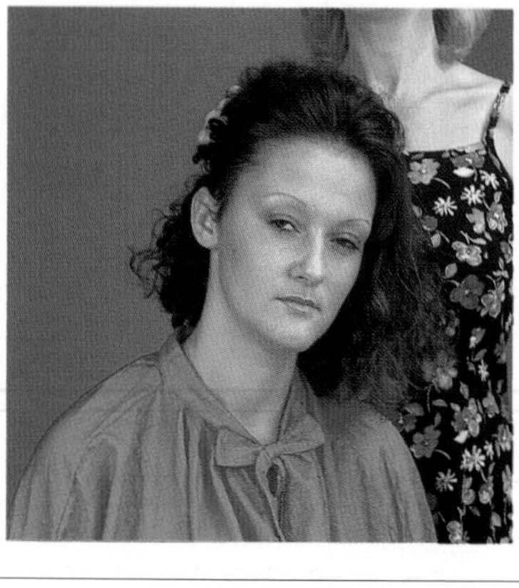

Figure 3.2 Gowned client

Gowning will normally be done following your initial consultation with your client; this may depend upon your salon's policy. During your consultation it is useful to be aware of the style of clothing that they wear, as this can give you a feel for their fashion sense, which in turn can guide you in your style suggestions. Note that, however, if your client has had previously damage to their clothing while visiting the salon, they may not be wearing their usual clothes. Clean gowning materials should be used so as to help prevent the spread of infectious disorders from one client to the next. Different salons' methods of gowning may vary, however all will endeavour to ensure that the client's clothing is protected.

Your choice of styling technique

The choice of techniques you will use to achieve the result discussed with your client will depend upon a number of factors. These include:

- The finished style required – some techniques are better suited to particular hairstyles,
- The hair texture – fine hair may require more support in the drying technique, whereas thick, strong, coarse hair will require less and will produce much of its own volume.
- The hair type – curly hair may require more tension when drying to control or reduce the natural curl.
- Strong hair growth patterns – for example, a 'double crown' may require more control in the drying process.

> ***TIP*** To enable you to select the most appropriate product for use on the client, you should understand the features of all of the styling aids used within your salon.

STYLING AIDS

Liquid styling aids

Liquid styling aids have the following properties:

- they help to make the hair more manageable during the drying process
- they prolong the life of the hair style (by excluding atmospheric moisture)
- they give the hair the necessary stiffness to enable the production of the required hair-style
- they help to condition and moisturise the hair
- they compensate for the damaging effect that heat can have on the hair. Liquid styling aids are usually applied to wet hair that has been towel dried.

Your choice of styling aid will be determined by the client's hair type, the required hair-style, the features of the particular product, your personal preference and the salon's policy.

> ***TIP*** The Control of Substances Hazardous to Health (COSHH) Regulations 1992 provides for your employer to ensure that you are trained in the safe handling of products and that suitable personal protective equipment is provided if identified as necessary. You should follow these guidelines and use equipment provided in the way indicated.

This information can be obtained by following the manufacturer's guidance notes. The trainee stylist may also follow guidance and ask advice from the stylist.

Blow-dry lotions are available in liquid form, as a single application phial and multi-application bottles, as well as aerosol and pump action. Liquids are applied by sprinkling onto the hair, spreading throughout using both your fingers and comb. Aerosols may be applied by directing the spray onto the hair, ensuring distribution by directing the spray throughout the head of hair and by combing. Take care: avoid applying too much of the product that will then run onto the client's neck, weigh down the hair and cause waste.

Mousse is a blow-dry lotion produced in foam form, making the product easier to apply and distribute by hand throughout all the hair or on specific areas of the hair. Apply by hand a sphere of mousse the size of a golf ball, distributing it throughout the hair using the fingers, followed by a wide-toothed comb (see Figure 3.3). Take care when first applying the mousse as it can be inclined to roll off the hair.

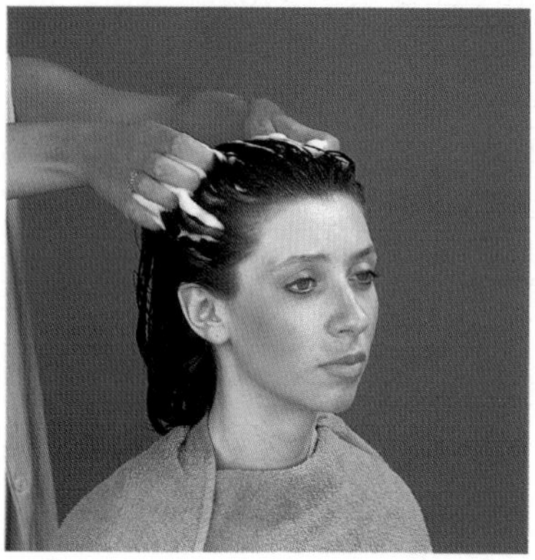

Figure 3.3 Applying mousse to the hair

> ***TIP*** If you are unfamiliar with any product you use on a client's hair, always read and follow the manufacturer's instructions.

Gel is a styling aid that has a heavier consistency than mousse or blow-dry lotions. Applied from the palms of your hands, it is distributed throughout the hair. The gel may also be applied to specific parts of the hair using the pads of your fingers. Gel can be available in both a normal dry look when dry, and a wet look. The crisp finish left on the hair, if the gel is left to dry undisturbed, makes gel very suitable for sculptured/slick looks.

These products are often available for a variety of hair types and degrees of hold, normal and firm.

Curl activators and moisturisers are usually available as a pump action spray. Spray this onto curly hair to gave a more controlled, defined curl. Direct the spray throughout the hair and distribute using a wide toothed comb and the fingers. These products are particularly useful on hair that is dry, difficult to control and fragile.

> ***HEALTH AND SAFETY*** If you are uncertain about how to use a particular hairdryer, follow the manufacturer's advice or ask your line manager or trainer.

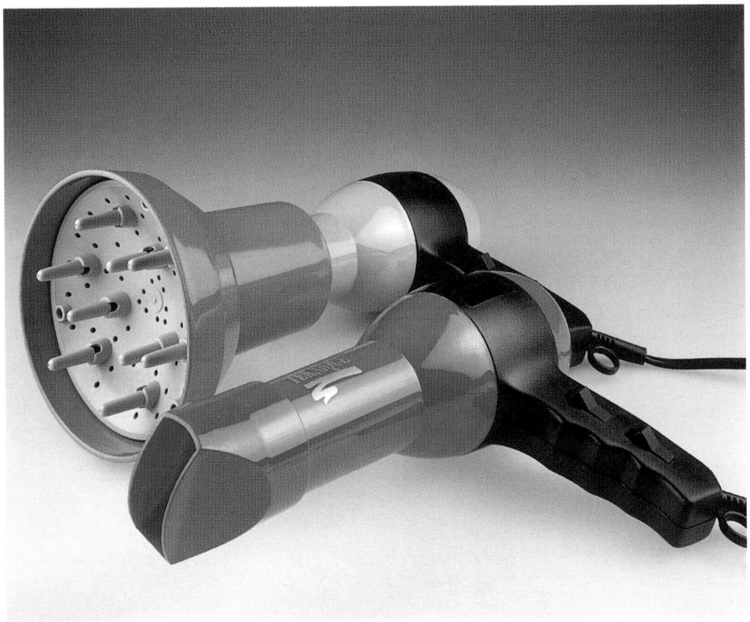

Figure 3.4 Fishtail and diffuser nozzles fitted to hairdryers

Styling tools

Your choice of blow-dryer may depend upon your personal preference, what is available and the type of style to be produced. 1

Hairdryers are available with a range of controls including differing air speeds and heat settings. For controlled drying a 'fishtail'-style nozzle can be fitted to concentrate the air flow to a narrow band. Diffusers may be fitted to many dryers to reduce the disruption to the hair caused by the air flow (see Figure 3.4).

> ***TIP*** Remember, do not handle electrical appliances with wet hands.

Select styling tools that will not be adversely affected by the levels of heat used in the drying process. Remember that many plastic- and nylon-based tools will distort if exposed to heat for too long. The fine nylon bristles of brushes may soften or the teeth of plastic combs may bend. Vulcanite (hardened rubber) combs have a slightly higher heat resistance. Metal tools, such as aluminium combs, may be used when controlling short hair or producing waves of raised partings, *but they can become very hot, and if then touched on the client's scalp may burn the skin.* Bone combs have a high resistance to heat.

There are a number of brushes designed specifically for use when blow drying, including 'vent' style brushes which are designed to aid air flow and thus speed up hair drying, and radial brushes of a variety of diameters which enable you to dry the hair into curved or rounded shapes (see Figures 3.5 and 3.6). Watch hairstylists, demonstrators and your instructors drying hair and the range of drying tools that they use. This may guide you in your choices.

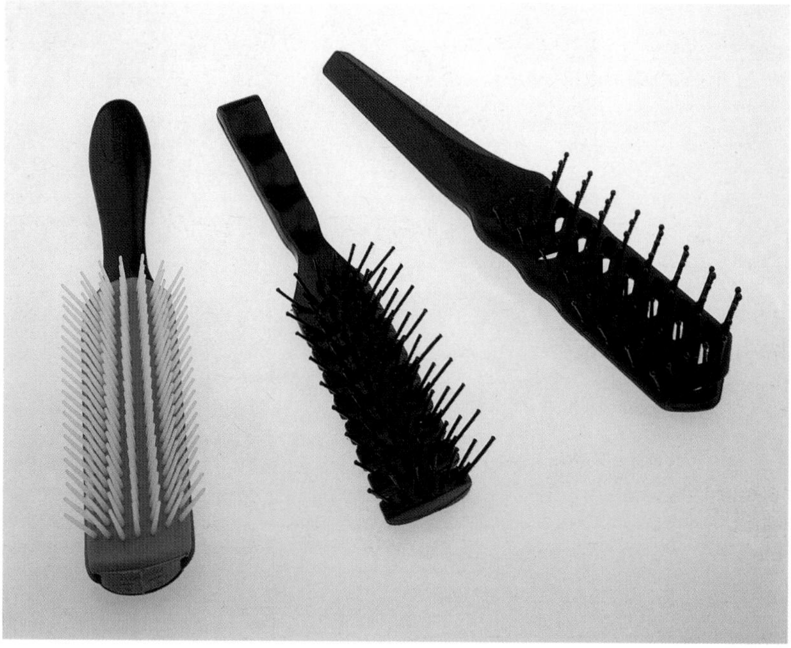

Figure 3.5 Blow drying brushes

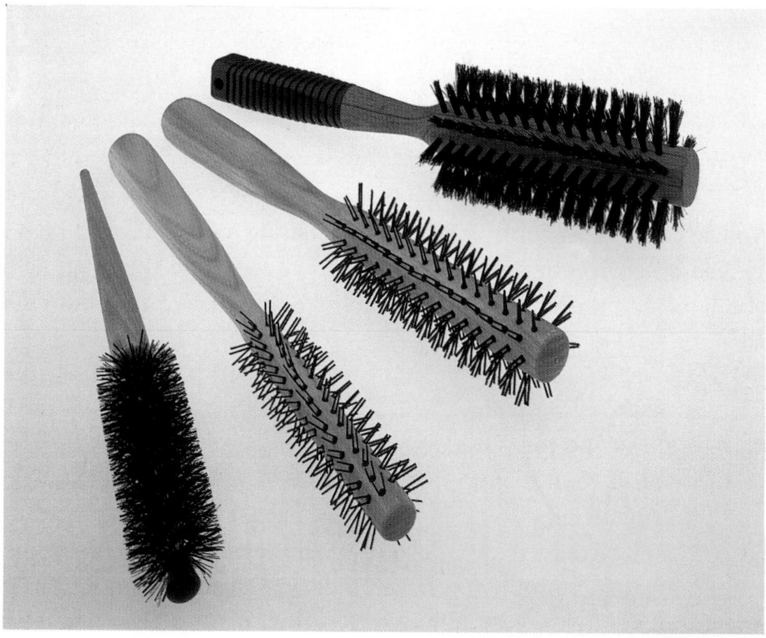

Figure 3.6 Radial brushes

TIP The Electricity at Work Regulations 1989 requires that all portable electrical equipment used in the salon is regularly electrical safety checked.

Take care that you do not use electrical equipment that you or a colleague has brought into the salon that has not undergone these safety tests.

TIP Remember before using to visually check all electrical equipment for any external damage. If damage is detected this should be reported to the responsible person and the equipment labelled and put out of use.

BLOW DRYING

This technique is suitable for a wide range of hairstyles on a variety of hair types and hair lengths. The hair dryer is used together with a variety of tools, including hands, combs and brushes, the choice of which depends on the style required.

Your best results will be achieved on hair that is freshly shampooed. Shampooing prepares the hair by cleansing the hair and enabling it to be stretched into a new shape. The hair can then be dried into this new shape, delaying elastic recoil, which it will retain until the hair is moistened again.

Following the shampoo, remove the excess moisture from the hair by towel drying. Remove any tangles from the hair using a wide-toothed comb, taking care not to cause discomfort to the client, or damage to the hair, by excessive tension on the hair. Fine porous hair is very easily damaged and broken while wet.

HEALTH AND SAFETY Never use electrical appliances when the cable is damaged or frayed in any way. Report any damaged equipment to your line manager or person responsible for maintenance.

Apply appropriate styling aids to the hair, taking care not to allow the product to spill onto the client's face or neck, and comb the hair into the direction of the style. Take care to avoid overheating the hair, as excessive heat can damage the hair and excessive heat on the scalp will cause your client discomfort. Avoid directing the air flow against the hair in one place for too long, as this may cause excessive heating and subsequent damage to the hair.

Having removed excess moisture start your blow dry at the lower parts of the hairstyle, those areas that will be on the underneath of the style (see Figure 3.7). If there is an area of the head or a part of the style that is likely to be particularly resistant to styling, this is often best dried first. Ensure that each mesh of hair is dried before moving on to the next, as meshes which are left damp will affect others which lie adjacent.

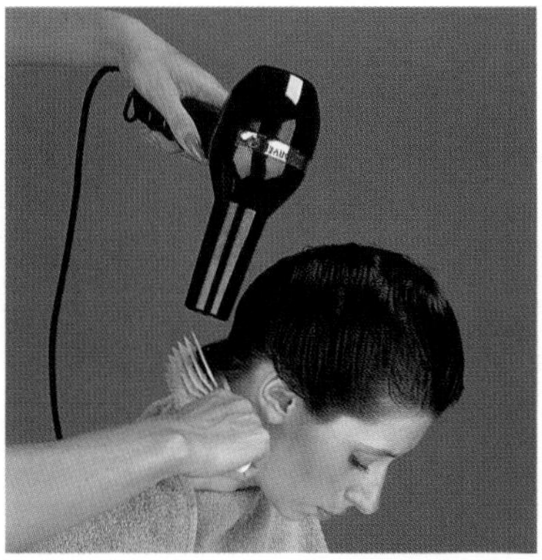

Figure 3.7 Blow drying at the nape

For smooth results the air flow should be directed with the direction of the hair. When achieving lift and volume, hold up meshes of hair in turn and direct the dryer into the upheld root area (see Figure 3.8).

Use the dressing mirror to check the shape and balance of the hair style being developed.

Using the radial brush

Using the radial brush will enable you to dry the hair into curls or waves. Your choice of brush will depend upon a number of factors:

- The strength of curl achieved will depend on the radius of the brush that you use: the larger the radius, the softer the curl; the smaller the radius the tighter the curl. Curl strength may also depend on the amount of hair wrapped around the hairbrush when drying.
- The length of hair may determine the size of brush, as the hair will need to be long enough to be wrapped around the brush.
- Differing types of bristle material have differing characteristics. Fine, closely-set bristle tends to grip the hair; widely-spaced bristle may control the hair more easily and remove tangles.
- Your choice will often be personal choice. If in doubt, check with your supervisor.

Use the radial brush as follows:

Using the fingers, section off a mesh of hair and place it on the brush. Rotate the brush to smooth the ends of the hair into the direction of movement. Wind the hair around the brush and direct the air flow from the hairdryer in the direction in which the hair is lying (see Figure 3.9). Directing the air flow against the direction of the hair will produce a messy result as the shorter hair within the mesh will be dried without control and may produce a fuzzy appearance in the style.

To avoid damage to the hair by excessive heat do not direct the airflow at one place all the time. Keep the airflow moving over the hair. Rotate the brush to ensure that the hair is dried into a smooth finish around it. When working with long or very thick hair, drying can be more effective if you dry the ends of the hair first, gradually winding the hair around the brush and drying it progressively, working towards the root area. Take care when drying very long hair that the brush does not become entangled in it.

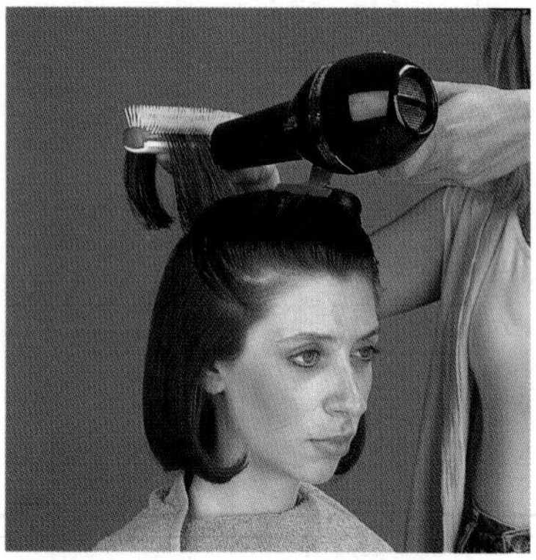

Figure 3.8 Blow-drying to achieve root lift

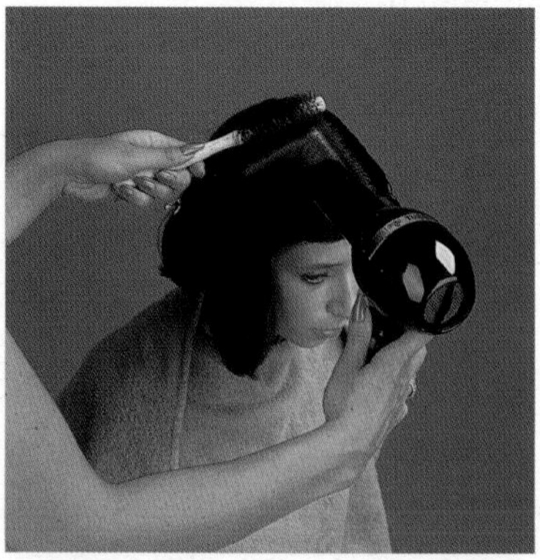

Figure 3.9 Blow-drying with a radial brush

When drying fine hair (that drops the curl easily) or hair that is resistant to curl, leaving the brush in place as the hair cools will enhance curl retention.

> ***TIP*** For safety, do not direct the airflow directly at the scalp as this may burn the client's skin.

To achieve lift at the roots, lift the mesh away from the head. The higher the mesh is lifted (over directed) the greater the lift achieved with the particular brush. Larger diameter brushes will produce more root lift. Flatter results will be produced by using root drag or incorporating the use both of the radial and flat brush on the hair.

Using the flat brush

Using the flat brush will enable you to produce smooth, straight hair styles. There are two main styles of flat brush:

- brushes with closely set, fine bristles, which can be very useful when styling very short hair that may not be long enough to lie easily on the brush
- brushes with widely spaced, thick bristles, which are ideal when styling smooth straight styles where the hair length is sufficient to lie on the brush.

Generally the differences between brushes of these categories lie in their size, the number of rows of bristles and the style of base. Your choice should be the one that is most comfortable for you to use. The styles of base available are rubber cushioned back, solid back or vented back. The rubber cushioned back allows the bristles to move slightly and therefore flex with the hair. Both this and the solid back give smoother results on straight hairstyles. The vented back aids speedy drying of the hair.

Using your fingers, take small meshes of hair and lay them onto bristles of the brush. With the air flow of the hair dryer directed onto the mesh of hair and in the direction of the hair, draw the brush from the roots to the points of the hair (see Figure 3.10). You will produce a smooth, straight result in this manner. When straightening wavy hair, slight tension must be maintained on the hair. If a slight movement is required, for example to turn the ends of a bobbed hairstyle either out or under, then roll the brush in the appropriate direction and direct the air flow onto the corner of the brush.

You may use either a brush or comb to control wet hair while blow waving:

- use a brush on long hair
- use a comb on short hair.

Shape the hair and direct the airflow into the trough of the wave.

FINGER DRYING

This technique is best suited to hair that falls into style easily, has some natural volume and movement and where an *informal* look is required. Your hands become the tools that guide the hair into position during the drying process. In many cases the body heat from your hands aids the drying of the hair. Drying is often aided by the use of the hair dryer. Your fingers will draw the

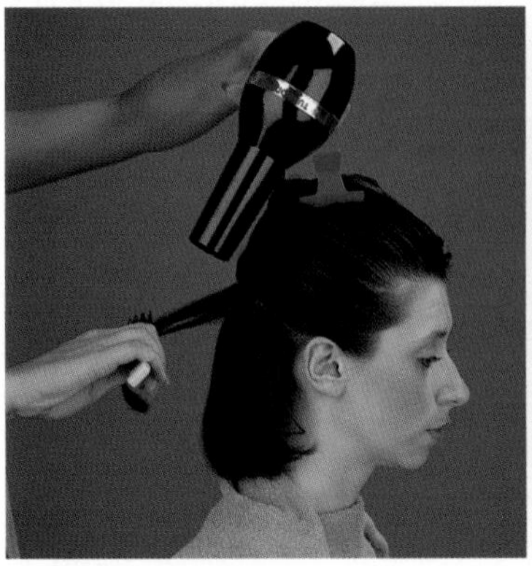

Figure 3.10 Blow-drying for smooth bob with vent brush

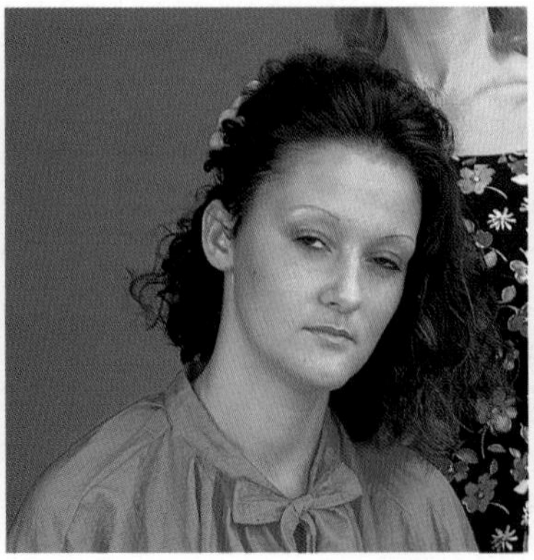

Figure 3.11 Finger drying curly hair into style

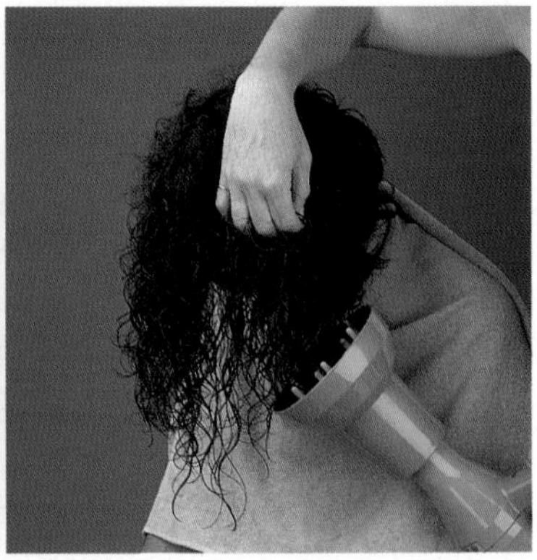

Figure 3.12 Scrunch drying in the hand

hair into place either in a 'claw-like' fashion, the fingers taking on the role of a wide-toothed comb or brush, or will mould the hair by wrapping it around the fingers to produce movement in the hair (see Figure 3.11). Lift and volume at the roots is achieved by rotary movements of the hair at the root, using either finger pads or the palm of your hand and lifting the hair away from the scalp. Your client's head is normally maintained in an upright position except when producing volume in medium-length and long hair, when the head may be inclined downwards and then brought upright when the root area is dry.

SCRUNCH DRYING

This technique is used when a full curly style is required, usually on medium or long hair lengths. Compress the wet hair, into its curled shape in the hand and direct the air flow onto the palm of the hand, opening the hand to allow the access of the warm air and then closing to scrunch (see Figure 3.12). Continue to scrunch the hair as the hair cools after the heat has been removed. This will improve retention of movement.

When dressing a finished hairstyle you may use this scrunching technique to encourage movement in the hair. Place a small amount of styling aid, mousse, gel or wax onto the palms of your hands and then, without added heat, scrunch the hair.

NATURAL DRYING

As we have seen, wet hair stretches more easily than dry hair. During most drying processes the hair is stretched into shape and position and dried into this form. Elastic recoil is delayed when the hair is dried and remains in this shape until the hair is made wet again, either when shampooed or as moisture is absorbed from the atmosphere, when it returns to its natural shape and direction.

When drying naturally, the hair remains in its unstretched state, having been gently put into shape and dried undisturbed either without heat or by applying radiant heat.

TIP When introducing a new hairstyle to your client, provide them with guidance on how to maintain their look between visits to the salon.

WHAT THE EXPERT SAYS Hair fashions today require a wide variety of drying techniques. With so many hair fashion leaders introducing their 'looks' for the season, your clients have a great wealth of creativity to call upon. At one time clients depended upon their hairstylist to inform them of current and emerging fashion. Today's business is consumer lead, and the consumer is informed by the media of what is available and what is emerging. This media takes the form of consumer magazines, some of which are related to the broad issues of fashion and others which are specific to their hair. These usually have features and designs from professional hairdressers. The media of television has realised the potential interest in fashion and several hairdressers now present their 'looks' on a variety of television productions.

This information coming to the consumer means that they will come to you, the professional hairdresser, with a number of preconceived ideas about how they wish to look. In extreme cases, due to the volume of differing ideas being presented via the media, they may come to you confused and wanting your professional guidance.

To be able to fulfil their expectations you need to be aware of current and emerging fashion trends and to be able to produce a range of looks for your clients. How do you do this?

The answers

As a professional hairdresser you must take the initiative to maintain your awareness of the fashion scene. Professional trade magazines can be one useful source of information and ideas. Often these magazines give you step by step guides in producing these styles as well as ideas for hair colour and other aids to enhance these looks.

Attending briefing seminars, often promoted by manufacturing houses or artistic groups, will enable you to maintain this awareness. There are a number of 'platform' shows, where well-known stylists or styling groups demonstrate techniques as well as presenting completed looks. Just as for many designer fashion exhibitions, much of the work demonstrated is not designed as 'street fashion'. However, ideas and concepts can be obtained from these and adapted for use with your clients.

New products or tools that enable you to produce specific fashion effects are often demonstrated at trade exhibitions, which occur throughout the year at a variety of venues.

Finding out

Information about forthcoming events is often given in professional trade magazines. Membership of a trade organisation can often be another source of this information.

Commitment

As hairdressers we should never stop learning new techniques or developing new skills if we wish to maintain a vibrant and growing clientele. Our clients seek a service that makes the most of their attributes in a fashionable way. As a successful professional you must be aware of this.

CREATING THE FINISHED LOOK

Having dried the hair in a controlled manner it will require dressing to give the finished look (see Figure 3.13).

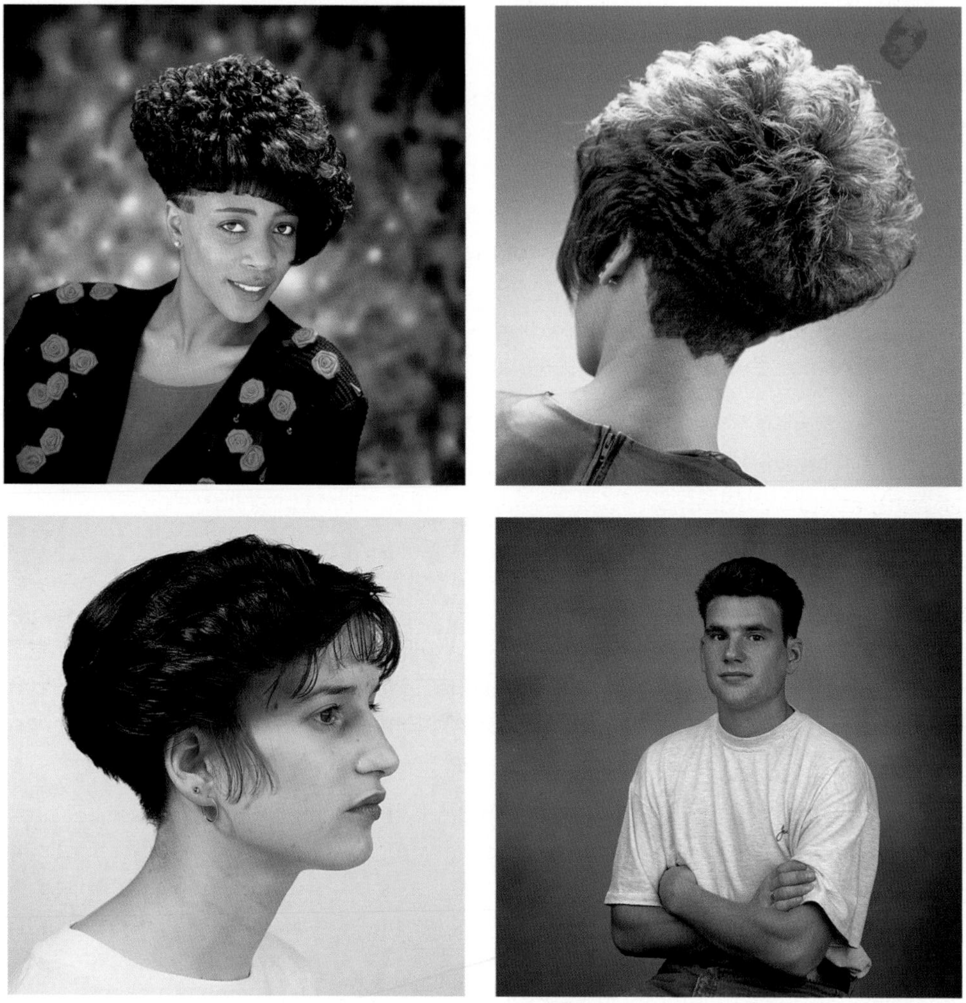

Figure 3.13 Finished fashion hairstyles

Depending upon the result that you require this dressing may consist of brushing the hair into place using a brush of either closely tufted or widely spaced bristle.

For heavy, smooth, one-length looks the hair is usually brushed with a widely spaced, thick-bristle brush, brushing in the direction of the hair fall. To add texture to the finish, the hair may be brushed at 90 degrees to the direction of fall, usually back from the front hairline, and then allowed to fall into place. To add volume to heavy, smooth one-length styles the brush may be placed into the hair, which already lies in the direction of fall, and slowly lifted up allowing the hair to fall gradually. The surface should be smoothed gently, taking care not to dig the teeth of a widely spaced, large-toothed comb or the bristles of a brush into the volume of the hair.

For textured shorter looks the hair may be textured by drawing the fingers through the hair, in a claw-like fashion, either in or across the direction of the hairstyle. The 'vent' brush may be used in a similar way.

For controlled curly/tousled looks the hair may be scrunched in the hands, your hands may be used to position hair, to separate strands of hair, to add height by rotating the roots or by back-combing the hair, pushing back towards the roots on small meshes of hair.

To produce many fashion effects combinations of techniques must often be used. Be prepared to learn and adapt your techniques to suit emerging fashions. If you are uncertain of the technique to use ask your stylist/instructor for advice and guidance.

Techniques of back combing or back brushing may be used when dressing these styles, to achieve more height or control over the hair.

Finishing products can be used to assist you in dressing the hair, to enable you to produce the desired look and to prolong the duration of the finished look.

Back combing, page 228

Back brushing, page 230

Some products are applied to the hair from the palms of the hands. They may also be applied, using the fingers, to particular areas of the style or to particular strands of hair. Others are applied as an aerosol directed at the hair.

To enable you to select the correct products for the hair texture and for the required result you must learn about the features of the products available in your salon.

The sprays available include hair fixing sprays that hold the hair in place. Some are available for particular hair types and conditions, and they are often available providing differing degrees of hold. In selecting, you will consider the required finished look and whether the style should move or if it should stay fixed in place. Gel spray offers an alternative to hair spray on dry hair, often being firmer. It is designed for use as a sculpting lotion, an aid to dressing the hair into position.

Gel may be used not only when drying wet hair but also as a dressing aid, using small quantities scrunched through the hair to create volume as well as on specific strands of hair to enable them to be moulded into place. Wet look results may be achieved using these products.

Wax may be used to give separation and definition to the hair and curl. It may be used throughout the hairstyle, having applied a small amount worked through the hair from the palms of the hands. Wax may also be applied to individual strands of hair using the fingers. Fly-away hair may be calmed using a little wax. On fine, soft, hair wax can sometimes be too heavy a product for use.

Dressing creams/mousses give control to hair and enables the hair to be sculpted and moulded into shape. These products are available in a range of strengths and are suitable for differing hair textures and style effects.

Gloss, usually a fine oil is available in liquid and aerosol forms. These give shine to the hair. Over-generous use of these products can result in a greasy look to the hair.

When applying hair-fixing spray to the finished look, avoid wetting the hair by holding the spray too close or by holding the spray in one place for too long. When using aerosol on fine, soft hair, the pressure of the spray may move or flatten the hair. Shield the client, their skin and clothing from the products being used.

TIP When you use finishing products on the hair, if you are unfamiliar with the product study the manufacturers instructions and always follow these instructions. Remember, many finishing products are inflammable and must be used with care.

FURTHER STUDY

- Find out what the emerging fashions are in hairstyling and how these styles are created.
- Read the consumer trade press to find out about current and emerging hair fashion.
- To increase your range of skills practise a variety of drying techniques.
- Find out what effect the Control of Substances Hazardous to Health Regulations have on the use of styling products within your salon.

REVIEW QUESTIONS

1. Which bonds, located within the hair's cortex, are broken down and then reformed during the blow-dry process?
2. (1) How much styling mousse is normally required when styling hair?
3. How should hair fixing spray be applied to the finished hairstyle?
4. What effect will moisture have upon the finished hairstyle?
5. Which factors will affect your choice of styling technique to be used?
6. (1) How may height be achieved in the hairstyle through blow-drying?
7. When blow-drying, how is a smooth effect achieved?
8. Which blow-dryer attachment should be used when scrunch-drying hair?
9. What styling product should be used to help achieve separation and definition in a finished hairstyle?
10. What may be the result of applying too much gloss spray to the hair?

CHAPTER 4

Haircutting

This chapter provides the essential knowledge of the basic techniques you will use to cut hair.

Level 2	
Unit 201	
Element 201.1	Consult with and maintain effective relationships with clients
Element 201.2	Advise clients on salon products and services
Unit 204	
Element 204.1	Maintain effective and safe methods of working when cutting hair
Element 204.2	Cut hair to achieve a variety of one length looks
Element 204.3	Cut hair to achieve a variety of layered looks
Unit 209	
Element 209.2	Support health, safety and security at work
Unit 210	
Element 210.1	Maintain effective and safe methods of working when using barbering techniques
Element 210.2	Cut hair to achieve a variety of looks with different neckline shapes

Contents

INTRODUCTION

This aspect of hairstyling has, arguably, the highest profile with your clientele. Clients appear to think haircutting more important than any other hairdressing skill. Such is the profile of haircutting that there are a number of emerging salon groups specialising in haircutting, often to the exclusion of any of the chemical hairdressing processes.

Haircutting skills are acquired through a thorough understanding of the shapes and effects that may be produced in hair using a range of techniques with a variety of cutting tools. These skills may be developed through practice, initially on wefts of hair (hair attached to a band or thread), then on training heads (lifelike heads with implanted hair, usually human). These tools will enable you, as a trainee hairdresser, to develop the basic techniques and manual dexterity required to create shapes in hair in a controlled manner. Eventually these skills must be applied to a live model. This will provide you with experience of a number of critical influencing factors, including a variety of hair textures, hair growth patterns, head and face shapes and lifestyles.

Learning to cut a number of individual haircuts without an understanding of the principles and processes which lie behind them will produce a skill which may not adapt to suit changing hair fashions and haircutting trends.

TOOLS USED FOR HAIRCUTTING

The quality and selection of tools is important in order for you to accomplish a good haircut. However, good tools will not produce a good haircut unless they are used in the correct manner. To do your best work you should use tools of good quality. However, as improper use will quickly destroy the efficiency of any implement, no matter how perfectly it might have been made in the factory, when starting to learn to cut hair it may not be advisable to purchase tools of a too high a cost until you have developed the skills to use them correctly.

Haircutting scissors

Scissors come in a variety of sizes, shapes and finishes. The sizes of scissors are measured from the points to the opposite end at the finger grip (see Figure 4.1b). The size is described in inches and may range from 3" through to 10" in $\frac{1}{2}$" stages. Your choice will depend mainly upon two factors:

- What feels comfortable to use. The third finger and thumb should fit comfortably, and the thumb should be easily removed from the grip when palming the scissors. Plastic inserts can be obtained for certain scissors, allowing the size of the finger and thumb grips to be varied to suit the user.
- The technique of cutting to be used. Scissor-over-comb techniques normally require a longer pair of scissors than would be used to produce more textured looks.

The shape of the blade may be straight or curved, the curved shape being used when club cutting curved shapes in hair. The surface of the cutting edges may be smooth, or one or both of the edges may have micro-serrations. This helps to prevent hair sliding along the length of the blades as they are closed onto the hair (see Figure 4.3a).

The scissors may be made of metals of differing hardness. The harder metals retain the keenness of the edge for longer, but are more brittle. Scissors are available in stainless steel, chrome-plated steel and plastic-coated steel. Ceramic blades are also available.

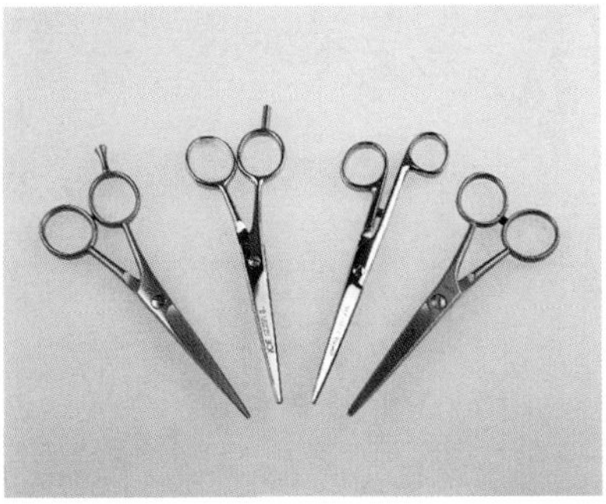

Figure 4.1a Range of scissors

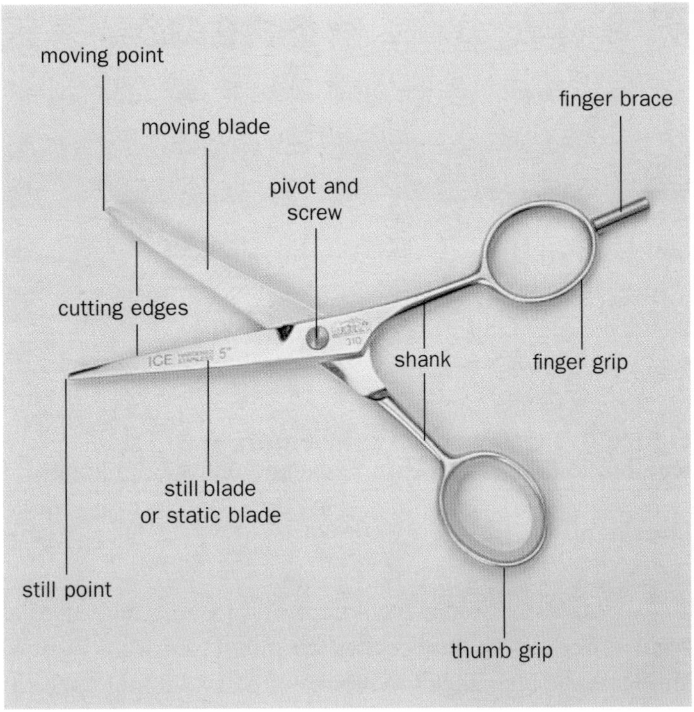

Figure 4.1b Haircutting scissors: the parts

Care of your scissors

- After use, always wipe you scissors dry and place them in their case.
- Use a light oil on the surfaces at the pivot.
- Always keep scissors sharp; the cut of the end of the hair is then much cleaner.
- Your scissors have blades which are finely ground; they require specialist sharpening.

> ***HEALTH AND SAFETY*** Don't keep haircutting scissors in your pocket, unless they are in a specialised wallet.

Thinning scissors

There are many types of thinning scissors, the main distinction between types being the serrations on the blade. When the blade is closed, hair slides into the serrations and is not cut. The hair which does not slide into the gap is cut, and this action thins the hair. The more serrations, the less hair that will be removed. The wider the serrations and teeth of the scissors, the bolder the cut will be. Closely set, fine teeth will remove much finer strands; a pair of scissors with a single serrated blade will remove a greater bulk of hair than they would if both blades were serrated (see Figures 4.2 and 4.3).

When used on wet hair, thinning scissors remove more bulk than when used on dry hair. Care must be taken not to over-thin the hair or to cause a definite line of demarcation, often the result if the scissors are closed only once on a strand of hair.

Razors/shapers

There are a number of razors and shapers that you may use on hair. You should only use them when the hair is wet. Traditionally the open razor was used for this, but its use has declined due to the highly specialised sharpening (honing and stropping) process needed and the risks associated with contagious blood-related disorders.

Shaving and face massage, page 256

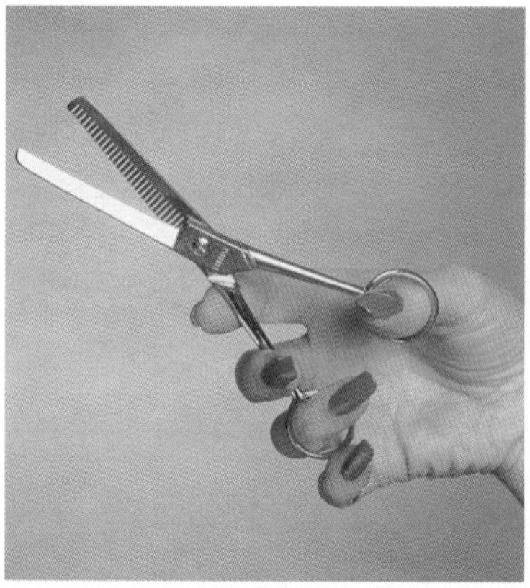

Figure 4.2 Thinning scissors with one serrated blade

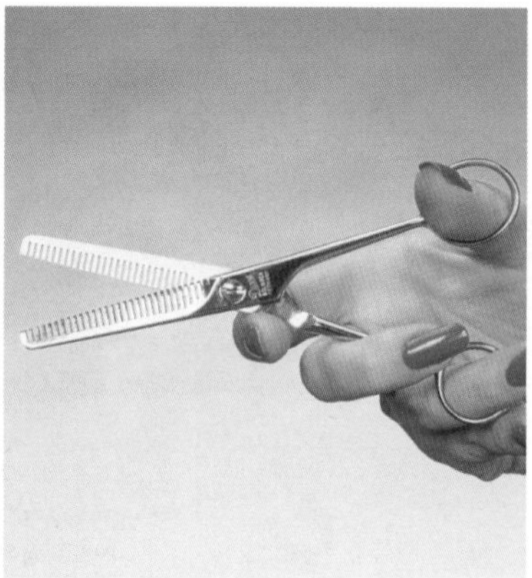

Figure 4.3 Thinning scissors with two serrated blades

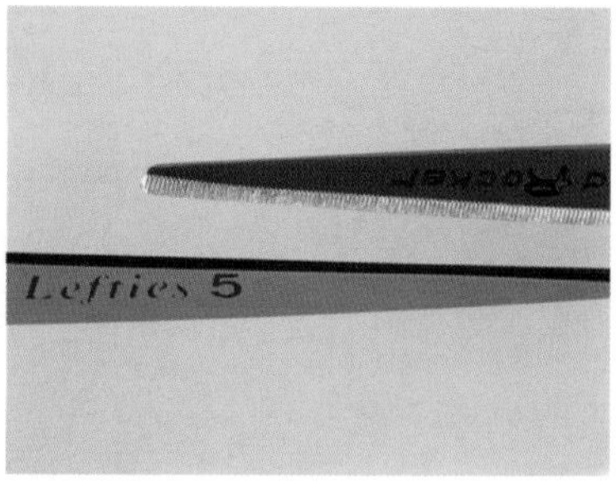

Figure 4.3a Smooth blade and blade with micro-serrations

Razors and shapers accept replaceable blades of a variety of types, some of which are highly specialised. Others may be purchased from most retail chemists and personal grooming shops. Some are shaped to replicate the traditional open razor (see Figure 4.4); others are shaped to fit the hand.

Hair clippers

The traditional hair clippers are operated by hand. They come in a variety of sizes, the size indicating the closeness of the cut achieved. In current use electric hair clippers are more commonly used.

Electric hair clippers

Cordless clippers may be safely used on moist and dry hair, although the battery requires recharging at frequent intervals. They come in a variety of sizes, which varies the closeness and the width of the cut.

➤Barbering, page 236

Corded clippers may be operated for longer periods. Some types are available with variable degrees of cut and others accept a variety of differently sized cutting heads.

Combs

A variety of combs are required when cutting hair (see Figure 4.4). Combs with a variety of teeth sizes allow tangles to be removed and then use the finer teeth to control the hair when cutting. The comb must be small enough to be held easily while also palming the scissors (see Figure 4.5).

Combs that have 'saw cut' teeth are less likely to damage hair than the cheaper, moulded combs, which may have rough surfaces between the teeth.

Holding haircutting tools

Scissors

Haircutting scissors are handled correctly by inserting the third finger into the finger grip of the still blade and placing the little finger on the finger brace (if provided). Insert the thumb into the thumb grip of the moveable blade. The tip of the index finger is braced near the pivot of the scissors in order to give better control (see Figure 4.6).

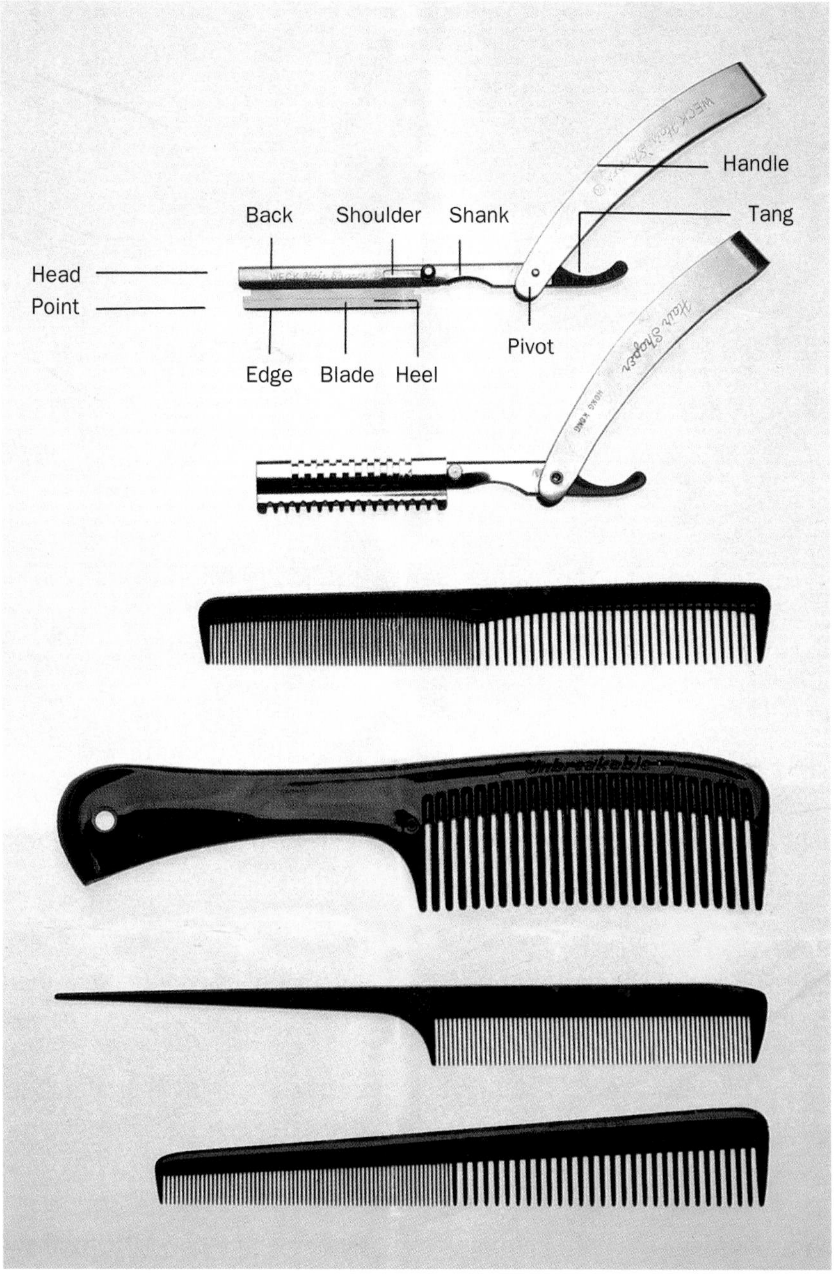

Figure 4.4 Top to bottom: Replacement blade open razor; open razor with safety guards; all purpose comb; large-tooth comb; tail comb; hair shaping comb

Holding comb and scissors

While cutting hair, you will be holding both comb and scissors in the same hand. Practise closing the blades of the scissors, removing the thumb from the grip, and resting the scissors in the palm. Hold the scissors securely with the ring finger. The comb is held between the thumb and fingers, 'palming the scissors' (see Figure 4.5).

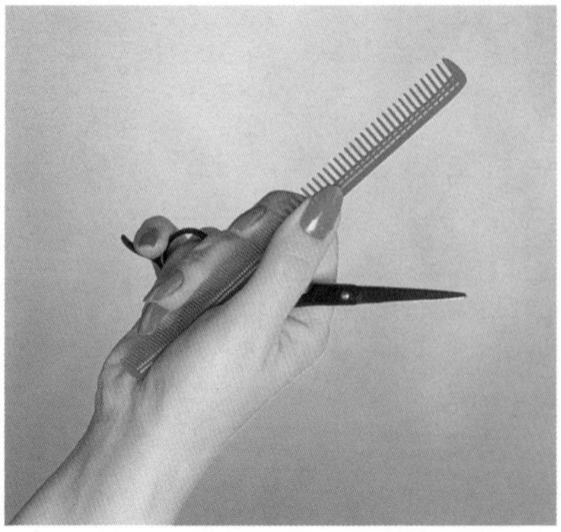

Figure 4.5 Holding comb and scissors together (palming)

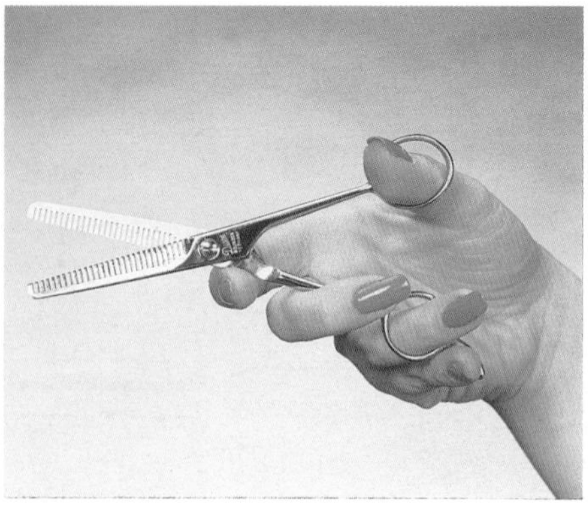

Figure 4.6 Hold scissors

TIP When combing the hair, hold the comb and scissors in the right hand as shown in Figure 4.5. When cutting the hair, hold the comb in the left hand. To save time, do not put the comb or scissors down during shaping.

Razor/shapers

Finger wrap hold

Place the thumb in the groove part of the *shank* and fold the fingers over the handle of the razor. The *guard* faces the hairstylist while working (see Figure 4.7).

Three-finger hold

Place three fingers over the shank, the thumb in the groove of the *shank*, and the little finger in the hollow part of the *tang* (see Figure 4.8).

When using the razor, keep the hair moist to avoid pulling the hair and to prevent dulling the razor.

TIP When combing the hair, hold the razor and comb in the right hand (see Figure 4.9). When cutting the hair with a razor, hold the comb in the left hand. Do not put down the comb or razor.

CLIENT CONSULTATION AND PREPARATION

A good haircut is the foundation of every hairstyle and can change a client's view of themselves and their image.

Client consultation

In order to be aware of the required hairstyle, you must assess your client's needs and requirements and negotiate how these may be best implemented. Effective communication is essential, there are a variety of tools to help you ensure that this takes place. These include style books,

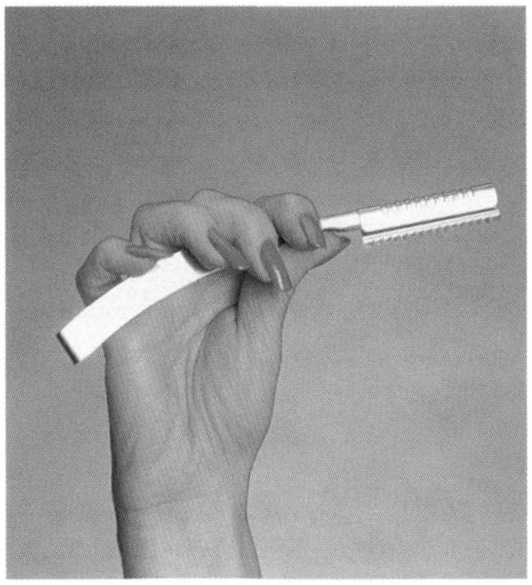

Figure 4.7 Finger wrap hold

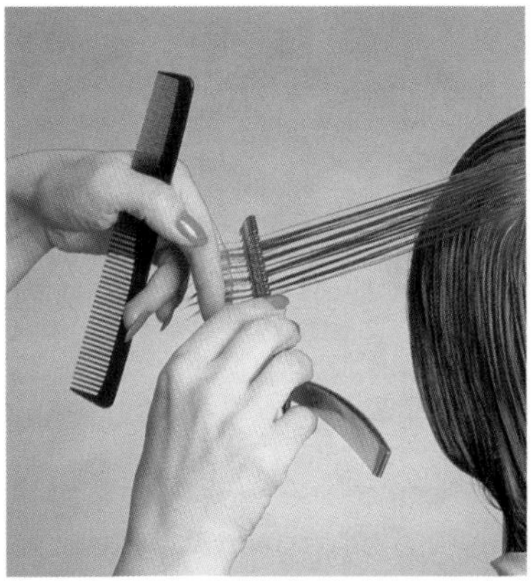

Figure 4.8 Three-finger hold

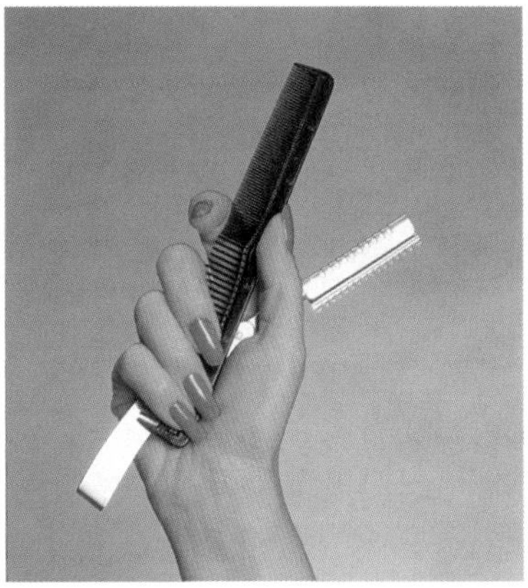

Figure 4.9 Razor and comb

video imaging systems and wigs. Confirmation of the agreed hairstyle should be achieved before commencing the haircut, although this may be reviewed during the cutting process as it progresses. Consultation should normally take place before any work is commenced on your client. The following checklist of factors to bear in mind will help you to assess and advise your client:

- your client's requirements, personality, life-style
- your client's face and head shape
- your client's body proportions
- your client's hair type, texture, thickness and length
- any strong directions of hair growth (hair growth patterns)
- the suggested hairstyle
- your client's ability to cope with their hair.

Head and face shapes, page 7

Check the hair and scalp for any contraindications to the cutting process, these may include contagious scalp disorders, open cuts or sores on the scalp.

> ***TIP*** When providing guidance to your client remember to be honest, tactful and sincere. Your client will respond to factual information provided in a clear, understandable and direct manner.

Gowning and protecting your client

The purpose of gowning your client prior to undertaking a haircut is to protect them and their clothing from hair clippings and any products used by you on their hair. Any method of gowning is acceptable provided that it protects your client and their clothing and is hygienic. Differing salons may have their own procedures for gowning the client. If in doubt consult with your line manager or trainer.

All items used should be clean, freshly laundered or disposable. Gowns and towels not laundered before re-use may pass infection from one client to the next. All gowning should be secured so that it does not come loose or fall during the cutting process.

A gown that is large enough to cover the client's clothing should be used, towels may be required when cutting wet hair, hairs embed themselves in towels, it may be considered more hygienic to towel dry the hair and use disposable plastic shoulder capes to protect the client. To prevent cut hairs from falling down between the client's neck and their clothing, insert a strip of clean cotton wool or a neck tissue around the neck area. These items are disposable and should be used only once.

> ***TIP*** Hair clippings from around your clients neck may be removed by blasting with the hair dryer. Take care, however, that hair clippings do not fly into your client's eyes.

Throughout the cut, loose hair clippings should be removed from the neck area using a clean neck brush. These brushes should be regularly washed, dried and sterilised. Do not allow quantities of hair clippings to build up around the client's neck during the cut, as this will easily become trapped in clothing. The application of talcum powder to the surface of the skin from a powder blower prior to brushing will help to remove clippings easily from the skin.

1. Having discussed the style with your client and assessed the hair for quality, quantity and length, gown the client and then shampoo or wet the hair, unless the hair is to be cut dry. The quality or condition of the hair will determine its elasticity and how well it will retain the dried shape. Hair that is dry or porous will lack shine and will not appear smooth and shiny once dried.
2. When wet the natural fall and movement of the hair may be determined. If this is assessed before wetting, the fall may be confused with the style introduced during the previous styling.
3. Check the hairline (front and back) for unusual hair growth patterns or characteristics that may affect the finished style.

The hair and scalp, page 278

HAIRCUTTING TECHNIQUES

There are three basic techniques in cutting hair. These techniques may be achieved with a variety of haircutting tools used in a variety of ways. Their selection will depend on the required outcome, the preferred technique and salon policy.

> ***TIP*** While the risk of cutting your client is slight, the risk is always there. Ensure that you are aware of your salon procedure in dealing with this, the location of the first aid box within the salon, and any reporting procedures.

Club cutting hair

Club cutting involves cutting of the hair so that all of its thickness is retained, reducing length but not volume (see Figure 4.10).

This technique is ideal when producing heavy, smooth hairstyles where curl or movement is not being encouraged. As all of the hair's natural volume is retained, it is ideal for use on thin, fine hair, where maximum volume is required (see Figure 4.11).

Thinning hair

Cutting the hair to reduce volume but not length (see Figure 4.12). This may be used to thin hair when it is too thick. It may be carried out over the whole head or just in localised areas (fringes and other hairline areas). Methods of thinning may be used to achieve lift, height or spiky effects in fashion styles. Thinning the point ends of the hair will encourage wavy hair to curl.

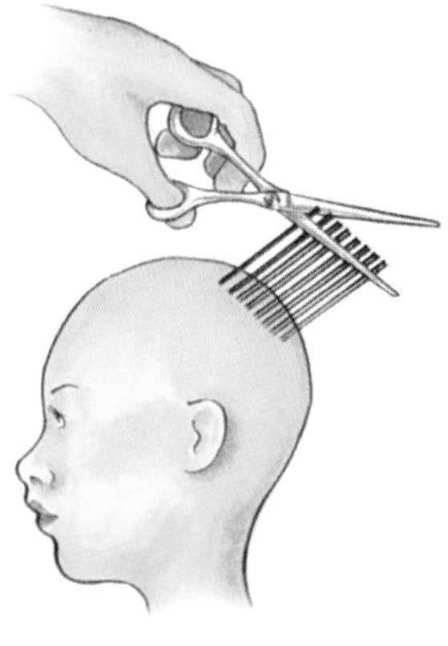

Figure 4.10 Club cutting

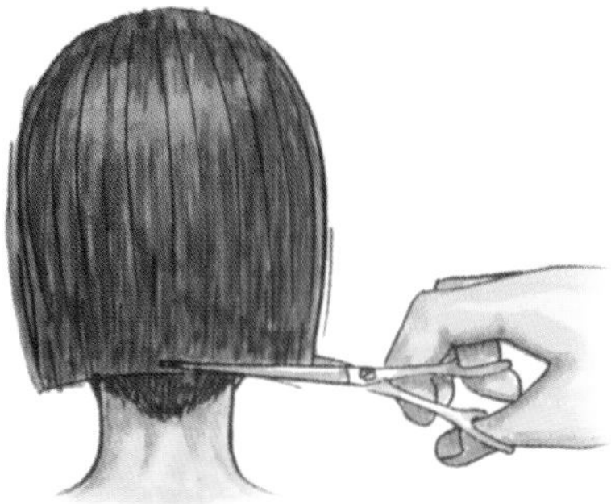

Figure 4.11a Maximising volume by club cutting

Taper cutting hair

Cutting the hair to reduce length as well as thickness. This may be carried out in a single operation (see Figure 4.15a) or may be carried out as a two-step process, with a club cut followed by thinning. This technique of cutting hair can produce a natural taper to the hair, making it appear more natural for softer shapes. It will encourage wavy hair to curl, therefore being ideally suitable for hairstyles which require movement or curl. Straight hair is going to be scrunch dried to curl will curl more easily if taper cut or thinned.

➤Scrunch drying, page 48

Taper cutting will make winding thick hair onto perm rods easier and will also aid the process of back combing.

➤Back combing, page 228

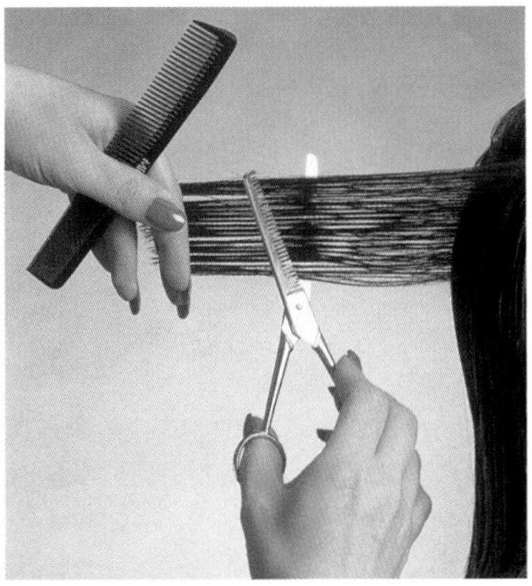

Figure 4.12 Thinning hair with thinning scissors

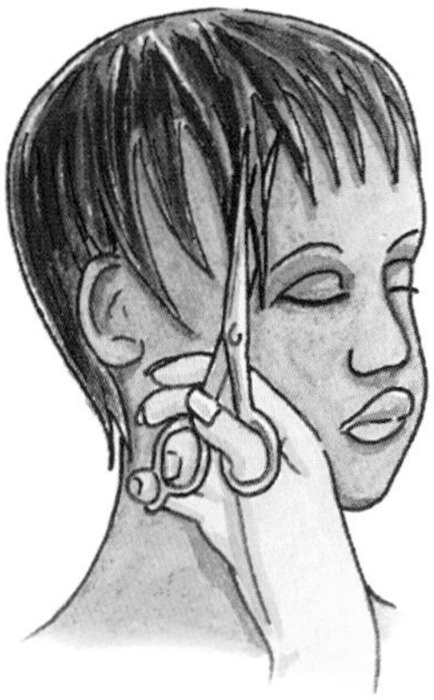

Figure 4.13 Point thinning a fringe section

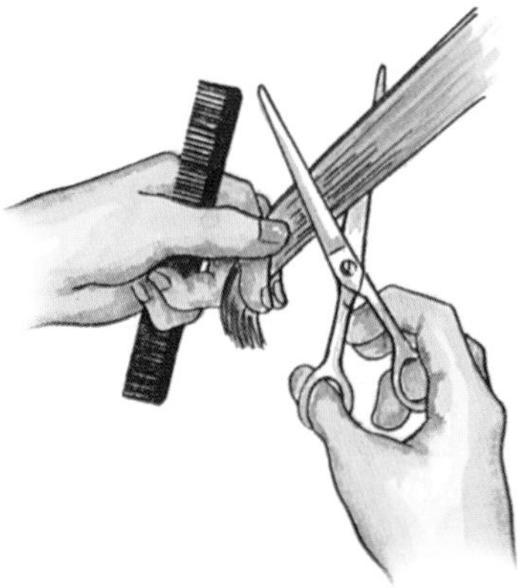

Figure 4.14 Thinning with haircutting scissors

ACHIEVING TECHNIQUES USING HAIRCUTTING TOOLS

Club cutting can be carried out using either scissors (on wet or dry hair) or with clippers (on dry hair). The method of cutting using scissors or clippers over a comb is a method of club cutting the hair, achieving a graduated shape in very short hair (see Figure 3.13c, page 50).

Thinning can be carried out with thinning scissors, haircutting scissors or a razor/shaper. When using thinning scissors, note that if used on wet hair more hair will be removed than when used on dry hair. The term *texturising* is often applied to the technique of thinning the hair to achieve strong fashion effects, where the thinning gives the hair movement often associated with heavily defined changes in hair length.

Taper cutting can be carried out in one step using either a razor/shaper or scissors. Razor/shapers should be used on wet hair only and scissors on dry hair (wet hair does not separate so readily to facilitate the taper with scissors).

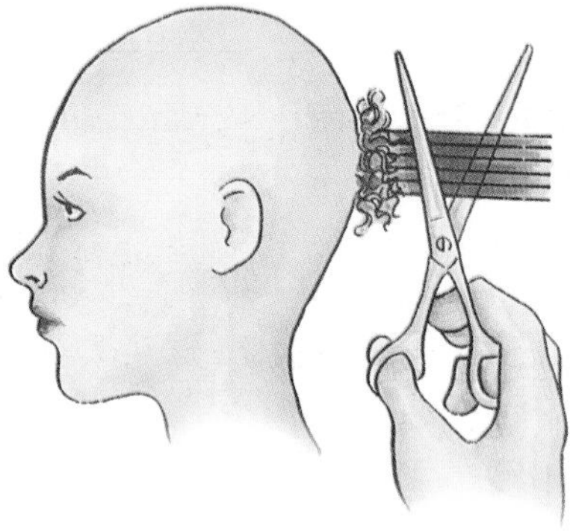

Figure 4.15a Taper cutting to aid back combing

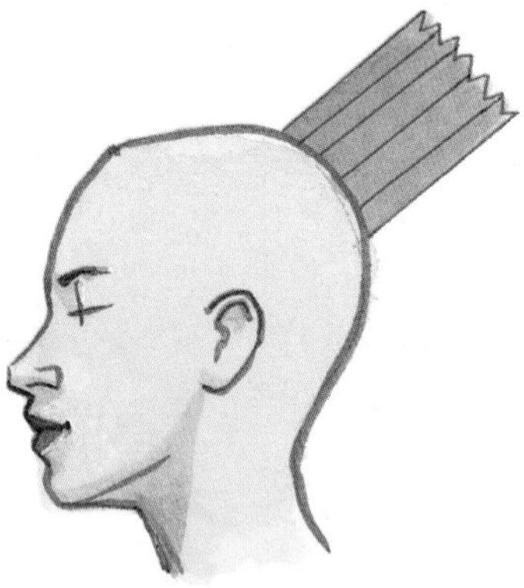

Figure 4.15b Taper out effect by cutting into the mesh of hair using the points of the scissors

The critical factors that can affect your hair cut:

- Very wavy hair is likely to appear much shorter when dry. Allowance should be made for this apparent reduction in length when planning the hair cut.

Strong directions of hair growth, in particular double crowns and cow licks, may cause hair to spring up when the length is removed. This can be problematic when creating a straight fringe in the presence of the cow lick as, if the hair is cut while held down, it may not lay flat when released.

- Strong nape whorls may be easier to control when slightly longer or closely graduated into the neck. Additional length provides weight in the hair to hold the hair down rather than moving sideways as it usually does in the whorl. Close graduation removes the hair length to an extent that any sideways direction is not perceived.
- Reducing the bulk, thinning, very wavy hair can make the control of the wave easier. It may be blow dried straight more readily.
- Very thick hair may appear too thick when cut to a one length bob. The hair ends may require thinning.
- Baby fine hair may often show cutting marks if club cut.

- When club cutting hair that is lightened on the top, often due to sunlight, apparent weight lines or cutting marks may appear at the point where the hair colour changes. Tapering or thinning the hair at these points may reduce this appearance.
- During consultation review the hairs' suitability to retain the style required. Consider if the hair has sufficient length, at the relevant points to enable the style to be produced. The texture of the hair will influence the style choice, fine hair may not produce the required volume unless chemical treatments are used. For example permanent wave style supports. You should remember that your client must be able to maintain their hairstyle between salon visits. The potential of very strong hair may be realised by using this strength to produce lift and volume within the style. This volume may be facilitated by dressing the hair against the direction of hair growth. Lift may be induced by cutting sections of hair within the mesh shorter so as to lift and support the surrounding hair.
- Creating sudden, definite changes in hair length will normally cause the hair to separate at this change point. You may use this to enhance a style where separation, possibly, of a fringe from the remainder of the hair style is required. Wherever there is to be a change in length without causing separation the length changes should be blended by 'overdirecting', that is drawing the hair at 180° to the direction in which it will fall and connecting to the shorter length that is also drawn in the same direction.

PRODUCING SHAPES IN HAIR

Hairstyles are three-dimensional and when cutting hair it is not just the hair's length and outline shape that is changed, but the internal shape as well. There are four basic shapes that may be cut into hair. These may then be used in isolation from each other or may be used in combination, often to achieve fashion effects.

TIP Sharp cutting tools can be dangerous if used in confined areas, where there is a real risk that you will be knocked while working. Razors should not be left open on the work top, but closed and placed in a case or protective cover.

One-length or solid shapes

All of the hair within the style extends to the design line (the base line) of the hairstyle. This style produces the volume of the style around the design line, the weight line. If used on its own the hairstyle will tend to be flat on the top, smooth and weighty around the perimeter. If used on wavy or curly hair the result can be a very full effect.

Uniform layered shapes

All of the hair within the style is cut to the same length. The shape achieved in the style is the same as the head shape. As all the hair is cut to the same length there is no localised build up of volume in areas of the head, so the hair in the design line (the base line) will be wispy.

Layered: internal hair length greater than hair length at hairline (graduation)

The hair at the nape and side design line is the shortest in the hairstyle, gradually getting longer to the top of the hairstyle. Maximum volume is created at the point where the point ends of the

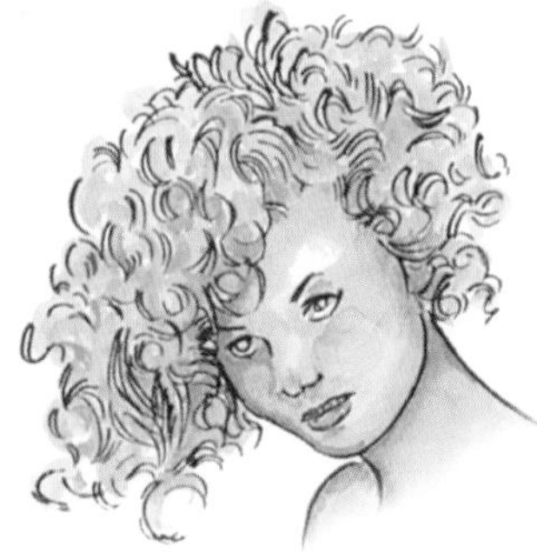

Figure 4.16 Achieving a full effect in wavy hair

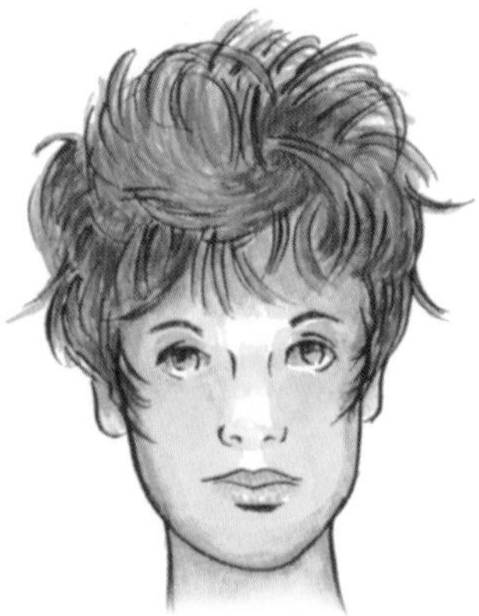

Figure 4.17 Achieving uniform layered shapes

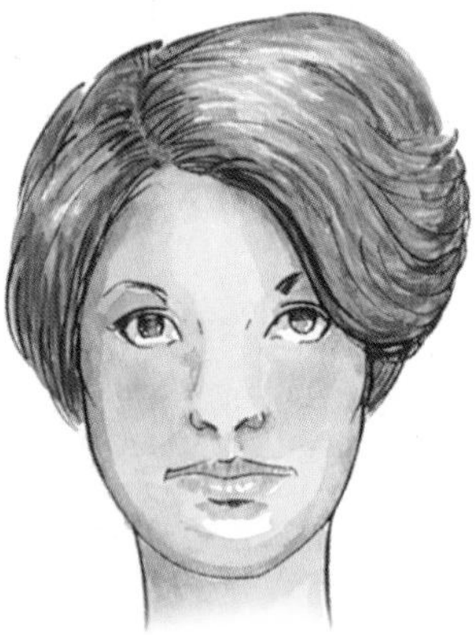

Figure 4.18 Layered hair: graduation where internal hair length greater than at hairline

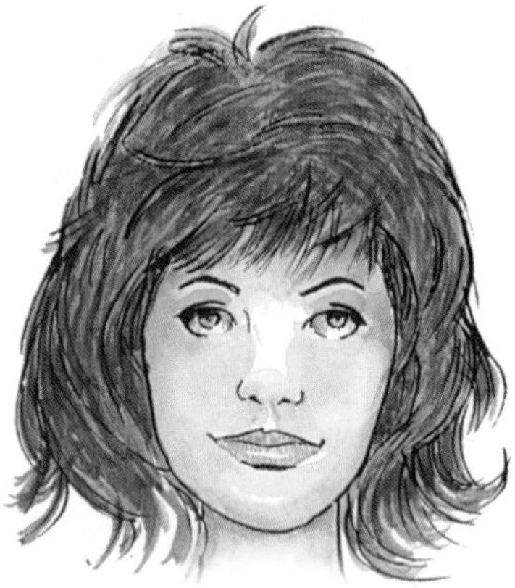

Figure 4.19 Layered hair: graduation where internal hair length shorter than at hairline

top layer reach. This is the weight line within the style. This shape enables the hairdresser to adjust the apparent shape of the head.

Layered: internal hair length less than hair length at hairline (reverse graduation)

The hair on the top of the hairstyle is the shortest in the hairstyle, gradually getting longer towards the style's design line. This enables a long-hair effect to be produced but with volume and movement within the internal structure of the style. The volume is created not by creating a weight line within the style but by producing shorter hair which may lift, and hair ends within the style which may curl.

> ***TIP*** When cutting wavy and curly hair wet, you must allow for elastic recoil as it dries. The extent of this will depend upon the degree of curl.

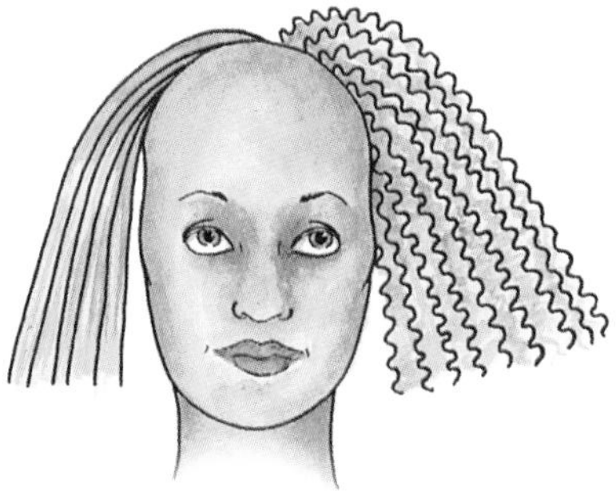

Figure 4.20 The one-length hairstyle

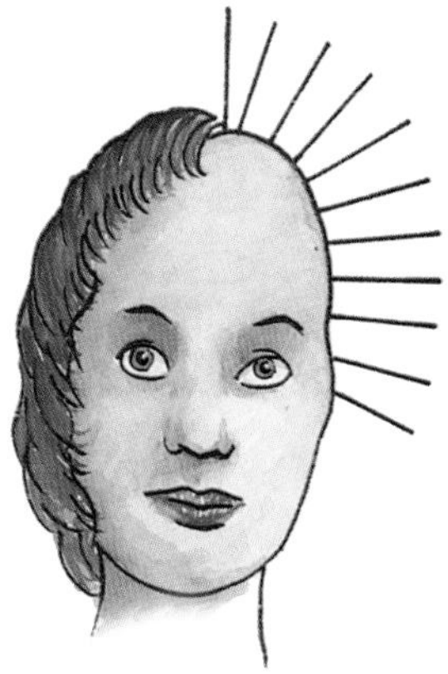

Figure 4.21 The uniform layered hairstyle

The one-length hairstyle (method of cutting)

This style requires that the weight be kept at the design line (base line) of the hairstyle, so the club cut technique should be used. The hair is best cut when wet as this gives maximum control over the hair. Very long hair will stretch while under tension, so take care not to place too much tension on it when cutting, as when released the hair will retract and the weight line will be lost. The process is:

1. Having sectioned the style, to control the hair the cutting of this style usually commences at the nape. Take small sections of hair, which may be easily controlled. Comb smooth and hold down flat to the head or shoulders and cut to the required length, allowing for elastic recoil. When cutting hair that will extend below the level of the nape hairline, it is advisable to keep your client's head upright or inclined forward slightly. The client's head should be central and not allowed to tilt to the side as this may lead to an unbalanced effect.
2. Bring down fine meshes of hair, in controllable sections, hold flat against the head and neck and cut to the position of the design line. The meshes of hair should be combed downwards to remove tangles and to control the hair. Keep the hair evenly wet while cutting so that you achieve an even level of hair stretch.
3. As you progress up the back of the head, taking fine sections of hair, holding in a downwards direction, the side sections of the head should be incorporated. This will help to ensure that there is no break or step between the back and sides. Hold the hair downwards, first cutting the design line. Allow for the additional hair length required to cover the ears and yet produce an even line at the design line.
4. Check the balance of the sides of the haircut by:
   a) Drawing hair from identical areas of each side of the head. If the hair is of even length, the points should meet centrally.
   b) Drawing the fingers down strands of the hair from both sides of the head, and check for level using the dressing position mirror.
5. Continue to progress up the head to the parting area. When directing the hair at the top of the head, comb it into the position into which it will fall when dry.
6. Check the cut when it is dry to ensure that all hair extends to the design line. This will allow for any uneven elastic recoil.
7. A fringe may be cut as an integral part of the style, or if it is not to be blended it may be separated off and cut.

8. Hard, solid design lines may be softened (thinned) by freehand cutting. This is cutting with scissors, pushing the scissors from within the hair-style, in the direction of the hairstyle and closing the blades. To remove more hair the scissors may be angled slightly across the line of hair fall. Soft wispy effects on the sides may also be produced in this way.
9. Once completed, or if your client is to be consulted on the progress of the cut, show them the style using the back view mirror.

> ***TIP*** When cutting hair that will extend past your client's shoulders, ensure that your client is upright. It may be more effective for the client to stand, so that their back is in an upright position and your view is not obscured by the chair back.

The uniform layered hairstyle

This hairstyle does not produce any weight lines in the hairstyle; it follows the shape of the wearer's own head. Additional shape and volume may be added to the style by perming and/or drying in a variety of ways. The hair-style may be cut on either wet or dry hair and may be either club cut or taper cut, depending on how much volume is required in the style, and on whether the style is to have movement (curl or wave). The process is:

1. This shape may be cut in hair starting at any point of the head. This is normally either at the nape or at the top front of the hairstyle.
2. Take small meshes, which can be easily controlled. Having established the desired length, comb adjacent sections of hair out at 90 degrees to the scalp and, using the adjacent cut section as a guide, cut the hair to the same length. Failure to hold the hair out at 90 degrees can result in the hairs' length either becoming longer or shorter than that previously cut.
3. The hair may be tapered or thinned, using scissors or a razor/shaper in a specific area, as required for the hairstyle.
4. Ensure that your client's head is upright when checking for evenness and balance. Use the dressing point mirror to check the balance of both sides, placing the fingers through the hair and drawing the hair outwards.

> ***TIP*** While cutting hair, watch your client's body language for any indications of discomfort, as this may indicate concern about the progress of the haircut. If this is the case reassure them and address their concerns.

The graduated hairstyle

The inner hair length is longer than the outline hair length but the inner hair does not reach to the design line. Graduation creates weight lines in the hairstyle. Figure 4.22 indicates the location of the design line, the weight line, the outline hair length and the inner hair.

The outline hair length or design line may be varied in length and shape depending upon the desired finished hairstyle. The location of the weight line can be varied by the angle of graduation, the weight line will be located at the top of the graduation, where the end of the longest hair reaches in the finished hairstyle.

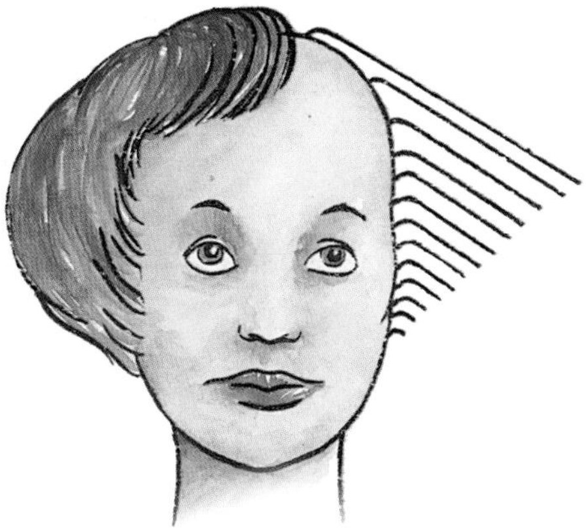

Figure 4.22 The graduated hairstyle

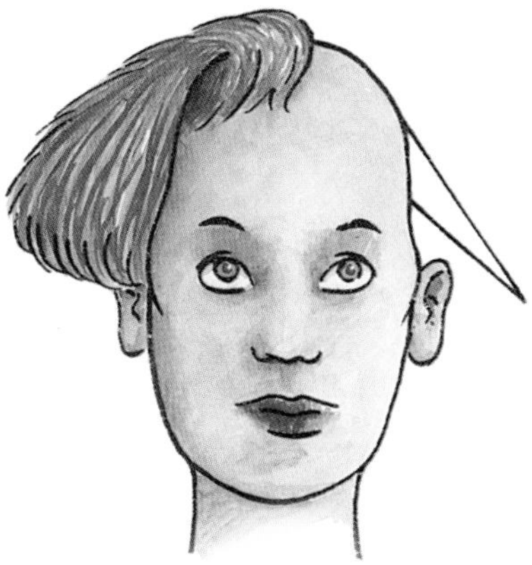

Figure 4.23

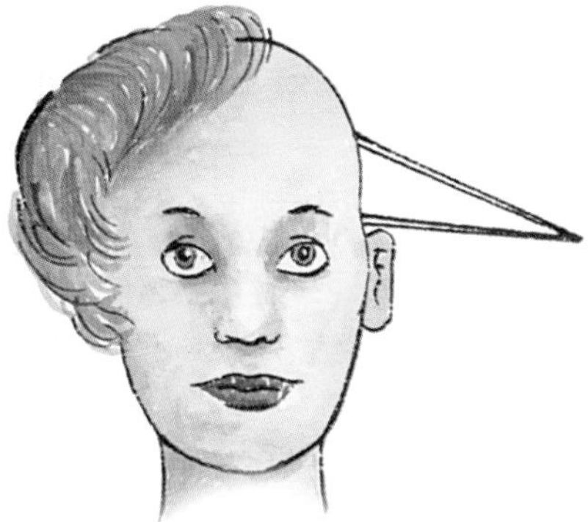

Figure 4.24

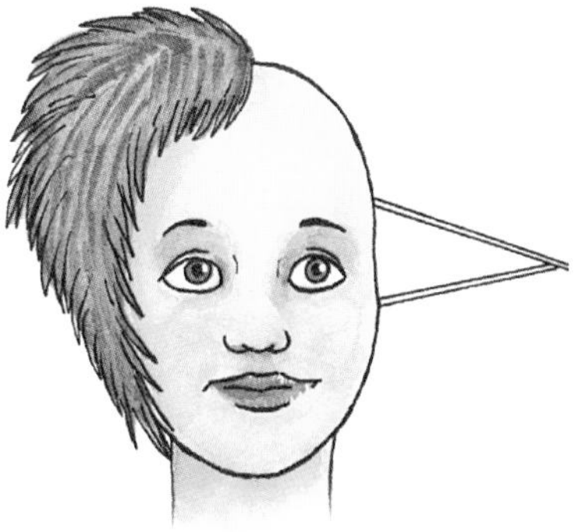

Figure 4.25

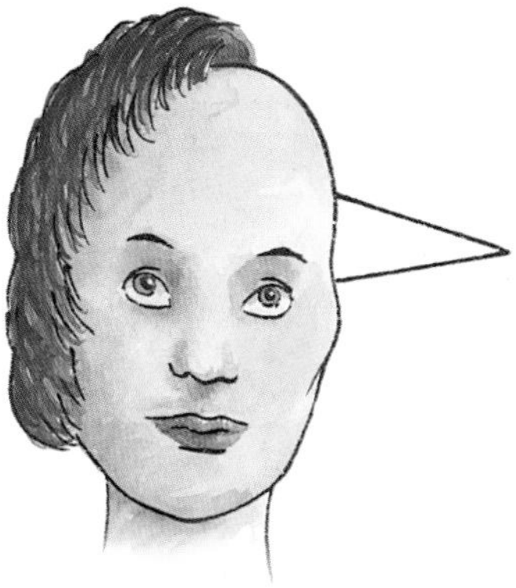

Figure 4.26

A graduation may be cut by taking sections that are at 90 degrees to the design line (vertical sections) or by taking sections that are parallel to the design line. Your choice of technique will depend upon:

- the technique with which you are most familiar
- the technique used in your salon.

Cutting the graduated hairstyle usually commences at the design line, this being the shortest area of the hairstyle. The actual start point may vary: it may be the nape or the sides or around the ear, depending on the finished hairstyle that is required and personal preference. Take small sections that may be controlled easily, comb the hair to remove tangles and then hold it at the required angle. If taking horizontal sections, parallel to the design line, the section of hair should be held at between 1 degree and 90 degrees, depending upon the required angle of graduation and the position of the weight line. The smaller the angle, the lower the graduation and the lower down the head that the weight line will be located. By enlarging the angle, the weight line will be raised. Figures 4.23 to 4.26 will show this.

Scissor-over-comb graduation

When a close graduation is required, the hair length being shorter than can be held between the fingers, a graduated result may be achieved by holding the hair in the teeth of the comb and cutting the hair. The comb is pushed upwards from the shortest length, into the longer hair. The cutting point is where the comb's teeth join the back of the comb. The comb's teeth should be angled to reflect the required angle of graduation. The comb should be moved in a steady

Barbering, page 236

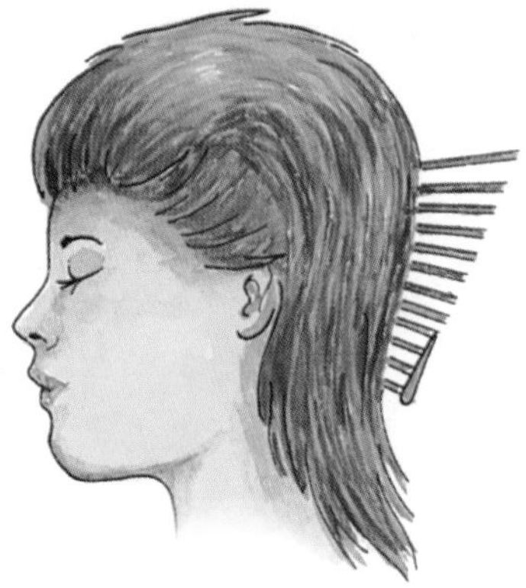

Figure 4.27 Scissor-over-comb graduation

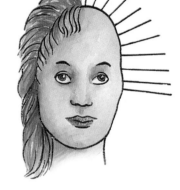

Figure 4.28 Reverse graduation

continuous movement, the teeth angled outwards and the static blade of the scissors in line with the back of the comb. Electric clippers may also be used with this technique (see Figure 4.27).

> ***TIP*** Maintaining weight and volume in hair will often produce straight smooth looks. Reducing volume and layering hair usually encourages hair to curl and lift.

The reverse graduation

The outer hair length is longer than the inner length. *Reverse graduation* does not create weight lines within the hairstyle, it does, however, allow height and movement within the framework of a longer hairstyle effect (see Figure 4.28).

The outline hair length or design line may be varied in length and shape, depending upon the desired completed hairstyle. The degree of reverse graduation, how much shorter the inner hair length is compared to the outline hair length, may be varied to suit the hairstyle.

The technique of cutting usually starts at the shorter areas of the hairstyle, taking sections that are parallel to the design line. The hair is overdirected at more than 90 degrees to produce the reverse graduation. The greater the angle the greater the degree of reverse graduation (see Figures 4.29 and 4.30).

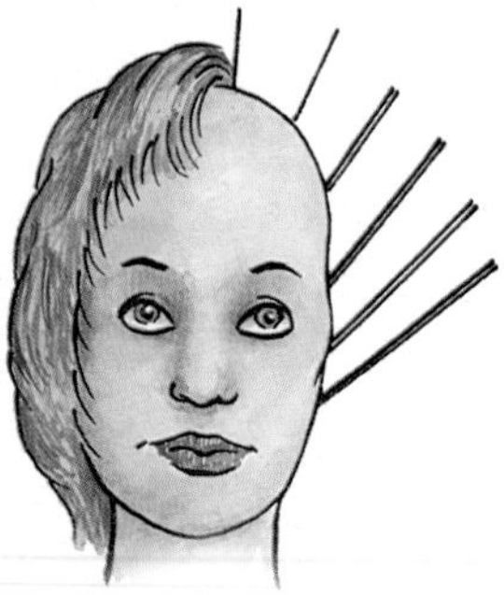

Figure 4.29 Producing reverse graduation (1)

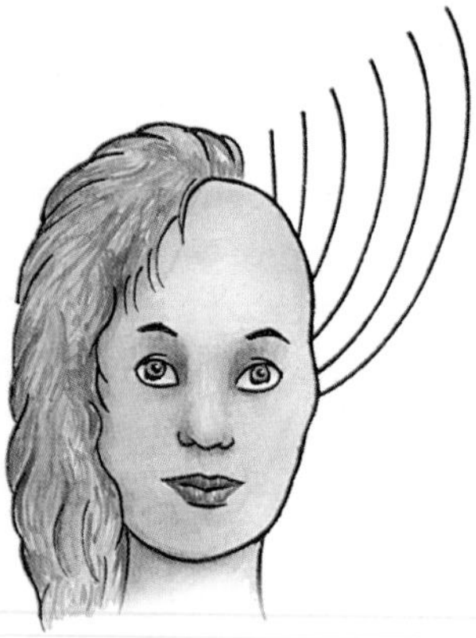

Figure 4.30 Producing reverse graduation (2)

TIP Hair cuttings should be swept away as soon as possible and placed in a covered bin. Do not allow hair cuttings to remain on your client or the floor longer than necessary.

COMBINATION AND FASHION TECHNIQUES

Most hairstyles today require a combination of cutting shapes and cutting techniques to achieve their look. Examples of these are shown in the following illustrations. Figure 4.31 shows the use of graduation at the sides and back, linked with a uniform layer on the top.

Often a shape can be linked with a specific cutting technique for selected areas of the head. Figure 4.32 shows a technique for producing a one length cut linked with a fringe which has been texturised to produce a contrasting spiky effect.

You can give separation to those areas that lie onto the skin at the hairline by the use of freehand cutting (see Figure 4.33). When ever the hair is cut while it is in a free unrestrained situation it may be termed freehand.

- This style of hair cutting can be advantageous when cutting very wavy hair that is likely to retract when released if held taut and it is required to lay in a specific point on the head. By cutting in situ there is less risk of the elastic recoil moving the cut line.
- Carefully stroking the points of the scissors into strands of hair while closing the scissors will reduce volume and encourage curl/wave and a natural effect to hair.
- Twisting small sections of short hair and particularly closing the scissors onto the mesh will produce a texture effect as some hair will be different lengths so that which is adjacent.

When using any cutting technique it is essential to view the progress of the style and respond to any effects that you did not at first expect, particularly when cutting a client's hair for the first time, when it may not always be possible to predict precisely how the hair will respond to the technique, method and length of the cut. Consult your client, explain what is happening and gain their confidence and agreement through your responsiveness.

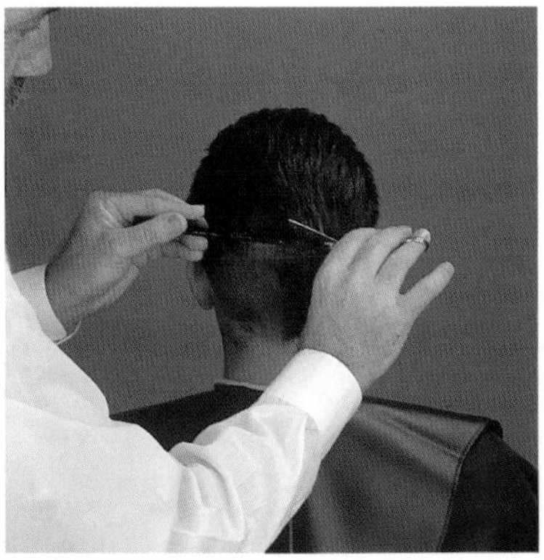

Figure 4.31 Graduated haircut

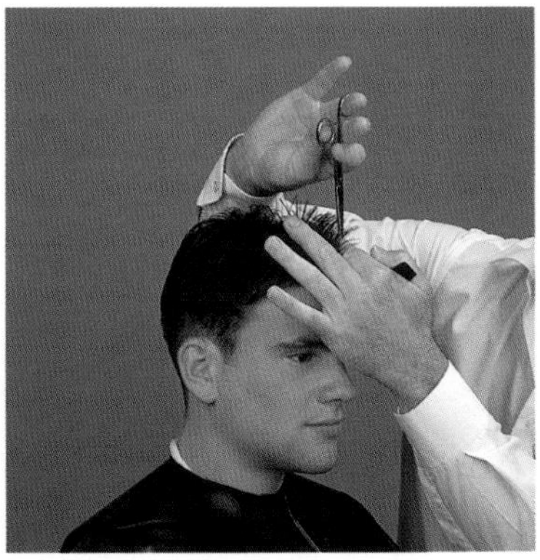

Figure 4.32 One length cut with spiky fringe

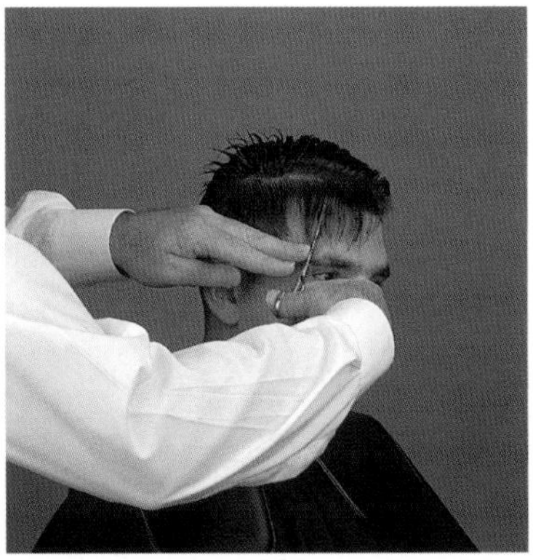

Figure 4.33 Effect of freehand cutting on hairline

FURTHER STUDY

- Find out about fashion cutting techniques and what effects they may produce in hair. Use trade magazines, videos and demonstrations to do this.
- All hair cutting techniques fall into one of the three categories: clubbing, thinning or tapering. Try to place the methods that you know into the appropriate technique category.
- Build a portfolio of current and emerging hairstyles and the techniques and methods used to achieve these. This will form a useful reference document for you in your work.

REVIEW QUESTIONS

1. Suggest two factors that may affect your choice of haircut for a client.
2. What is the purpose of gowning your client for a haircut?
3. For control, how should hair cutting scissors be held?
4. What is the name given to the hair cutting technique that reduces length but retains all of the hair's natural volume?
5. Which hair cutting technique will encourage wavy hair to curl?
6. Give another name for a layered look where the inner hair lengths are longer than the outer hair lengths.
7. What is a weight line?
8. How may the balance of the haircut be checked?
9. What advantage does scissor-over-comb graduation have over other methods of graduating?
10. Should a haircutting razor/shaper be used on **wet** or **dry** hair?

CHAPTER 5A

Permanent waving

This section provides the essential knowledge needed to understand the permanent waving process. It describes the procedures for carrying out a range of basic perms and guides you in selecting appropriate techniques and products.

Level 1	
Unit 101	
Element 101.1	Maintain effective and safe methods of working when shampooing
Element 101.2	Shampoo and surface condition hair
Unit 102A	
Element 102A.1	Maintain effective and safe methods of working
Element 102A.2	Neutralise hair as part of the perming process
Unit 102B	
Element 102B.1	Maintain effective and safe methods of working
Element 102B.2	Neutralise hair as part of the perming and relaxing process
Unit 104	
Element 104.1	Develop effective working relationships with clients
Element 104.2	Develop effective working relationships with colleagues
Element 104.3	Develop yourself within the job role
Unit 105	
Element 105.2	Support health and safety at work

Level 2	
Unit 201	
Element 201.1	Consult with and maintain effective relationships with clients
Element 201.2	Advise clients on salon products and services
Element 201.3	Advise clients on after-care procedures
Unit 202	
Element 202.1	Maintain effective and safe methods of working with shampooing and conditioning hair
Element 202.2	Shampooing hair and scalp
Element 202.3	Condition hair and scalp
Unit 5	
Element 205A.1 + 205 5B.1	Maintain effective and safe methods of working when perming, relaxing and neutralising hair
Element 205A.2 + 205B.2	Perm hair using basic techniques
Element 205A.3 + 205B.4	Neutralise hair
Unit 208	
Element 208.1	Develop and maintain effective team work and relationships with colleagues
Element 208.2	Develop and improve personal effectiveness within the job role
Unit 209	
Element 209.2	Support health, safety and security at work

Contents

INTRODUCTION

Chemical processes, including permanent waving, enable you to offer a wide range of hairstyles and effects to your clients. This in turn enables you to satisfy your clients' needs and from a business point of view is very important.

The wide variety of products and techniques available enable you to produce many differing effects, from those that are subtle but support the style to those which have a dramatic, obvious effect. The properly completed perm provides many valuable benefits, including:

- long-lasting style retention
- easy manageability for your client when styling at home
- additional volume and fullness for styling soft, fine hair textures
- greater control in styling hair that is naturally coarse, wiry and hard to manage.

These processes must be carried out with due care, as the chemicals used when permanently curling hair, if used incorrectly, may cause damage to the hair and even injury to your client and yourself. Always follow the manufacturer's directions for safe use.

HISTORY OF PERMANENT WAVING

Attempts to wave and curl straight hair date back to early civilisation. Egyptian and Roman women were known to apply a mixture of soil and water to their hair, wrap it on crudely made wooden rollers, and then bake it in the sun. The results, of course, were not always permanent.

The machine age of permanent waving

In 1905 Charles Nessler invented a heavily wired machine that supplied electrical current to metal rods around which hair strands were wrapped. These heavy units were heated during the perming process. They were kept from touching the scalp by a complex system of counterbalancing weights suspended from an overhead chandelier mounted on a stand (see Figure 5A.1).

Two methods were used to wind hair strands around the metal units. Long hair was wound from the scalp to the ends, a technique called spiral winding (see Figure 5A.2). After World War 1, when many women cut their hair into the short bobbed style, the croquignole winding technique was introduced (see Figure 5A.3). Using this method, shorter hair was wound from the ends towards the scalp. The hair was then styled into deep waves with loose end curls.

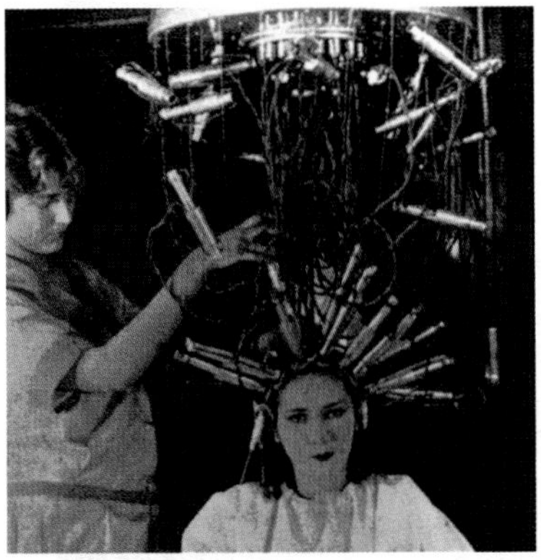

Figure 5A.1 Machine permanent wave

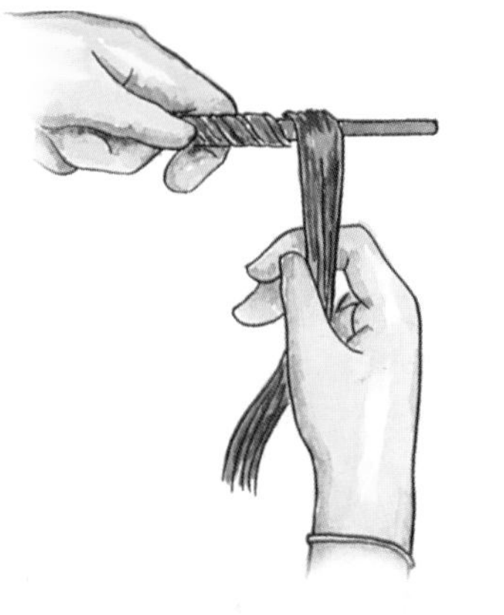

Figure 5A.2 Spiral flat wind

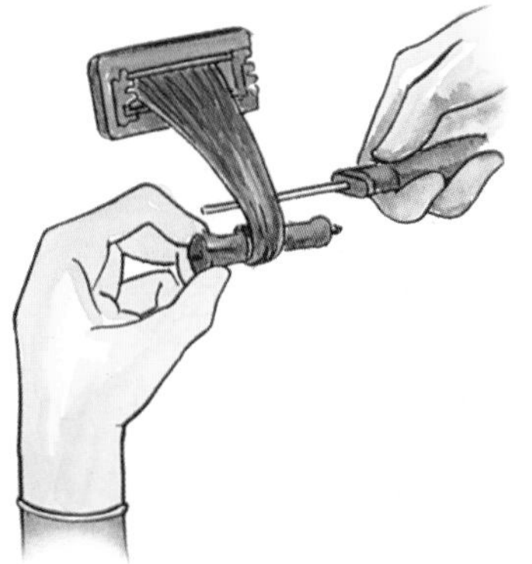

Figure 5A.3 Croquignole wind

The client's fear of being 'tied' to an electrical contraption with the possibility of receiving a shock or a burn led to the development of alternative methods of waving hair. In 1931, the pre-heat method of perming was introduced. Hair was wrapped using the croquignole method, and then clamps, pre-heated by a separate electrical unit, were placed over the wound curls. This was known as the falling heat or wireless system.

The first machineless perm

An alternative to the machine perm was introduced in 1932 when chemists Ralph L. Evans and Everett G. McDonough pioneered a method that used external heat generated by chemical reaction. Small, flexible pads, called exothermic pads, containing a chemical mixture including calcium oxide, were wound around hair strands. When the pads were moistened with water, a chemical heat was released. This process created long-lasting curls. Thus the first machineless permanent wave was born. Salon clients were no longer subjected to the dangers and discomforts of the Nessler machine.

Cold waves

In 1941 scientists discovered another method of permanent waving. They developed the waving lotion, a liquid that softens and expands the hair strand. After the waving lotion has done its work, another lotion called a neutraliser is applied. The neutraliser hardens and shrinks that hair strand, allowing it to conform to the shape of the rod around which the hair is wrapped. It also stops the action of the waving lotion.

Because this perm does not use heat, it is called a 'cold wave'. Cold waves replaced virtually all predecessors and competitors, and cold waving and permanent waving became almost synonymous terms. Modern versions of cold waves, usually referred to as alkaline perms, are still very popular today.

> ***NOTE*** The word 'perm' is now popularly used to indicate permanent waving with either alkaline- or acid-balanced solutions.

Acid-balanced perms

For many years, manufacturers sought to develop a permanent wave solution that would minimise hair damage and permit hair that had been damaged by lightening or tinting services to receive a perm. To achieve these goals, they developed a waving lotion that was not as highly alkaline as earlier lotions.

Ph scale, page 75

Acid-balanced permanent waves with pH levels ranging from 4.5 to 7.9 were introduced in 1970. They did not contain strong alkalis and therefore were less damaging to the hair. Acid-balanced lotions were, however, slow to penetrate hair, and processing time was longer. To overcome this problem, the client is placed under a pre-heated hood dryer to shorten the processing time. Often the curl pattern achieved from acid-balanced perms is softer than that achieved from an alkali wave, therefore a size smaller perm rod is often advised.

MODERN PERM CHEMISTRY

Perm chemistry is constantly being refined and improved. Perms are available today in many differing formulas for a wide variety of hair types. Waving lotions and neutralisers for both acid-balanced and alkaline perms are being formulated with new conditioners, proteins and natural ingre-dients that help to protect (or 'buffer') and condition the hair during and after perming.

Stop-action processing is incorporated in many waving lotions to ensure optimum curl development. The curling takes place in a fixed time without the risk of over processing or damaging the hair. Special pre-wrapping lotions have also been developed to compensate for hair that is not equally porous all over and therefore protect the hair.

Virtually all permanent waves are achieved with a two-step chemical process:

1. Waving lotion, which softens or breaks the internal structure of the hair.
2. Neutraliser, which re-hardens or re-bonds the internal structure of the hair.

There are some perming systems that have wrapping lotions which help to pre-soften the hair making it easier to wind and ready to receive the perming agent.

The pH scale

This 14 point scale is used to indicate the acidity or alkalinity of a substance. The symbol pH (potential Hydrogen) refers to the quantity of hydrogen ions present. The centre of the scale (7) is neutral and is a point which is neither acid nor alkali. The further from the central point the higher the level of either acidity (pH of less than 7) or alkalinity (pH of over 7). The diagram (see Figure 5A.4) indicates the relative pH of a number of hair-dressing-related substances.

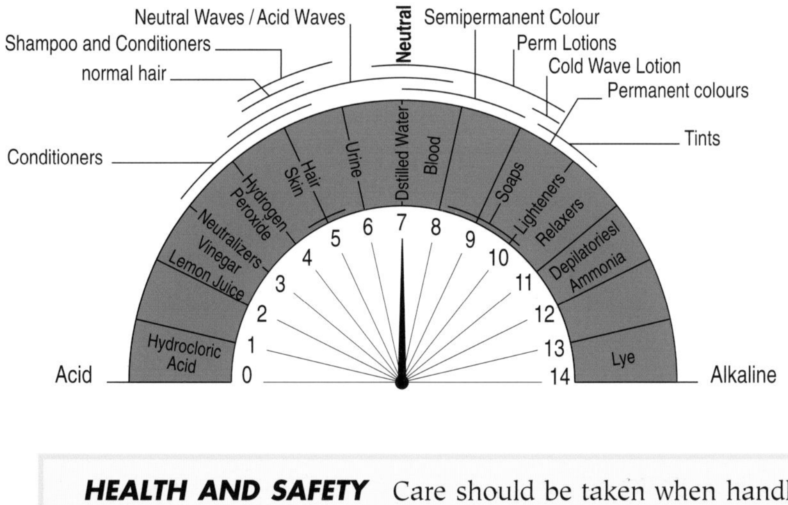

Figure 5A.4 Relative pH of hairdressing substances

HEALTH AND SAFETY Care should be taken when handling any substance the pH of that falls near the extremes of the scale, as it may cause injury to the skin.

Alkaline perms

The main active ingredient (or 'reducing agent') in alkaline perms, ammonium thioglycolate, is a chemical compound made up of ammonium hydroxide and thioglycolic acid. The pH of alkaline waving lotions generally falls within the range 8.2 to 9.6, depending on the amounts of ammonium hydroxide present. Because the lotion is more alkaline, the cuticle layers swell slightly and open, allowing the solution to penetrate more quickly than acid-balanced lotions. Some alkaline perms are wound with perm lotion ('pre-damping'), others are wound with water, the perm lotion being applied after all the hair has been wound ('post-damping'). Some require a plastic cap (to retain scalp heat) for processing, others do not. Therefore, it is extremely important to read the manufacturer's instructions for use before beginning.

The benefits of alkaline perms are:

- strong curl patterns
- fast processing time (varies from 5 to 20 minutes)
- room temperature processing.

Generally, alkaline perms should be used when:

- perming resistant hair
- a strong/tight curl is desired
- the client has a history of early curl relaxation.

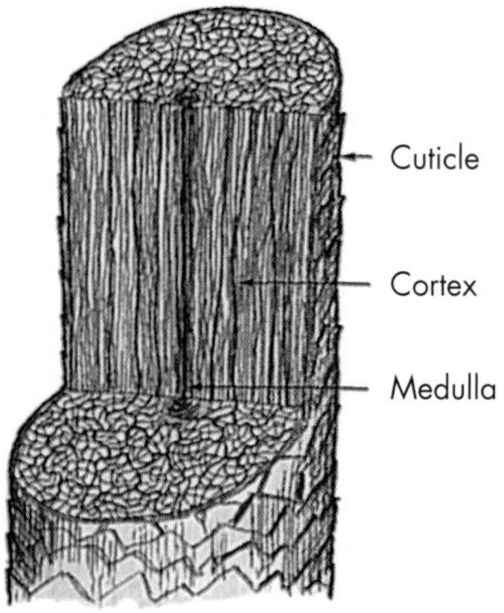

Figure 5A.4b Structure of a hair

Acid-balanced perms

The main active ingredient in acid-balanced waving lotions is glycerol monothioglycolate, which effectively reduces the pH. This lower pH is gentler on the hair and typically gives a softer curl than alkaline cold waves. Acid-balanced perms have a pH range of approximately 4.5 to 7.9 and usually penetrate the hair more slowly. Thus, they require a longer processing time and heat to develop curl. Heat is produced in one of two ways:

1. The perm is activated by heat created chemically within the product. This method is called exothermic.
2. The perm is activated by an outside heat source, usually a conventional hood-type hair dryer. This method is called endothermic.

TIP Your employer will have arranged a review of the risks associated with the use of chemicals in your salon. This is part of the Control of Substances Hazardous to Health (COSHH) regulations 1992. If personal protective equipment is provided you are advised to use this.

TIP Your employer will have arranged for training, if required, in the correct use of chemicals. You should follow the guidance provided in their correct use.

Recent advances in acid-balanced perm chemistry, however, have made it possible to process some acid-balanced perms at room temperature without heat. These newer acid-balanced perms usually have a slightly higher pH but still contain glycerol monothioglycolate as the active ingredient.

Most acid-balanced perms are water wrapped, require a plastic cap (to retain scalp heat), and may or may not require a pre-heated hood dryer for processing. Read the manufacturer's perm directions carefully before starting the perm.

The benefits of acid-balanced perms are:

- softer curl patterns
- slower, but more controllable processing time (usually 15 to 25 minutes)
- gentler treatment for delicate hair types.

Generally, acid-balanced perms are used when:

- perming delicate/fragile or colour-treated hair
- soft, natural curl or wave pattern is desired
- style support, rather than strong curl, is required.

The chemistry of neutralisers

Neutralisers for both acid-balanced and alkaline perms have the same important function: to 1
permanently establish the new curl shape. Neutralising is a very important step in the perming process. If the hair is not properly neutralised, the curl will relax or straighten after one or two shampooings. Generally, today's neutralisers are composed of a relatively small percentage of hydrogen peroxide, an oxidising agent, at an acidic pH. An alternative oxidising agent is sodium bromate. As with waving lotions, there are slightly different procedures recommended for individual products. To achieve the best possible results, read and follow the manufacturer's directions.

HAIR STRUCTURE AND PERMING

Whether using an acid-balanced or alkaline formula, all perms subject the hair to two different actions:

- physical action – wrapping sections of hair around a perm rod
- chemical action – created first by reducing agent (waving lotion) and second by an oxidising agent (neutraliser).

Since both of these actions work together to create a change in the internal structure of the hair, it is important to understand the composition of hair and how it is affected during perming.

The physical structure of hair

Each strand of hair is structurally subdivided into three major components:

- The cuticle or outer covering normally consists of seven or more overlapping layers. Although it comprises a small percentage of the total weight of hair, the cuticle possesses unique structural properties that protect the hair. During perming, the waving lotion raises the cuticle layers and allows the active ingredients to enter the cortex.
- The cortex, the major component of the hair structure, accounts for up to 90% of its total weight. The cortex gives hair its flexibility, elasticity, strength and resilience, and

contains the colour. It is in the cortex that the physical and chemical actions take place during the perming process to restructure the hair into a new curl configuration.

- The medulla is the innermost section of the hair structure. The function of the medulla, if any, is unknown. In fact, it is not at all unusual for an otherwise normal, healthy hair to be without a medulla.

The chemical composition of hair

The chemical composition of hair consists almost entirely of a protein material called keratin, which is made up of approximately nineteen amino acids. When many acids are bonded together, they form a polypeptide chain. These chains twine around each other in a spiral fashion to assume a helical shape very similar to a spring. Hair contains a high concentration of the amino acid cystine that is joined together crosswise with disulphide linkages or bonds. Disulphide bonds add strength to the keratin protein, and it is these bonds that must be broken down to allow the perming process to occur.

Processing

The chemical action of a waving lotion breaks the disulphide bonds and softens the hair. When the chemical action softens the inner structure of the hair enough, it can mould to the shape of the rod around which it is wound (see Figure 5A.5a–c).

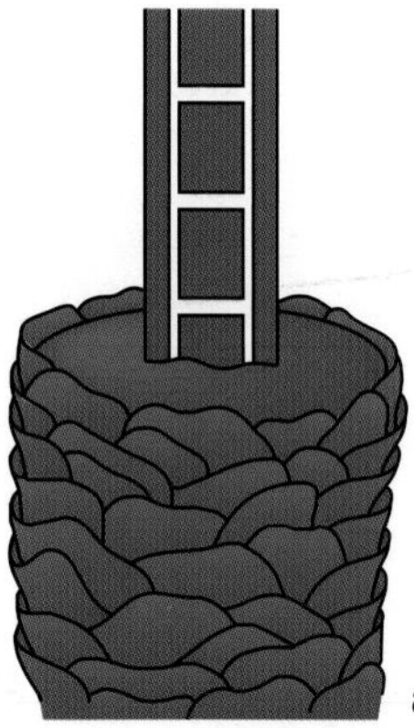
a

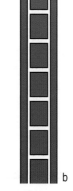

Figure 5A.5a Each hair strand is composed of many polypeptide chains. This series of illustrations shows the behaviour of one such chain

b

Figure 5A.5b Hair before processing. Chemical bonds (links) give hair its strength and firmness

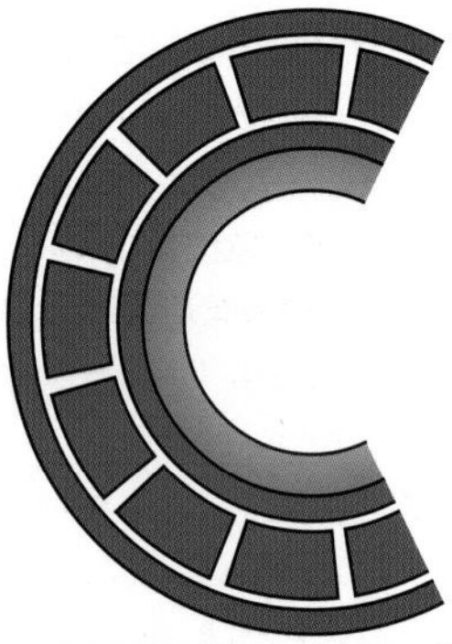
c

Figure 5A.5c Hair wound on rod. The hair bends to the curvature and size of the rod

Neutralising

When the hair has assumed the desired shape, the broken disulphide bonds must be chemically rebonded. Neutralising rehardens the hair and fixes it into its new curl form. When the neutralising action is completed, the hair is unwrapped from the rods, and you have a new curl formation (see Figure 5A.6a and b).

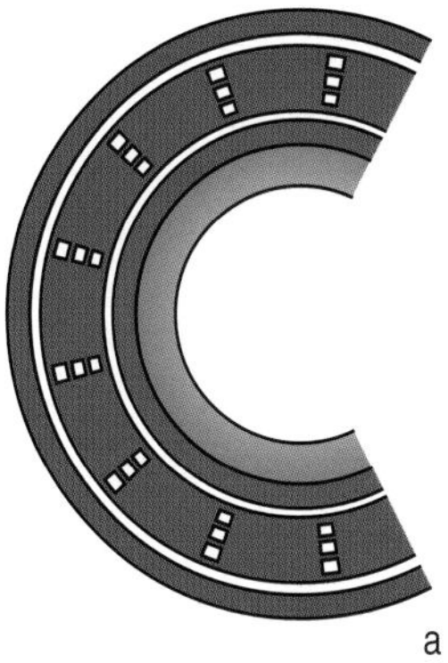

a

Figure 5A.6a During processing, waving lotion breaks the chemical cross-bonds (links) permitting the hair to adjust to the curvature of the rod while in this softened condition

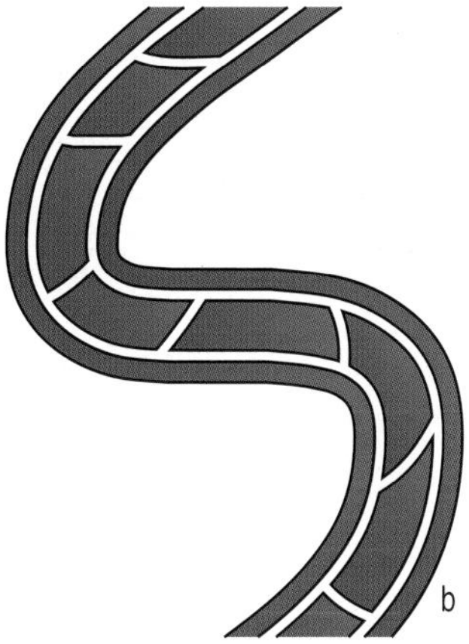

b

Figure 5A.6b The neutralizer reforms the chemical bonds (links) to conform with the wound position of the hair, and rehardens the hair, thus creating the permanent wave

CHOOSING THE RIGHT PERMING TECHNIQUE

The stages of perming are:

1. client consultation
2. selection of equipment and products
3. preparation of the hair
4. the perm wind/wrap
5. application of perm lotion
6. processing
7. neutralising.

In order to decide which perming technique is right for your client you must be able to evaluate and analyse your client's hair. You will consult with your client to establish what they expect to accomplish with a perm – a tight, curly look or a loose, wavy look. This information helps you to select the correct perm product and technique.

Basic manual perming skills

Successful perming requires manual dexterity. With practice, your skills in handling and manipulating hair will improve. Before actually applying a perm lotion, you will probably spend considerable time practising pre-perming skills like pre-perm sectioning, curler sectioning and winding/wrapping. Your ability to give successful perms depends on mastering these important skills.

Client consultation

Every perm client has a different idea of how he or she wants the perm to look. The only way to meet your client's expectations is to determine what those expectations are. Talk to your client in a friendly but professional way. Take a few minutes to discuss:

- What hairstyle and how much curl your client wants. Photos or magazine pictures help to make this clearly understood by both of you.
- Your client's life-style. Does he or she have a lot of leisure time, or a demanding schedule that requires a low-maintenance style?

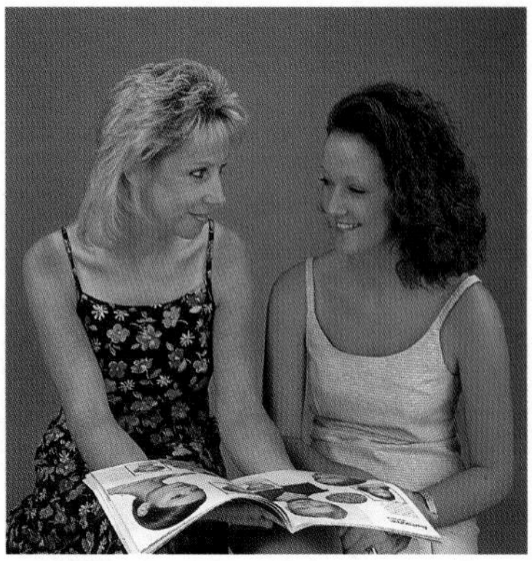

Figure 5A.7 Pre-perm consultation

- How your client's hairstyle relates to overall personal image. Is your client concerned about current fashion trends?
- Your client's previous experience with perming. What did he or she like or dislike about past perm services?

Once you learn what questions to ask and how to ask them, the consultation with your perm client takes only a few minutes. It is time well spent, however, because the consultation helps establish your credibility as a professional. It inspires your client's confidence in your technical and creative abilities, and makes the perming experience more satisfactory for both of you.

TIP If the presence of previous, unknown chemical treatments is apparent, carry out an incompatibility test to test for the presence of metallic salts on the hair. See page 158 for details of this test.

Keep the vital information you learn during the client consultation as a permanent record, either written or computerised, along with other important data, including the client's address and both home and business telephone numbers. Here is an example of an organised format for maintaining client records:

TIP As your salon retains information relating to clients it will be registered with the Data Protection Commission. Your salon will have rules regarding who has access to client information, this information's security and to what purpose the information may be used. Familiarise yourself with these as you have a responsibility to comply with these.

WHAT THE EXPERT SAYS A major contribution to the financial success of the salon is based upon the provision of chemical services. A satisfied client will make return visits to the salon. Perming can enable you to provide a full and satisfying service for your clients.

No matter what your role within the salon, you can help to provide the service. At reception the correct booking and phasing of appointments supports a

PERMANENT WAVE RECORD

Name .... Tel. ....

Address ....

....

DESCRIPTION OF HAIR

Length	**Texture**	**Type**		**Porosity**	
☐ short	☐ coarse	☐ normal	☐ very porous	☐ slightly porous	
☐ medium	☐ medium	☐ resistant			
☐ long	☐ fine	☐ tinted	☐ moderately porous	☐ resistant	
		☐ highlighted			
		☐ bleached	☐ normal		
Condition					
☐ very good	☐ good	☐ fair	☐ poor	☐ dry	☐ oily

Tinted with ....

Previously permed with ....

TYPE OF PERM

☐ alkaline ☐ acid ☐ body wave ☐ other

No. of rods .... Lotion .... Strength ....

Results

☐ good ☐ poor ☐ too tight ☐ too loose

Date	Perm used	Stylist	Date	Perm used	Stylist

Other side of Record, continue with:

Date	Perm used	Stylist	Date	Perm used	Stylist

Figure 5A.8 A client record sheet

smooth delivery of the service. As an assistant, the preparation of the working area and the provision of the correct tools, in the correct place at the appropriate time will support the service. The stylist's skill will come about as a result of full product knowledge and extensive practice in all aspects of the perming process, including client consultation as well as the actual winding/wrapping of the perm.

Remember that in order to satisfy your client's expectations, you must provide the relevant support for them to care for their new perm between visits. This will include advice and guidance on drying techniques and the frequency of salon visits. Home haircare products should be suggested and their method of use described. If your client is willing to incur the expense of this chemical service they will want their hair to look good at all times.

PERM PREPARATION

Pre-perm analysis

After the client consultation, you must analyse the overall condition of your client's hair and scalp. This analysis is essential for you to determine:

- If it is safe and advisable to proceed with the perm service. The hair must be in good condition and have the necessary strength to accept a chemical alteration to achieve a successful perm.
- Which perm product should be chosen for the best results on the particular hair type.
- Which perm technique should be used: curler/rod and parting sizes and winding/wrapping pattern.

First, examine the scalp for abrasions, irritations, open sores or contagious disorders. If any of these exist, do not give the perm. Minor abrasions may be protected by using petroleum jelly BP as a barrier between the skin and the lotion. Next, judge the physical characteristics of the hair with regard to these important criteria: porosity, density, texture and length. Finally, determine the overall condition of the hair. Observe if the hair has been previously treated with chemicals: perm, tint, bleach, highlighting (frosting, dimensionally coloured). This will guide you in choosing the appropriate perm.

Incompatability test, see page 158

Check with your client for the previous use of products on the hair that may be incompatible with the perming process. Products that contain metallic salts, (compound Henna, hair colour restorers, progressive hair dyes and metallic coloured hair sprays) leave traces of salts on the hair which react with the process. If the presence of these salts is detected it is not safe to proceed with the perming process until all traces are removed. If you are in doubt of the presence of salts, carry out an incompatibility test on a sample of the hair.

CAUTION If pre-perm analysis is not correct, poor curl development or hair damage can result.

Check any existing salon records regarding previous treatments and their outcomes.

Determining porosity

Porosity refers to the hair's capacity to absorb moisture. There is a direct relationship between the hair's porosity, the type of perm (acid-balanced or alkaline) you will use, and the strength of waving lotion you will choose.

The processing time for any perm depends more on hair porosity than any other factor. The more porous the hair, the less processing time it takes, and the milder the waving solution required. Hair porosity is affected by such factors as excessive exposure to sun and wind, use of harsh shampoos, tints and lighteners, previous perms and use of thermal styling appliances.

Porous hair may be dry – even very dry. If hair is tinted, bleached, or has been exposed to the sun or was over-processed by a previous perm, it will absorb liquids readily. Soft, fine, thin hair usually has a thin cuticle so it will absorb liquids quickly and easily. Rough, dull-looking hair and hair that tangles easily is also likely to be porous.

While the hair is dry, check porosity in three different areas: front hairline, in front of the ear and in the crown area. Select a single strand of hair, hold the end securely between the thumb and first finger of one hand and slide the thumb and first finger of the other hand from the hair end to the scalp.

If the hair feels smooth and the cuticle is dense and hard, it is considered resistant and will

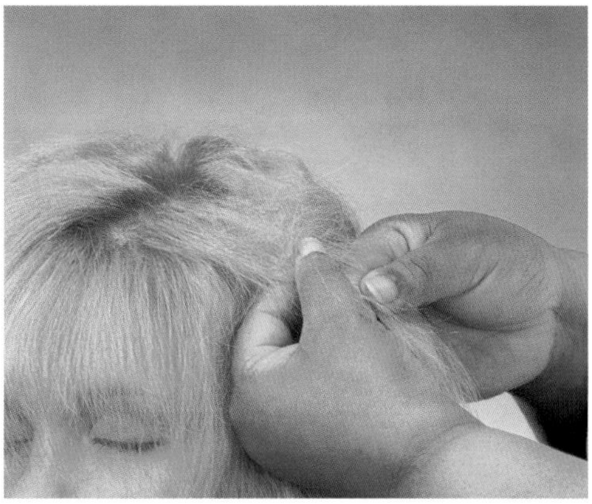

Figure 5A.9 Testing for hair porosity

not absorb liquids or perm lotion easily. If you can feel a slight roughness, this tells you that the cuticle is open and that the hair is porous and will absorb liquids more readily (see Figure 5A.9).

Poor porosity (resistant hair)
Hair with the cuticle layer lying close to the hair shaft. This type of hair absorbs waving lotion slowly and usually requires a longer processing time and/or a strong waving lotion.

Good porosity (normal hair)
Hair with the cuticle layer slightly raised from the hair shaft. Hair of this type can absorb moisture or chemicals in an average amount of time.

Porous (tinted, lightened or previously chemically treated) hair
Hair that has been made porous by various treatments or styling. This type of hair absorbs lotion very quickly and requires the shortest processing time. Use either an acid-balanced perm or a very mild alkaline wave.

Over-porous hair (a result of over-processing)
This type of hair is very damaged, dry, fragile and brittle. Until the hair has been reconditioned or the damaged part has been removed by cutting, it should not be permed.

If hair is unevenly porous (usually porous or over porous at the ends with good to poor porosity near the scalp), a pre-wrap lotion, specifically designed to even out the porosity, is recommended to achieve even curl results and help prevent over-processing porous ends (see Figure 5A.10a–d).

Determining texture

Texture refers to how thick or thin (in diameter) each individual hair is. Fine hair has a small diameter; coarse hair has a large diameter. You can feel whether hair is fine, coarse, or medium when a single dry strand is held between the fingers.

The texture and porosity together are used to determine the processing time of the waving lotion. Although porosity is the more important of the two, texture does play an important role in estimating processing time. Fine hair with a small diameter becomes saturated with waving lotion more quickly than coarse hair with a large diameter, even if both are of equal porosity. However, when coarse hair is porous, it processes faster than fine hair that is not porous.

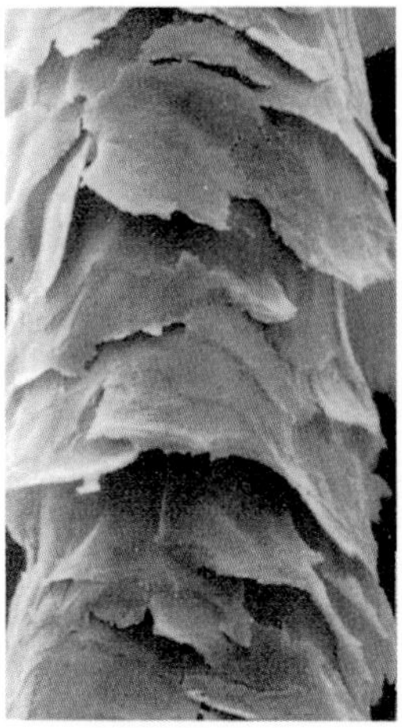

Figure 5A.10a Normal (moderate porosity)

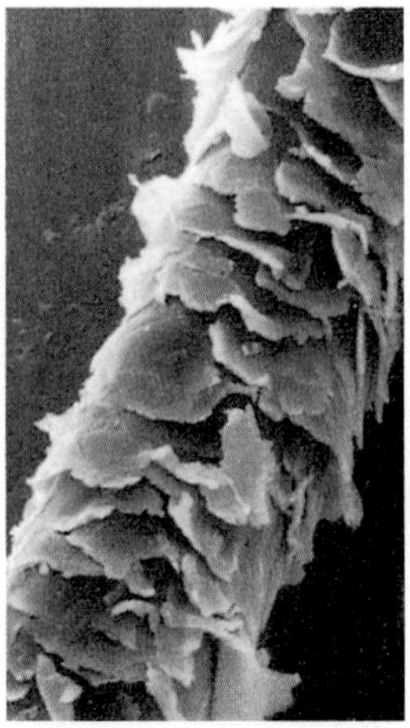

Figure 5A.10b Resistant (poor porosity)

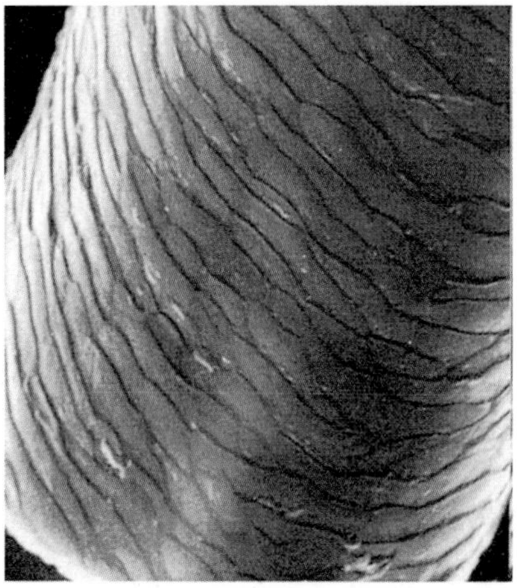

Figure 5A.10c Tinted (extreme porosity)

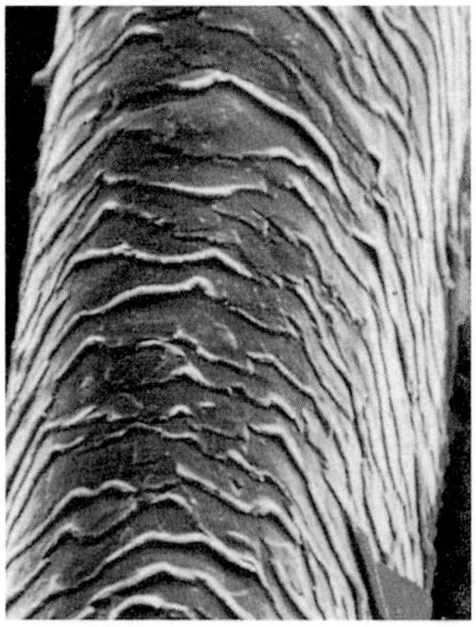

Figure 5A.10d Damaged (over-porous hair)

A perm adds body to hair that appears limp, lifeless, and does not hold a style very long. For coarse, wiry hair, a perm provides greater manageability in styling (see Figure 5A.11a–c).

Testing elasticity

Elasticity is the ability of hair to stretch and then return to its original length. To test for elasticity, stretch a single dry hair. If the hair breaks under very slight strain, it has little or no elasticity. Other signs of poor elasticity include a spongy feel when the hair is wet and/or hair that tangles easily. When hair is completely lacking in elasticity (for example, extremely damaged hair), it will not take a satisfactory permanent wave. The greater the degree of elasticity, the longer the wave will remain in the hair, because less relaxation of the hair occurs. Hair with good elastic qualities can be stretched by 20% of its length without breaking (see Figure 5A.12).

Assessing density

Density, or thickness, refers to the number of hairs per square centimetre on your client's head. Density is one characteristic that determines the size of the partings you will use. Thick hair

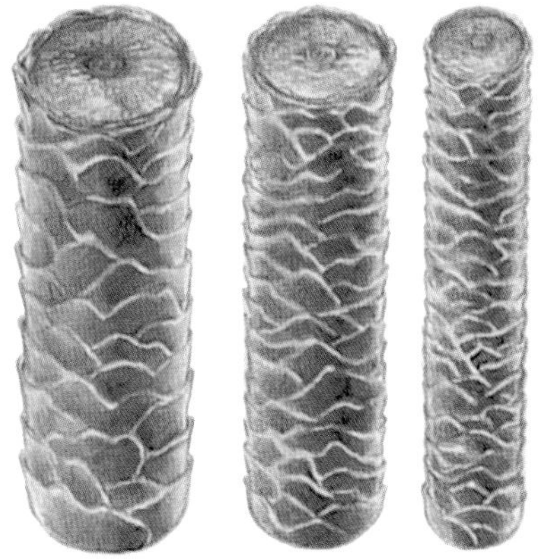

Figure 5A.11a Coarse; b Medium; c Fine

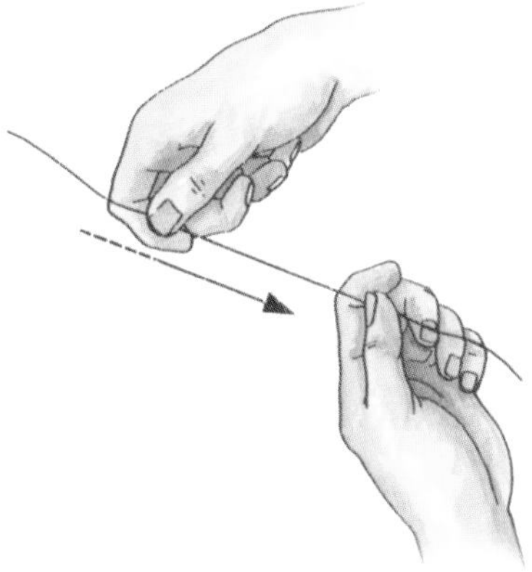

Figure 5A.12 Testing for elasticity

(many hairs per square centimetre) will require small partings on each rod. Too much hair on the rod can result in a weak curl, especially at the scalp.

If hair is thin (few hairs per square centimetre), slightly larger partings can be used, but avoid stretching or pulling the hair towards the rod because this can cause hair breakage or straight, misdirected hair at the scalp.

Hair length and perming

Hair that is 5 cm to 15 cm long is considered ideal for perming. Hair should be long enough to make at least 2.5 turns around the rod. To perm hair longer than 15 cm, smaller partings must be used to allow the waving lotion and neutraliser to penetrate more easily and thoroughly.

Perm lotion selection

The type of perm lotion you choose depends on the total evaluation of your client's hair and wishes during the consultation and pre-perm analysis. The following is a general guide to help you decide whether to use an alkaline or an acid-balanced perm.

Hair type	Type of perm lotion
Coarse, resistant	Alkaline lotion wind or alkaline post-damp
Fine, resistant	Alkaline lotion wind or alkaline post-damp
Normal	Alkaline post-damp or acid-lotion
Normal, porous	Alkaline post-damp or acid-lotion
Normal, delicate	Acid-lotion
Tinted, non-porous	Alkaline post-damp or acid-lotion
Tinted, porous	Acid-lotion
Highlighted/frosted/dimensionally coloured	Acid-lotion
Highlighted, tinted	Acid-lotion
Bleached	Acid-lotion

Today's perm products offer a wide selection of special features and formulas for all hair types. There are alkaline formulas for bleached hair and acid-balanced formulas for resistant hair. Each formula gives excellent results if you choose the perm carefully and follow the manufacturer's directions.

Pre-perm shampooing

1 Today, there are shampoos specifically formulated for pre-perm cleansing that thoroughly yet gently cleanse the hair. Use of these shampoos is recommended for optimal results.

When analysing a client's hair before perming, you may notice that the hair looks and feels coated. This coating might be the build-up of shampoo or conditioners, improper rinsing, resins from styling products or hair spray, or mineral deposits from hard water. This coating can prevent penetration of the waving lotion and interfere with perm results. It is very important for the hair to be free of all coatings before beginning any perm.

Begin the process by wetting the hair, applying the shampoo, and gently working into a lather. If the hair is extremely coated let the shampoo remain in the hair for several minutes before rinsing. Rinse thoroughly to remove all shampoo and dissolved build-up. Towel blot excess water from the hair. For more information about the shampooing procedure read the section headed 'Shampooing' on pages 21–26. If you are in doubt about the selection of the appropriate shampoo to use consult your supervisor or the stylist.

> ***NOTE*** While shampooing or undertaking any pre-perm preparation of a client's hair, you should avoid vigorous brushing, combing, pulling or rubbing that can cause the scalp to become sensitive to perm solutions.

Pre-perm cutting or shaping

If your client has chosen a hairstyle that is the same or very similar to the design he or she currently has, reshape the style using either scissors or a razor. If the finished style requires texturising or thinning of the ends, wait until after giving the perm to texturise. Over-tapered or thinned ends are more difficult to wrap smoothly and accurately. Irregular effects cut into hair can be difficult to wind without distortion of the hair. Lightly tapering thick hair before winding can aid the winding process.

If your client wants a completely new style, rough cut the hair into an approximation of the final shape. After the perm is completed, you can finish shaping the style more exactly.

Perm curlers and rods

Correct selection of perm curler or rod size is essential for successful perm results. The size of curler determines the size of curl created by the waving process. Perm curlers are typically made of plastic and come in varying sizes. They range in diameter (distance through the centre of the curler from side to side) from 0.3 to 1.9 cm. They are usually colour-coded to identify their size easily.

Perm curlers are also available in three lengths: short, medium and long (4.4 to 8.8 cm). Curlers of all diameters are available in long lengths. Medium and short lengths are not always available in all diameters. These shorter curlers are used for wrapping small or awkward sections.

As well as the traditional shape of perm curlers, there are a range of alternatives, some especially designed to achieve specific shapes in the hair. These include spiral curlers, rick-rack sticks, triangular curlers, flexible curlers and crimping shapers.

TIP When selecting perm rods for use with acid perms, choosing a size smaller than the required curl size can help to reduce the effect of curl drop, sometimes experienced with this type of perm.

Types of curlers

There are two types of curlers: concave and straight. Concave curlers have a small diameter in the centre area and gradually increase to their largest diameter at the ends, resulting in a tighter curl at the hair ends, with a looser, wider curl at the scalp. The diameter of the straight curlers is the same throughout their length, creating an even-sized curl from end to scalp.

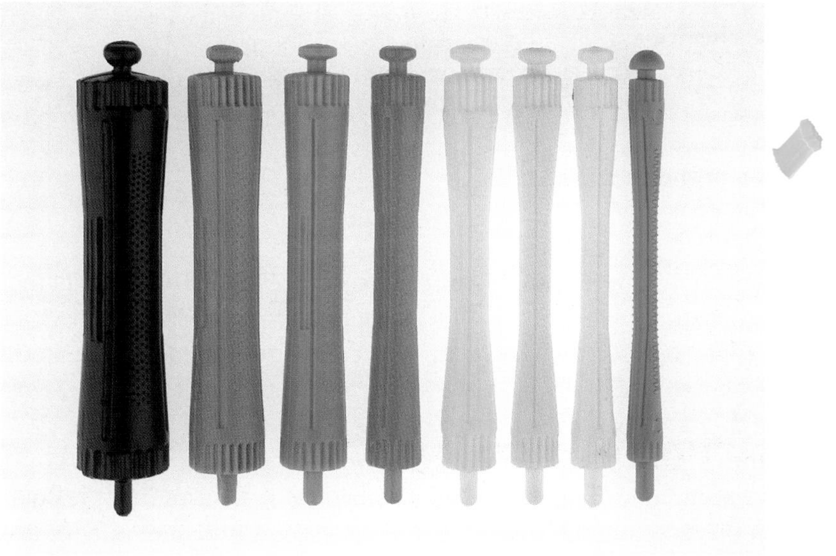

Figure 5A.13 Perm curlers, or rods, colour coded according to size

All curlers have some means of securing the hair on the curler to prevent the curl from unwinding. Usually an elastic band, with a fastening button or loop attached to the end, stretches across the wound hair and secures it when the button or loop is inserted into the opposite end of the curler. Rounded curler rubbers are less likely to mark and break hair than are the flat ones.

Selecting curler size

When selecting curler size, two things must be considered:

- amount of curl desired
- physical characteristics of the hair.

Curl desired: The amount of wave, curl, or body needed is determined between you and your client during the consultation. Your success in creating a style depends primarily on the curler sizes you choose, the number of curlers used, and where the curlers are placed on the head.

Hair characteristics: Of the hair characteristics described earlier, three are important to curler size selection:

- hair length
- hair elasticity
- hair texture.

Suggested hair sectioning and curler size

Although the hair length, elasticity, and texture must be considered in the choice of curlers, the texture should be the determining factor.

Coarse texture, good elasticity

Requires smaller (narrower) sections and larger curlers to permit better placement of curlers for a definite wave pattern.

Medium texture, average elasticity

Medium or average textured hair requires sections that are the same size as the size of the curler.

Fine texture, poor elasticity

Requires smaller sections and curlers wound without any tension on the hair.

Hair in nape area

Use short sections and short curlers.

Long hair

To permanently wave hair longer than 15 cm, use small sections. This permits the waving lotion and neutraliser to penetrate more easily and thoroughly. Spiral winding, piggy back or double winding techniques may be used to achieve an even curl pattern from points to roots.

Sectioning and parting

Pre-sectioning is the division of hair into uniform working areas at the top, front, crown, sides, back and nape. Pre-sectioning makes the winding easier as it ensures that the curlers will fit onto the client's head in the direction that you intend. It also secures the hair out of the way and keeps it off your client's face while winding.

Parting, also known as blocking, is the overall plan for the curler placement. You block so that you know where to place the curlers in order to give the design the support, direction, and curl pattern it needs. It is important that the blocking is done in uniform sections. You should use the following guidelines to help you:

- Uniformly arrange sections.
- Equally subdivide sections (blockings).
- Create clean and uniform partings (length and width).
- The average parting should match the diameter (size) of the curler being used.
- The length of the blocking should be the same as or a little shorter, but never longer, than the length of the curler (see Figures 5A.14 – 5A.16). Blocking is carried out as you wind the perm.

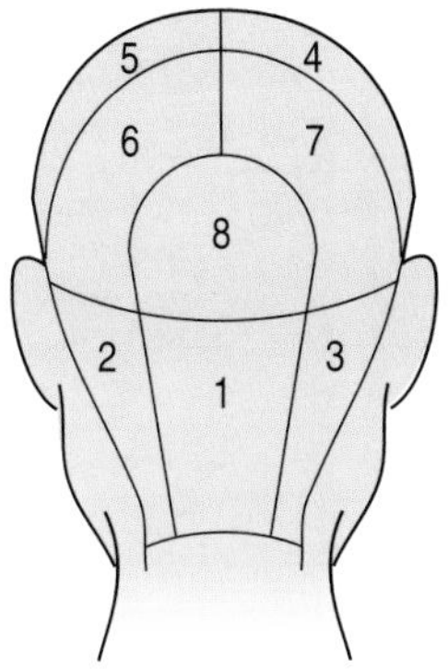

Figure 5A.14 Sectioning

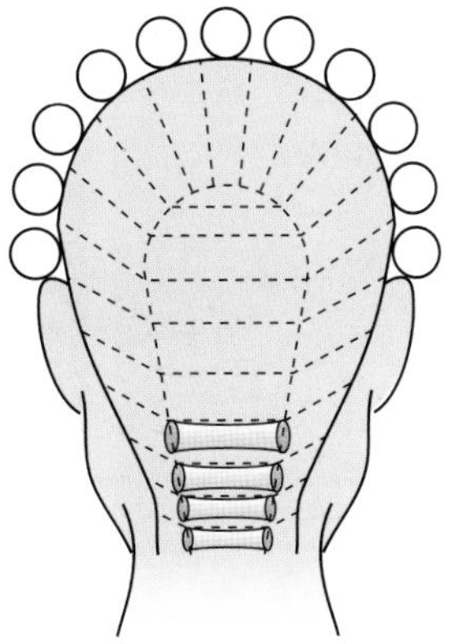

Figure 5A.15 Blocking

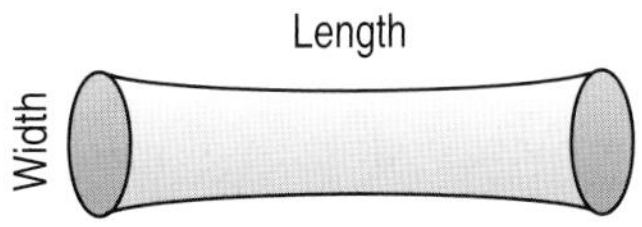

Figure 5A.16 Length denotes span of blocking. Width refers to the depth of the blocking.

WINDING

Winding patterns

Just as the curler size and sectioning size determine the size of the curl, the winding pattern determines the direction or flow of the curl.

Six popular winding patterns are:

- orthodox wind (nine-section)
- directional wind
- spiral wind
- brick wind
- carousel wind
- stack wind

All winding patterns may be adapted to suit particular head shapes and to allow the blocking to follow the direction of the required hairstyle or the natural fall of the hair.

Orthodox (conventional) wind

This traditional sectioning pattern is perhaps the most widely used when perming. The hair is divided into nine sections to allow the curlers to fit easily on the head. This allows the curlers to be wound in a downward direction, following the natural fall of the hair and back off the face. The top/front section may also be wound in a forward direction if required to follow the direction of the hairstyle or to follow the natural fall of the hair on the top.

Brick wind

This technique does not use pre-sectioning. The curlers are located on the head in a staggered brickwork pattern. This technique prevents the occurrence of continuous partings in the end curl pattern and this makes the technique very suitable for use when perming hair which will be naturaly dried, especially short hair.

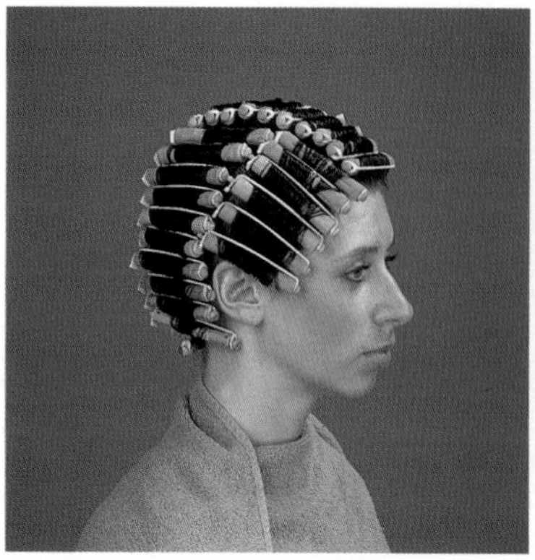

Figure 5A.17 Orthodox wind

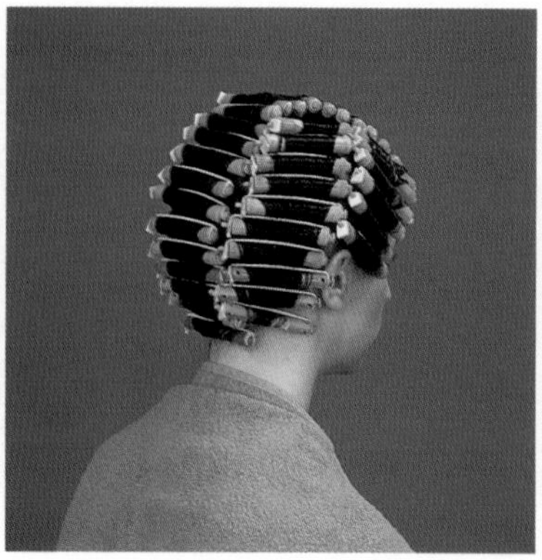

Figure 5A.18 Orthodox wind

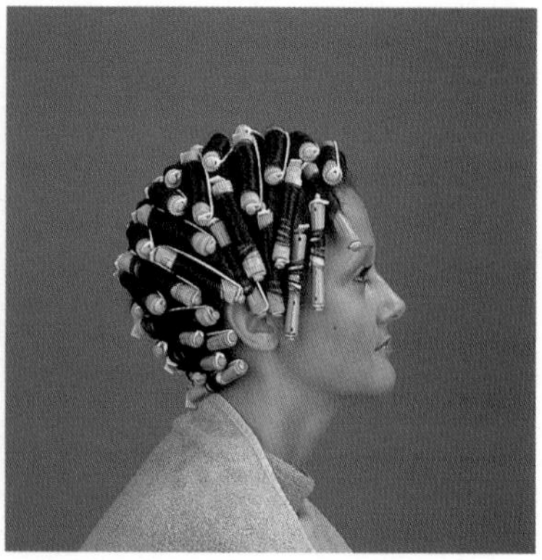

Figure 5A.19 Brick wind

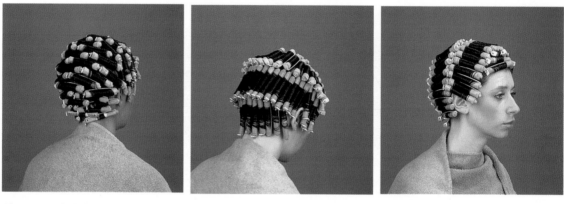

Figure 5A.20 Brick wind

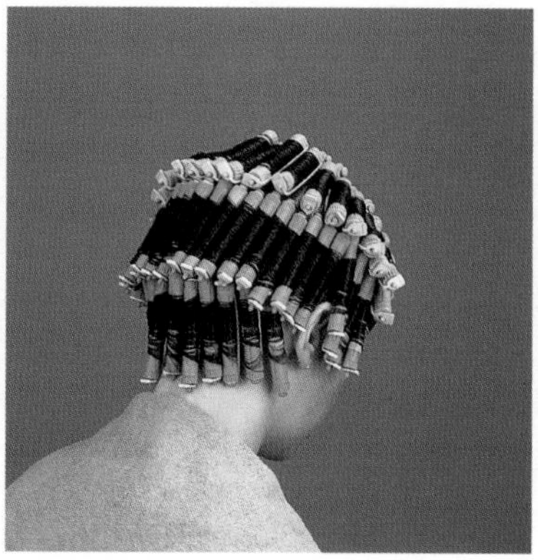

Figure 5A.21 Directional wind

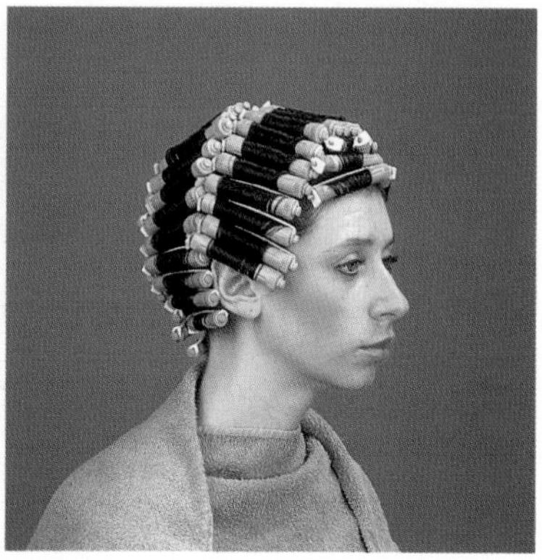

Figure 5A.22 Directional wind

The wind commences at the focal point of the hairstyle, usually at the front. The skill of the hairdresser is to position the curlers in a brickwork pattern that will follow the direction of the required hairstyle without placing the hair under tension.

Directional wind

Sectioning patterns may be devised to enable the curlers to fit onto the head in directions that will support the direction of the hair style. Pre-sectioning will ensure that all curlers fit onto the head without placing the hair under tension.

Carousel wind

This pattern will enable long hair to be wound on the ends, without perming the root area. This produces a wavy look in the hair without producing too full a look to the head.

Spiral wind

This technique is used when a continuous curl is required along the length of long hair, without root lift. Pre-sectioning is essential when spiral winding as the wrap will hang down and obscure the scalp area below. For this reason the wind works from the lower areas of the head first. Without sectioning, the hair will be difficult to control.

Stack wind

This technique may be used to produce curl at the ends of the hair. It may be used to produce a large volume at the ends of the hair, with a definite flatter area at the top of the head.

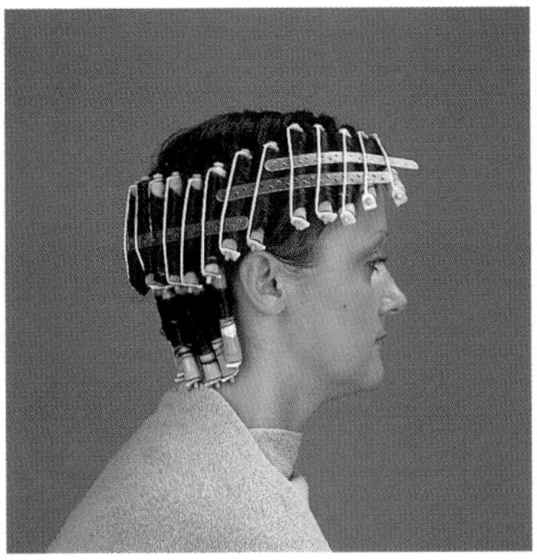

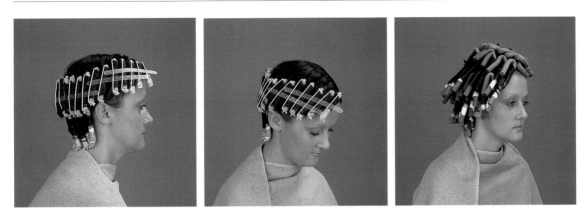

Figure 5A.23 Carousel wind

Figure 5A.24 Carousel wind

Figure 5A.25 Spiral wind

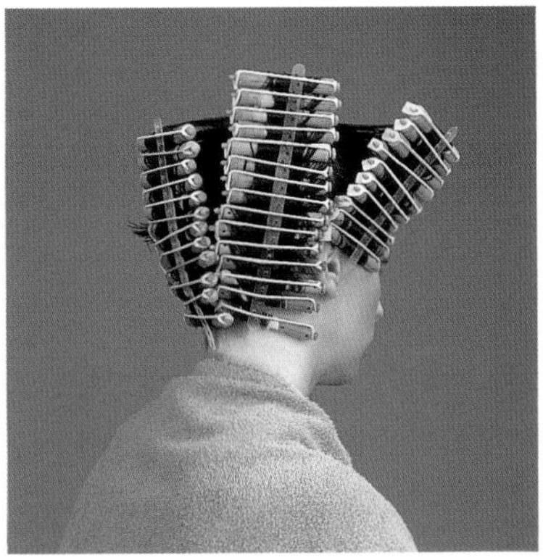

Figure 5A.26 Stack wind

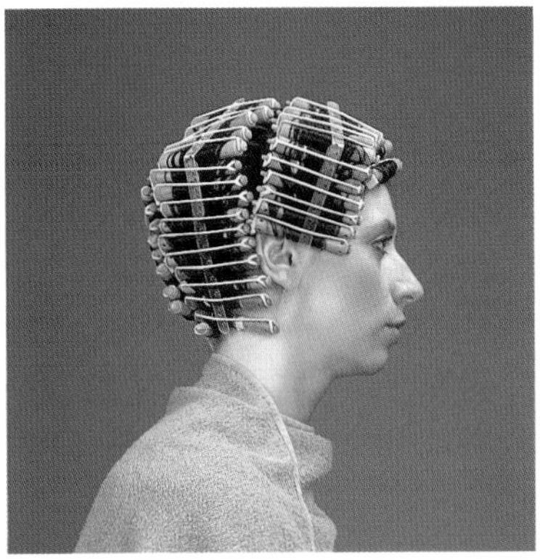

Figure 5A.27 Inverted stack wind with stacking sticks

If the technique incorporates an inverted stack on the top of the head, an overall curl effect may be produced without producing a large level of volume on the top. It is very suitable for thick, plentiful hair.

Winding the hair

To create a uniform wave or curl pattern, the hair must be wrapped smoothly and cleanly on each perm rod without stretching. As noted earlier, the action of the waving lotion expands the hair. Hair that is tightly wound interferes with this action: the hair may be damaged, and the tight wind may prevent penetration of the waving lotion and neutraliser.

When winding with acid wave a slight tension may be used.

Hair strand parting in relation to the head

The term 'base' refers to the area of the head or scalp where the curler is placed in relation to the head. The curlers can be wrapped on-base, off-base, or one-half off-base. Each of these curler positions creates a slightly different scalp wave direction, which will influence the overall curl pattern results.

Curl on-base

When the strand is held in an upward position (at 90 degrees to the head) and wound on the rod, the curl will rest on-base (see Figure 5A.28). Hair wound in this manner will produce curls that

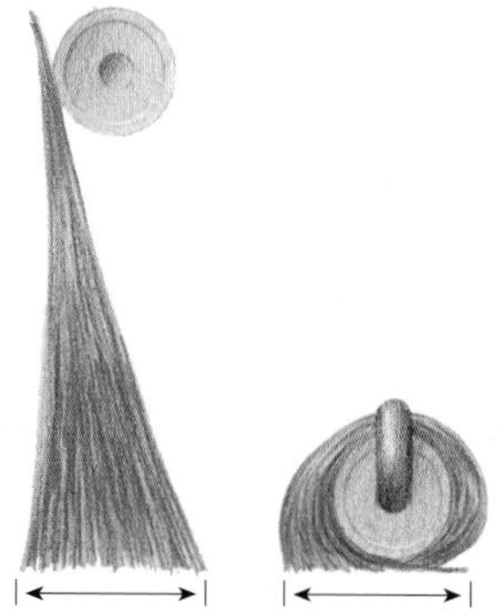

Figure 5A.28 Curl on-base

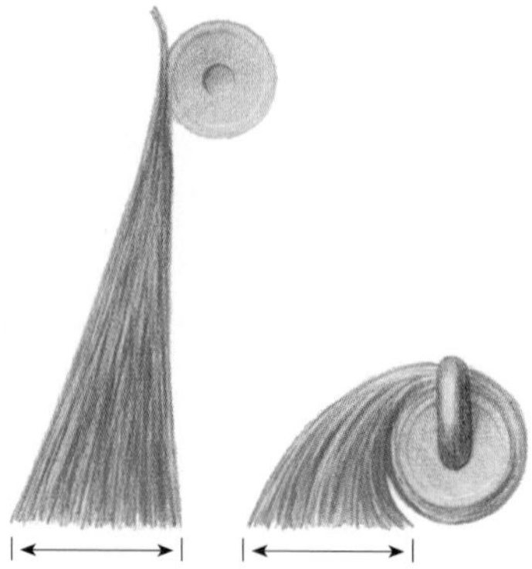

Figure 5A.29 Curl off-base

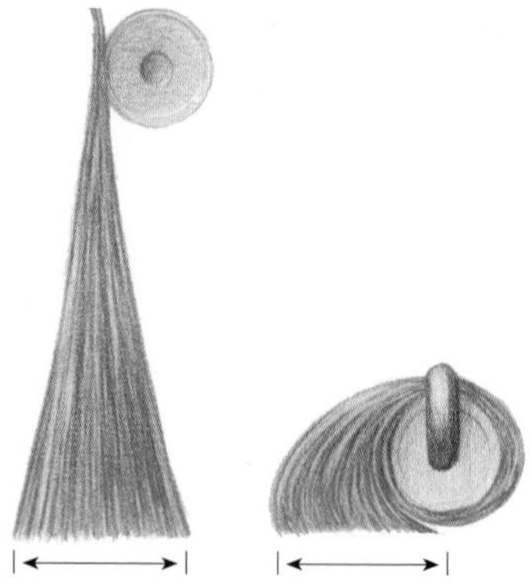

Figure 5A.30 Curl one-half off-base

start close to the scalp for hairstyles that require fullness, height, and upward movement. When perming very curly hair, overdirecting the hair (holding the hair at more than 90 degrees to the head) will enable the perm to control the curl even closer to the scalp.

Curl off-base

When the strand is held in a downward position and wound on a curler, the curl will rest off-base (see Figure 5A.29). Hair wound in this manner will produce a curl that starts further away from the scalp than hair wound on-base. Off-base winding produces close-to-the-head hairstyles that do not require fullness of height.

Curl one-half off-base

When the strand is held straight out from the head and wound on a curler, the curl will rest one-half off-base (see Figure 5A.30). Hair wound in this manner will produce a combination of the previous two.

End papers

End papers or end tissues are porous papers used to cover the ends of the hair to ensure smooth, even winding. End papers minimise the danger of buckled or distorted ends and help to form smooth, even curls and waves. They are especially important in helping to wind uneven hair lengths smoothly.

There are three methods of end paper application in general use today. Each method is equally effective, if properly used.

- double-end paper wrap
- single-end paper wrap
- book-end wrap.

Hair should be shampooed and left moist (not saturated) for wrapping. Section hair, then begin by making your first parting (blocking). Remember, each parting should be no longer than the length of the curler. If the parting is too long, the hair will not wave evenly and hair may be placed under undue tension. If the hair should become dry while you are winding, moisten the hair lightly using water from a trigger spray.

Double end paper wrap

1. Part off and comb the parted hair up and out until all the hair is smooth and evenly distributed (see Figure 5A.31). Do not pinch the ends together.
2. Place one end paper under the hair strand so that it extends below the ends of the hair. Place the other end paper on the top (see Figure 5A.32).
3. With your right hand, place the curler under the double end papers, parallel with the parting at the scalp (see Figure 5A.33).
4. Wind the strand smoothly on the curler to the scalp without tension (see Figure 5A.34).
5. Fasten the band on the top of the curler.

> ***TIP*** To prevent breakage, the band should not press into the hair near the scalp or be twisted (flat rubbers) against the wound hair.

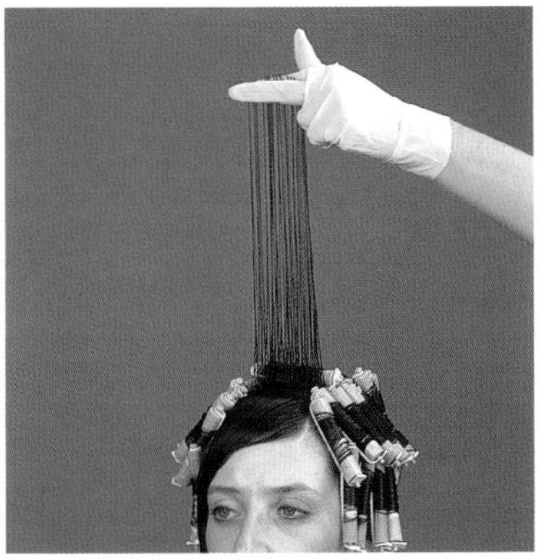

Figure 5A.31 Combed hair ready for end tissue

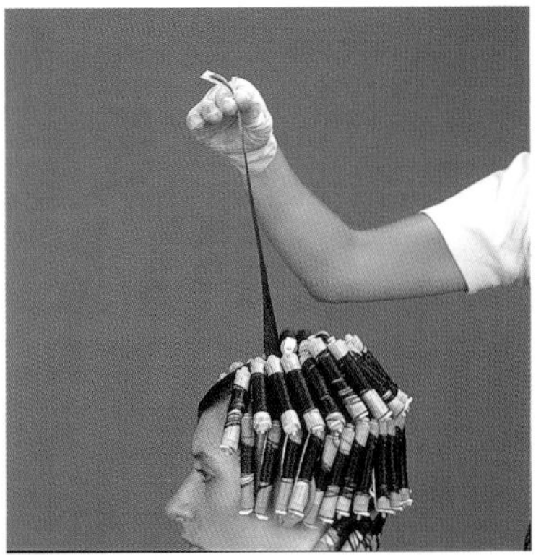

Figure 5A.32 Two-end tissues, one above hair, one beneath

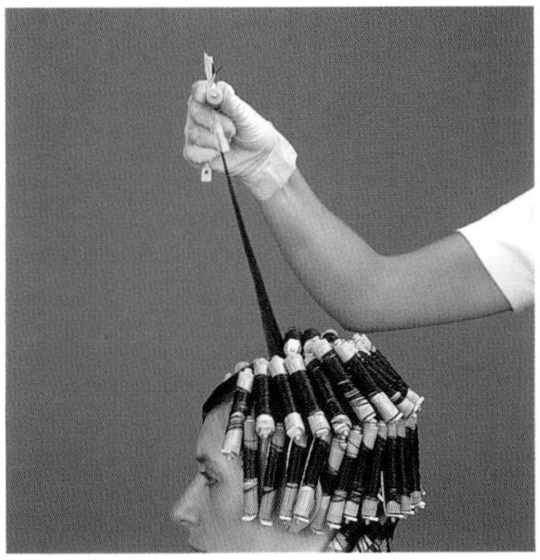

Figure 5A.33 Locating and winding perm rod at the hair ends

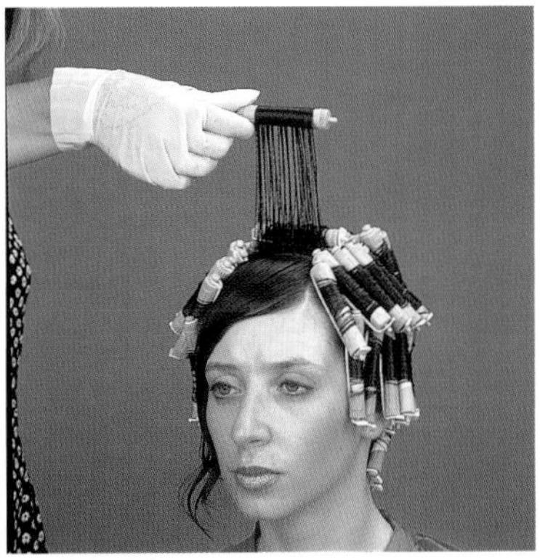

Figure 5A.34 Winding rod, middle length, smooth even tension

The preparation and winding of curls for a single end paper wrap and book-end wrap are the same as the double end paper wrap, with the following exceptions:

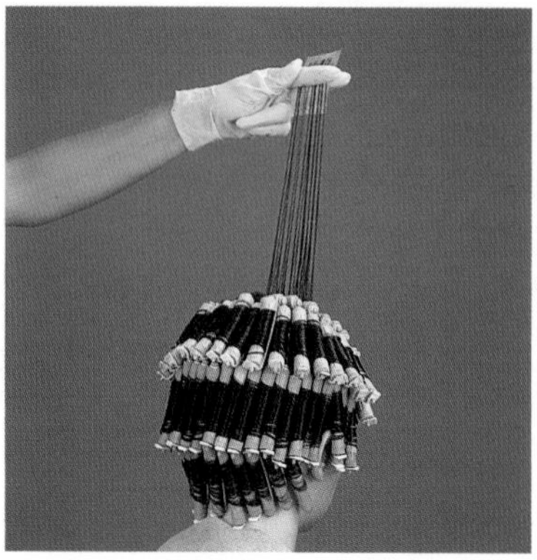

Figure 5A.35 Single-end tissue in place

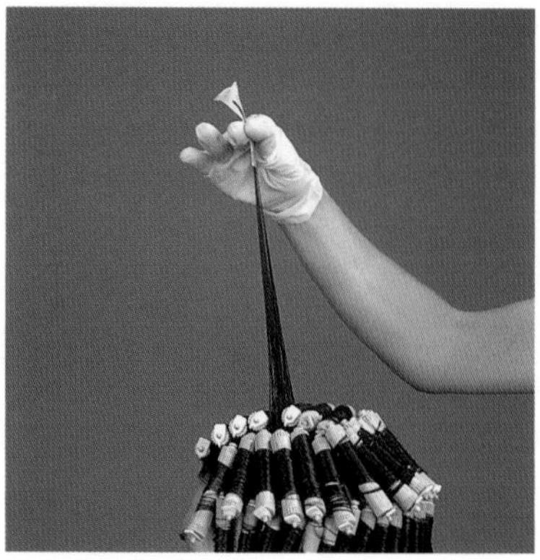

Figure 5A.36 Book-end wrap

Single end paper wrap

Place only one end paper on top of the hair strand and hold it flat between the first and second fingers to prevent bunching (see Figure 5A.35). The hair is wound in the same manner as the double end wrap.

Book-end wrap

Hold the strand between the first and second fingers; fold and place an end paper over the strand, forming an envelope. Take care not to indent into the hair with the folded side of the paper. Wind the curl as in the double-end wrap (see Figure 5A.36).

The piggy-back (double-curler) wind

The piggy-back (double-curler) method of winding is especially suitable for extra long hair. This wrapping technique permits maximum control of the size and tightness of the curl from the scalp to the hair ends. Control of the amount of curl can be exercised by the size of the curlers selected. Thus, the use of larger curlers will result in a loose, wide wave, while small or medium curlers will give tighter curls. The following is the procedure for wrapping in the piggy-back (double-curler) method:

1. Section the head in the usual manner (orthodox sectioning).
2. Select the desired size of curlers. The curlers used in the area from midpoint to the scalp should be at least one size larger than those used on the hair ends.
3. About halfway up the strand, place porous end papers one on top and one underneath (see Figure 5A.37).
4. Start at the midpoint part of the strand. Place the larger curler underneath the hair strand and start winding (see Figure 5A.38).
5. Roll the curler toward the scalp and, at the same time, control the hair ends by holding them to the left away from the rod.
6. Secure the wrapped curler at the scalp, leaving the hair ends dangling free from the rod (see Figure 5A.39).
7. Place an end paper on the hair strand covering the ends. Using the smaller sized curler, wind the hair ends up to the larger rod above.
8. Secure the second rod to rest against the first one in piggy-back fashion (see Figure 5A.40).
9. To maintain better control over the winding and processing, it is advisable to complete the winding of each strand before proceeding to the next one.
10. Test curls should be taken from the curlers closer to the scalp, because the hair in this area is more resistant and might require additional processing.

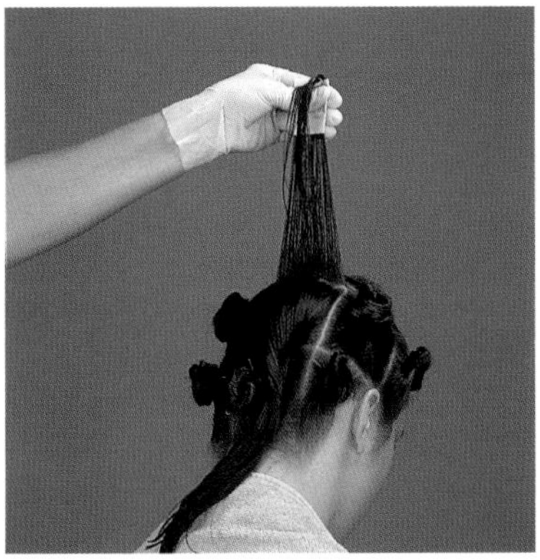

Figure 5A.37 Locating end tissue part way down for piggy-back wind

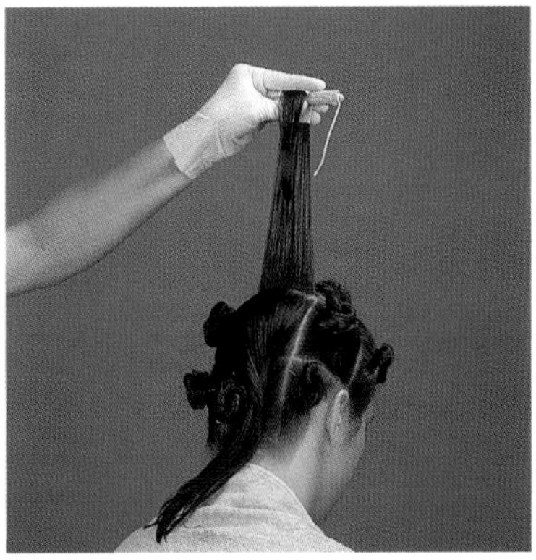

Figure 5A.38 Locating first perm rod for piggy-back wind

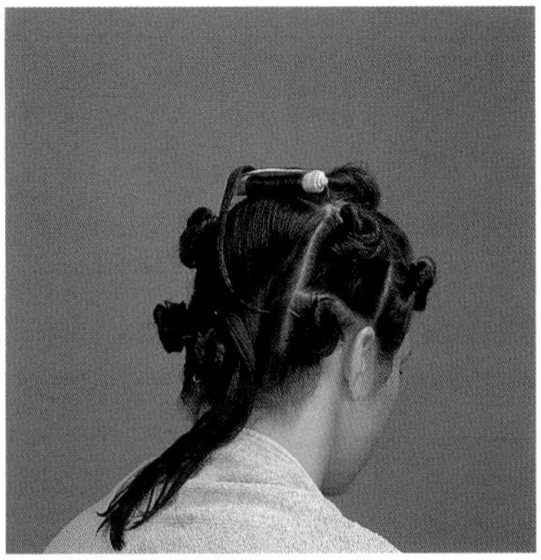

Figure 5A.39 First rod wound and in place for piggy-back wind

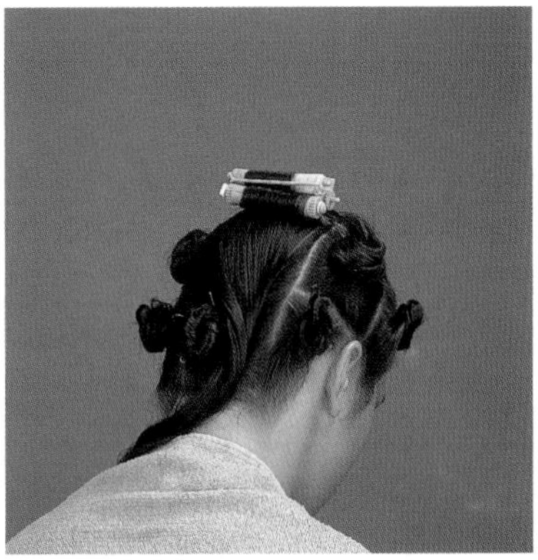

Figure 5A.40 Piggy-back curlers fixed in place

When winding hair, always avoid bulkiness on the rod. Bulkiness prevents the formation of a good curl because the hair cannot conform to the shape of the curler, and the waving lotion and neutraliser cannot penetrate evenly and thoroughly. To ensure a smooth wave formation and to avoid fishhook (buckled) ends, the first part-turn of the curler should be the end papers without any of the hair ends between them.

Piggy-back wind (alternative method)

This technique avoids the distortion of the hair that can at times occur in the area between the two curlers. It does, however, create an elongated curl on the area of the hair nearest the scalp.

1. Locate the end papers at the ends of the hair and wind the ends of the hair with the smaller perm curler.
2. Wind the curler to a mid point of the hair length and then insert a second perm curler.
3. Wind both curlers together to the scalp and secure.

PRELIMINARY (PRE-PERM) TEST CURLS

Preliminary test curls help determine how your client's hair will react to a perm. It is advisable to carry out a test on hair that is tinted, bleached, over-porous, or shows any signs of damage.

Preliminary testing gives you the following additional information:

- Actual processing time needed to achieve optimum curl results.
- Curl results based on the curler size and perm product you have selected.

> ***HEALTH AND SAFETY*** When applying perm lotion you should wear protective gloves or apply barrier cream to your hands.

Procedure

1. Shampoo the hair and towel dry.
2. Following the perm direction, wrap two or three curlers in the most delicate areas of the hair.
3. Wind a coil of lightly moist cotton wool around the curlers.
4. Apply waving lotion to the wrapped curls, being careful not to allow the waving lotion to come into contact with the unwrapped hair.
5. Set a time and process the hair according to the perm directions.
6. Check the hair frequently.

To check a test curl, unfasten a rod and carefully (remember – the hair is in a softened state) unwind the curl about $1\frac{1}{2}$ turns of the curler. Do not permit the hair to become loose or unwound from the curler completely. Hold the hair firmly by placing a thumb at each end of the curler. Move the curler gently towards the scalp so that the hair falls loosely into the wave pattern. Continue checking the curlers until a firm and definite 'S' is formed. The 'S' reflects the size of the rod used (see Figure 5A.41). Be guided by the manufacturer's directions.

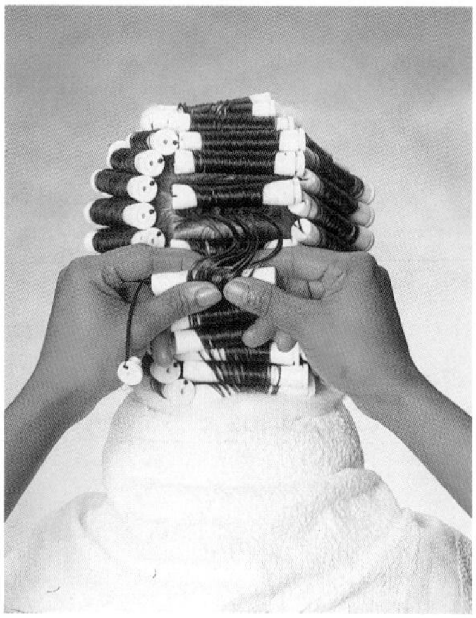

Figure 5A.41 Unwinding hair carefully, without pushing or pulling

When judging test curls, different hair textures with varying degrees of elasticity will have slightly different 'S' formations. Fine, thin hair is generally softer and has less bulk. The wave ridge might be less defined and more difficult to read. Coarse, thick hair has better elasticity and seems to reinforce itself, falling into the wave pattern more readily. The wave ridge will be stronger and better defined. Long hair may produce a wider scalp wave than short hair, because larger curlers are used and the diameter of the wave widens towards the scalp.

When the optimum curl has been formed, rinse the curls with warm water, blot the curls thoroughly, apply, process and rinse the neutraliser according to the perm directions and gently dry these test curls. Evaluate the curl results. If the hair is over processed (see page 97), do not perm the rest of the hair until it is in better condition. If the test curl results are good, proceed with the perm, but do not re-perm these preliminary test curls.

Overprocessing

Any lotion that can properly process the hair can also overprocess it, causing dryness, frizziness, or hair damage. Overprocessed hair is easily detected. It cannot be combed into a suitable wave pattern, because the elasticity of the hair has been excessively damaged, and the hair feels harsh after being dried. Reconditioning treatments should begin immediately.

Causes of over processing are:

- Lotion left on the hair too long.
- Improperly judged pre-perm hair analysis and/or waving lotion that was too strong.
- Test curls were not made frequently enough or were judged improperly.

Underprocessing

Underprocessing is caused by insufficient processing time of the waving lotion. After perming, underprocessed hair has a limp or weak wave formation. The ridges are not well defined, and the hair retains little or no wave formation. Typically, after a few shampooings, the hair will have no curl pattern at all (see Figure 5A.42).

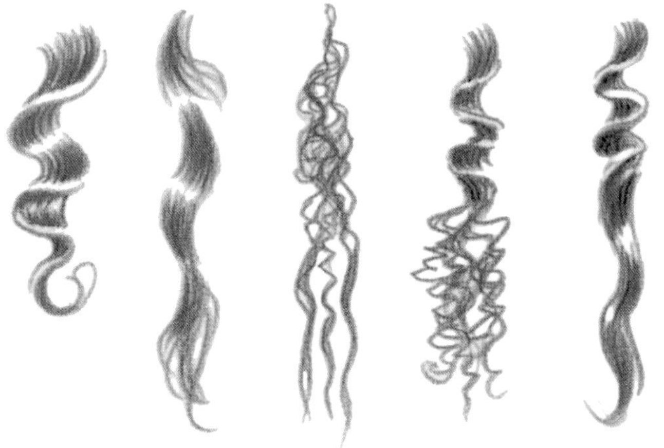

Figure 5A.42 a Good results; b Underprocessed curl; c Overprocessed curl; d Porous ends; e Improper winding.

Underprocessed hair, even if there is no curl, has been chemically treated. If, in your professional judgement, you decide the hair can be re-permed, condition it first, choose a milder lotion, and test the curls frequently.

IMPORTANT SAFETY PRECAUTIONS

Remember that the lotions used for perming contain chemically active ingredients and therefore must be used carefully to avoid injury to you and your client. The following precautions should always be taken:

- Protect your client's clothing with a plastic shampoo cape. 1
- Ask your client to remove glasses, earrings, and necklaces to prevent damage.
- Do not give a perm to a client who has experienced an allergic reaction to a previous perm.

- Do not save any opened, unused waving lotion or neutraliser. These lotions can change in strength and effectiveness if not used within a few hours of opening the container.
- Do not dilute or add anything to the waving lotion or neutraliser unless the product directions tell you to do so.
- Keep waving lotion out of eyes and away from the skin. If waving lotion contacts these areas, rinse thoroughly with cool, clean water.
- Do not perm and apply hair colour to a client on the same day. Perm the hair first, wait one week, then apply hair colour. There are products available today which combine perming and colouring within the one process.

PERMING TECHNIQUES

Before you begin perming, make sure you have all the necessary materials at hand. Good organisation and planning will help to develop precision and speed in completing a perm. At the perming station the following equipment should be laid out in an organised, easily accessible fashion:

- perm product
- client's record card
- towels
- curlers (organised by size)
- plastic hair clips and pins
- end papers
- pin tail comb
- cotton wool
- protective gloves
- perm lotion applicator.

> ***TIP*** Always read and follow the manufacturer's directions carefully.

Some alkaline perm product directions call for water winding, some are lotion wound, and others require pre-wind lotions. Some wave lotions come in two parts that must be mixed just prior to use. Some need dryer heat. (Note: the dryer should be pre-heated.) Some perms require that a plastic cap be placed over the curlers during the processing, others do not. Considering all the variables, it is not a good idea to trust your memory. Make it a practice to check the printed directions that accompany every perm each time you give a perm.

Partial perming

Perming only a section of a whole head of hair is called partial perming. Partial perming can be used on:

1. clients (male and female) who have long hair on the top and crown and very short, tapered sides and nape
2. clients who need volume and lift only in certain areas
3. designs that require curl support in the nape area but a smooth, sleek surface.

Partial perming uses the same techniques and wrapping patterns that have already been described. There are a few additional considerations:

1. When you are winding the hair and reach the area that will be left unpermed, go to the next larger curler size so that the curl pattern of the permed hair will blend into the unpermed hair.
2. After wrapping the area to be permed, place a coil of moist cotton wool around the wrapped curlers as well as around the entire hairline.
3. Before applying the waving lotion, apply a heavy, creamy conditioner to the sections

that **will not** be permed to protect this hair from the effects of the waving lotion (waving lotion softens and straightens unwrapped hair).

Applying perming lotion

The technique used in applying perming lotion will vary depending on a number of considerations.

HEALTH AND SAFETY Whenever winding with perm lotion, either pre-saturation or pre-damping, wear protective gloves to protect your skin.

Styles of application

Pre-saturation

May be used when perming strong straight hair. By applying the lotion to all of the hair before commencing winding, the hair begins to soften uniformly, and offers less resistance to winding.

Pre-damping

Wetting the hair with perm lotion as you wind. This enables more resistant areas, if wound first, to begin to soften before the less resistant, therefore producing an even curl development throughout the hair. This method may also be used when perming hair using winding patterns to which it may be difficult to apply the perm lotion after winding. In some cases a mild lotion strength may be used as a winding lotion, followed by a stronger lotion, post-damping. This is often used when perming hair with differing rates of porosity along the hair's length.

Post-damping

The hair is water wound, and then the lotion is applied after the wind is completed. This gives time for the winding process to take place. Care must be taken to ensure that lotion is applied to all wound curlers.

After shampooing, shaping, and wrapping the hair, place a coil or band of moist cotton wool around the entire hairline. To prevent skin irritation and for added protection, apply a barrier cream to skin around the hairline before applying the cotton wool band. This safety precaution prevents waving lotion from coming into contact with the skin and possibly causing irritation. If lotion is applied accurately there should be a minimum of dripping, but the cotton wool assures your client's comfort and safety. After the waving lotion has been applied, remove the cotton wool, gently pat the skin with water-soaked cotton wool, and replace with fresh.

Unless otherwise specified in the product instruction, apply waving lotion with care to the wound hair. Systematically apply lotion to each curler, in turn, using an applicator bottle. Run the nozzle along the top of the curler, releasing lotion onto the hair. Avoid allowing lotion to flood onto the scalp. Coverage will be assured by making three applications to the entire head, a little at a time. Remember, dry hair will not absorb moisture easily. By gradually adding lotion to the hair, it will be more readily absorbed ensuring thorough distribution and coverage (see Figure 5A.43).

HEALTH AND SAFETY Should perm lotion enter your client's eyes, rinse with sterile water from an eye bath. Should eye irritation continue inform your line manager and if required seek medical advice.

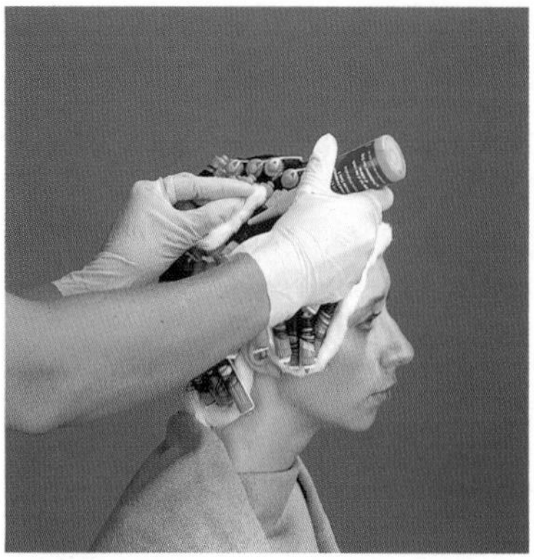

Figure 5A.43 Applying perm lotion to wound hair

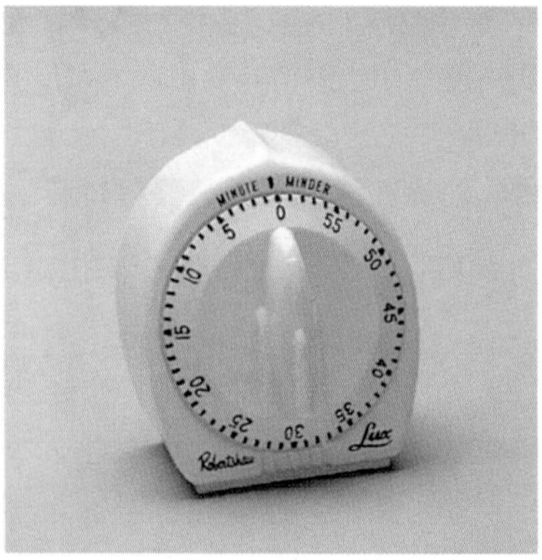

Figure 5A.44 Processing timer

Processing time

Processing time is the length of time required for the hair strands to absorb the waving lotion (softening). It depends on the hair type (porosity, elasticity, length, density, texture, and overall condition) and the specific perm lotion you are using. Again, follow the manufacturer's directions closely. It is usually safe to anticipate that the processing time will be less than suggested by the manufacturer or a client's previous record card. Some perms have stop-action processing so that all you have to do is set a timer (see Figure 5A.44). Some perms give you a general timetable to follow and require that you do a test curl during processing. It is very important to accurately time the perm process to help prevent over- or underprocessing.

The ability of the hair to absorb moisture may vary from time to time in the same individual, even when the same lotions and procedures are used. A record of the previous processing time is desirable, but should be used only as a guide.

It is sometimes necessary to saturate all the curlers a second time during processing. This might be due to:

- evaporation of the lotion or dryness of the hair
- hair poorly saturated by the hairstylist
- no wave development after the maximum time indicated by the manufacturer
- improper selection of solution strength for the client's hair
- failure to follow the manufacturer's directions for a specific formula.

A reapplication of the lotion will hasten processing. Watch the wave development closely. Negligence can result in hair damage.

Most manufacturers provide instructions with their product. Here are some you will encounter:

- 'Process at room temperature'. Make sure that your client is not sitting in a draught or too close to a heater. A room that is cool slows down the processing.
- 'Place a plastic cap over the wrapped curlers'. Be sure that the plastic cap covers all the curlers and that the cap is airtight. Secure the cap with a non-metallic clip. The cap holds in scalp heat. If it is too loose or if all the rods are not covered, processing might take longer A dry towel placed over the plastic cap will increase the effect and will reduce the influence of blasts of warm or cold air on parts of the head (producing uneven development).

- 'Use a preiheated dryer'. Turn the hood dryer to a high setting and medium air flow. Allow the dryer to warm up for approximately 5 minutes before placing your client under the dryer. Cover the wound curlers with a plastic cap secured in place, locate the hood to enclose all of the curlers and reduce the heat to a medium setting. (Note: Dryer filters should be cleaned frequently so that optimum heat and airflow will remain constant.) Take care not to overprocess the hair, in particular porous hair.
- 'Use an accelerator'. This may be used to aid the process of the perm. The curlers are not usually covered with a plastic cap. The accelerator must be located correctly and evenly around the head. Using the correct heat setting process, taking care not to allow the hair to become dry. In some cases these machines are programmable to particular lotions and hair types. Having located a sensor on the hair it will regulate the processing.

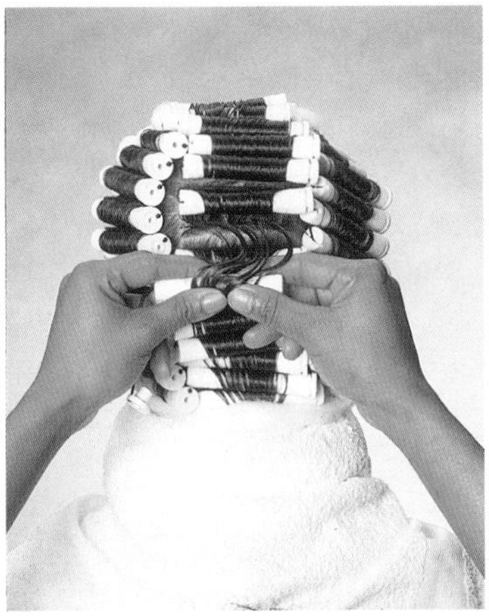

Figure 5A.45 Properly processed strand opens up into 'S' formation

Testing curls during processing

Optimum curl development occurs only once during the processing time. The ability to read a test curl 'S' formation and recognise proper wave development will help you avoid overprocessing and underprocessing. Three test curls should be taken: in the nape, on top of the head and on the side of the head. These three locations will allow you to judge the progress of curl development on the most resistant and the least resistant areas of the head. Follow the procedure for unwinding the curler and checking the 'S'-pattern formation described in the preliminary (pre-perm) test curl section on pages 95–97 (see Figure 5A.45).

Water rinsing

Rinsing the waving lotion from the hair is extremely important. Any lotion left in the hair can cause poor perm results. When your test curl indicates that the optimum curl has been achieved, remove the cotton wool from around the hairline. Rinse the hair thoroughly with a moderate force of warm water. The manufacturer's perm directions will indicate for how long you should rinse – usually 3 to 5 minutes. Always set your timer for the exact time. Remember, you are rinsing the lotion out of the internal hair structure, not merely off the surface. Make sure that all curlers are thoroughly rinsed. Pay particular attention to the curlers at the nape of the neck. They are a little difficult to reach, but they must be rinsed as well as all the other curlers. Long hair and thick hair usually require the maximum rinsing time (5 minutes) to make sure that all lotion has been removed from all hair wrapped around the curlers. Indicator papers are available which, when pressed to the hair, will indicate if any perm lotion remains in the hair. 1

Undesirable effects of improper or incomplete rinsing include:

- Early curl relaxation. Even if the perm has been processed correctly, any waving lotion left in the hair can interfere with the action of the neutraliser. If the neutraliser is not able to properly rebond the hair, the curl will be weak or will not last very long.
- Lightening of hair colour (natural or tint). Rinsing helps reduce the pH of the hair and helps to close the cuticle layer. If the hair is not rinsed properly, the hydrogen peroxide in the neutraliser can react with waving lotion left in the hair and cause the hair colour to lighten. This lightening effect is usually seen on the hair ends.
- Residual perm odour. If any waving lotion is left in the hair, it will become trapped inside the hair when the neutraliser is applied. This is especially true of acid-balanced perms. Unpleasant odours may be evident each time the hair gets wet or damp.

Blotting after water rinsing

1 Careful blotting ensures that the neutraliser will penetrate the hair immediately and completely: do not omit this important step. To obtain the best results from towel blotting, carefully press a towel between each curler, using your fingers. Do not rock or roll the rods while blotting. When the hair is in a softened state, any such movement can cause hair breakage. Change to dry towels frequently in order to remove as much excess water as possible. Excess water left in the hair can dilute or weaken the action of the neutraliser. If this happens the curl can be either weakened or relaxed.

After rinsing and blotting has been completed, place a fresh, clean band of moistened cotton wool around the hairline before applying neutraliser.

> ***HEALTH AND SAFETY*** Whenever handling perming chemicals, wear protective overalls and protective rubber gloves.

NEUTRALISING/NORMALISING

1 Neutralising procedures can vary according to the perm product you are using. Again, follow the manufacturer's directions exactly.

In general, the following procedure is the accepted method of neutralising:

1. Apply neutraliser to the top and underside of the rods. Apply to the top of the rod, then gently turn the rod up and apply to the underside of the rod in the same manner you applied the waving lotion. When using foam neutraliser, apply the neutraliser to the curlers and foam up.
2. Repeat the entire application a second time, to ensure complete coverage.
3. Wait 5 minutes to allow for optimum rebonding. Set a timer for accuracy (see Figure 5A.44).
4. Remove the curlers carefully and gently, unwinding without tension as this may straighten the hair.
5. Work remaining neutraliser onto the ends of the hair, pushing the neutraliser onto the hair so as not to drag the curl.
6. Rinse the hair thoroughly with warm water and apply an after-perm treatment if required.
7. Towel blot the hair and using a wide-tooth comb, gently comb the hair into place.

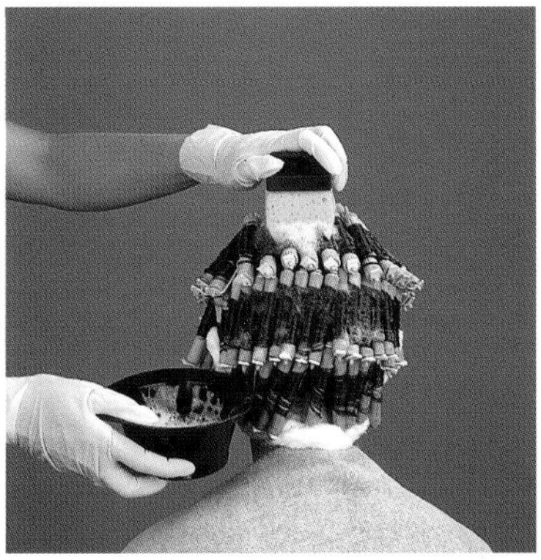

Figure 5A.46 Applying foam neutraliser

If you are uncertain of the procedure, or whether an after-perm treatment should be applied, consult with your supervisor or stylist.

Post-perm precautions

After blotting, your new perm is ready for final shaping and styling. It is important to avoid shampooing, conditioning, stretching or excessive manipulations of freshly permed hair. When styling, do not pull on the hair or use intense heat that could result in curl relaxation. Generally, hair should not be shampooed, conditioned, or treated harshly for 48 hours after perming. This special care will help to ensure that the perm does not relax. 1

TEN POINTERS FOR A PERFECT PERM

1. Consult with your client.
2. Analyse the hair and scalp carefully.
3. Select the correct curler size for the desired style.
4. Choose the appropriate perm product for the hair type and final design. Follow the manufacturer's directions carefully.
5. Section and make accurate partings for each curler. Wrap specifically for the style chosen.
6. Apply waving lotion to the top and underside of all wound curlers, one at a time. Ensure each curler is thoroughly wet with lotion.
7. If the perm product requires a test curl, be sure the result is a firmly formed 'S' shape.
8. Water rinse for at least 3 to 5 minutes and carefully towel blot each curler. 1
9. Apply neutraliser to the top and underside of all curlers. Saturate thoroughly. Wait 5 minutes, remove the curler carefully, without pulling. Apply remaining neutraliser, and gently work through the hair. Rinse with warm water.
10. Educate your client in how to care for their new look. Recommend hair care and styling products which are suitable. Instruct in how best to style the hair at home and remind your client not to shampoo the hair for at least 24 hours and to avoid getting the hair wet during that period.

> ***TIP*** Remember to promptly update your client's records to reflect the perm treatment provided.

Cleaning up

1. Discard all used materials.
2. Clean up the work area.
3. Thoroughly clean and sterilise the curlers and other tools used.
4. Wash and dry your hands.
5. Complete your client's record card.

FURTHER STUDY

- Find out more about the variety of machine and machineless perming systems once used.
- There are a wide variety of perm curlers, made from a variety of materials and designed to produce a number of fashion effects. Look at the trade press, visit trade exhibitions and consult manufacturers to find out about what is available to help you produce fashion perm effects on your clients.
- Find out your salon's procedures for dealing with accidental spillage of lotions onto your clients.

REVIEW QUESTIONS

1. Why is permanent waving beneficial to the client?
2. What is hair porosity?
3. What is hair texture?
4. What is hair elasticity?
5. What is hair density?
6. What is spiral wrapping?
7. What is croquignole wrapping?
8. What is the purpose of a) waving lotion, b) neutraliser?
9. What factor determines the size of perm curler to be used?
10. What is a test curl?
11. What two factors determine processing time?
12. What effect will a cold room have on the development time of a perm?
13. What is the likely result of overprocessing a perm?
14. What may incomplete neutralising cause?
15. Why do you rinse the hair before applying neutraliser to the hair?
16. What is the main active ingredient of a perm neutraliser?

CHAPTER 5B

Relaxing hair curl

This chapter will provide the essential knowledge to help you understand the hair relaxing processes that may be applied to very curly hair. Guidelines in the relaxing processes will help you perform these tasks.

Level 1	
Unit 101	
Element 101.1	Maintain effective and safe methods of working when shampooing
Element 101.2	Shampoo and surface condition hair
Unit 102B	
Element 102B.1	Maintain effective and safe methods of working
Element 102B.2	Neutralise hair as part of the perming and relaxing process
Unit 104	
Element 104.1	Develop effective working relationships with clients
Element 104.2	Develop effective working relationships with colleagues
Element 104.3	Develop yourself within the job role
Unit 105	
Element 105.2	Support health and safety at work

Level 2	
Unit 201	
Element 201.1	Consult with and maintain effective relationships with clients
Element 201.2	Advise clients on salon products and services
Element 201.3	Advise clients on after-care procedures
Unit 202	
Element 202.1	Maintain effective and safe methods of working when shampooing and conditioning hair
Element 202.2	Shampoo hair and scalp
Element 202.3	Condition hair and scalp
Unit 205B	
Element 205B.1	Maintain effective and safe methods of working when perming, relaxing and neutralising hair
Element 205B.2	Perm hair using basic techniques
Element 205B.3	Relax hair
Element 205B.4	Neutralise hair
Unit 208	
Element 208.1	Develop and maintain effective team work and relationships with colleagues
Element 208.2	Develop and improve personal effectiveness within the job role
Unit 209	
Element 209.2	Support health, safety and security at work

Contents

INTRODUCTION

Chemical hair relaxing is the process of permanently rearranging the basic structure of very curly hair into a straight form, and relaxing perms to reshape overly curly hair into a more clearly defined open curl shape. When done professionally, it leaves the hair straight and in a satisfactory condition, ready to be set or dried into almost any style. Due to the nature of the chemicals used for permanently straightening hair, it is essential that you have a thorough understanding of their correct use.

CHEMICAL HAIR RELAXING PRODUCTS

The basic products that are used in chemical hair relaxing are a chemical hair relaxer, a neutraliser, and a petroleum cream, which is used as a protective base to protect the client's scalp during the sodium hydroxide chemical straightening process.

Chemical hair relaxers

The two general types of hair relaxers are hydroxide, which does not require pre-shampooing, and ammonium thioglycolate, which may require pre-shampooing.

The hydroxide relaxers are divided into two groups: Sodium Hydroxide and Calcium Hydroxide.

Sodium Hydroxide relaxers, sometimes called Lye or caustic soda, generally have fast processing times and produce straightness that has a reduced likeness to revert following shampooing.

Calcium Hydroxide relaxers sometimes called no-lye. These are not caustic soda based.

Sodium hydroxide, a caustic relaxer often called a hair straightener, both softens and swells hair fibres. As the solution penetrates into the cortex, the sulphur and hydrogen cross-bonds are broken. The action of the comb, the brush, or the hands in smoothing the hair and distributing the chemical straightens the softened hair.

HEALTH AND SAFETY Because of the high alkaline content of sodium hydroxide, great care must be taken in its use: always wear protective gloves when handling and applying these products.

Manufacturers vary the sodium hydroxide content of the solution from 5% to 10%, and the pH factor from 10 to 14. In general, the more sodium hydroxide used the higher the pH, the quicker the chemical reaction will take place on the hair, and the greater the danger will be of hair damage.

Although ammonium thioglycolate (a thio-type relaxer often called a relaxer) is less drastic in its action than sodium hydroxide, it softens and relaxes overly curly hair in much the same manner. You may recall that this is the same solution used in permanent waving.

Neutraliser

1 The neutraliser is also called a stabiliser or fixative. The neutraliser stops the action of any chemical relaxer that may remain in the hair after rinsing. The neutraliser for a thio-type relaxer reforms the cysteine (sulphur) cross-bonds in their new position and re-hardens the hair.

Base and no-base formulas

Sodium hydroxide relaxers have two types of formulas, base and no-base. The base formula requires the use of a petroleum cream that is designed to protect the client's skin and scalp during the sodium hydroxide chemical straightening process. This protective base is also important during a chemical straightening retouch. It is applied to protect hair that has been straightened previously, and to prevent over-processing and hair breakage.

Petroleum cream has a lighter consistency than petroleum jelly, and is formulated to melt at body temperature. The melting process ensures complete protective coverage of the scalp and other areas with a thin, oily coating. This helps to prevent burning and/or irritation of the scalp and skin. Previously treated hair should be protected with cream conditioner during the straightening process.

'No-base' relaxers are also available. These relaxers have the same chemical reaction on the hair, although usually the reaction is milder. The procedure for the application of a 'no-base' relaxer is the same as for a normal relaxer except that the base cream is not applied. It is advisable to use a protective cream around the hairline and over the ears.

STEPS IN CHEMICAL HAIR RELAXING

All chemical hair relaxing involves three basic steps: processing, neutralising, and conditioning.

Processing

As soon as the chemical relaxer is applied, the hair begins to soften so that the chemical can penetrate to loosen and relax the natural curl.

Neutralising

1 As soon as the hair has been sufficiently processed, the chemical relaxer is thoroughly rinsed out with warm water, followed by either a built-in shampoo neutraliser or a prescribed shampoo and neutraliser.

Conditioning

Depending on your client's needs, the conditioner may be part of a series of hair treatments, or it may be applied to the hair before or after the relaxing treatment.

Hair treated with lighteners or metallic dyes must not be given a chemical hair relaxer, because it might suffer excessive damage or breakage.

> ***TIP*** Overly curly hair that has been damaged from heat appliances or other chemicals must be reconditioned before a relaxer service is performed.

RECOMMENDED STRENGTH OF RELAXER

The strength of relaxer used is determined by a strand test. The following guidelines can help in determining which strength relaxer to use for the test:

- fine, tinted, or lightened hair – use mild relaxer
- normal, medium-textured virgin hair – use regular relaxer
- coarse virgin hair – use strong or super relaxer.

ANALYSIS OF YOUR CLIENT'S HAIR

It is essential that you have a working knowledge of human hair, particularly when giving a relaxing treatment. You will learn to recognise the qualities of hair by visual inspection, feel, and special tests. Before attempting to give a relaxing treatment to overly curly hair, you must judge its texture, porosity, elasticity, and the extent, if any, of damage to the hair.

Permanent waving, pages 71–104

Your client's hair history

To help ensure consistent, satisfactory results, records should be kept of each chemical hair-relaxing treatment. These records should include the client's hair history and all products and conditioners used (see sample form on page 110). You should be sure to find out if your client has ever had hair-relaxing treatment before. If so, was there any adverse reaction? You must not chemically relax hair that has been treated with a metallic dye. To do so damages and destroys the hair. In addition, it is not advisable to use chemical relaxers on hair that has been bleached lighter.

Before starting to process the hair, you must know how the client will react to the relaxer. Therefore, the client must receive:

- a thorough scalp and hair examination
- a hair strand test.

Scalp examination

Inspect the scalp carefully for eruptions, scratches, or abrasions. To obtain a clearer view of the scalp, part the hair into 1 cm deep sections. Hair parting may be done with the first and second fingers or with the handle of a tail comb. In either case, you must exercise great care not to scratch the scalp. Such scratches may become seriously infected when aggravated by the chemicals in the relaxer (see Figure 5B.2).

If your client has scalp eruptions or abrasions, do not apply the chemical hair relaxer until the scalp is healthy. If the hair is not in a healthy condition, prescribe a series of conditioning treatments to return it to a more normal condition. Then you may give a strand test.

Strand tests

To help you estimate the results you may expect to get from chemical relaxing, it is advisable to test the hair for porosity and elasticity. This can be done using one of the following strand tests:

Finger test

A finger test determines the degree of porosity of the hair. Grasp a strand of hair and run it between the thumb and first finger of the right hand, from the end towards the scalp. If it ruffles or feels bumpy, the hair is porous and can absorb moisture.

Figure 5B.1 Relaxer record

RELAXER RECORD

Name..Tel. ....

Address ....

....

DESCRIPTION OF HAIR

Form	**Lenght**		**Texture**	**Porosity**	
☐ wavy	☐ short	☐ coarse	☐ soft	☐ very porous	☐ less porous
☐ curly	☐ medium	☐ medium	☐ silky	☐ moderately porous	☐ least porous
☐ extra-curly	☐ long	☐ fine	☐ wiry	☐ normal	☐ resistant

Condition

☐ virgin ☐ retouched ☐ dry ☐ oily ☐ lightened

Tinted with ....

Previously relaxed with (name of relaxer)..

☐ Original sample of hair enclosed ☐ not enclosed

TYPE OF RELAXER OR STRAIGHTENER

☐ whole head ☐ retouch

☐ retouch .... strength................ ☐ straightener............. strength................

Results

☐ good ☐ poor ☐ sample of relaxed hair enclosed ☐ not enclosed

Date	Operator	Date	Operator
....	....	....	....
....	....	....	....
....	....	....	....

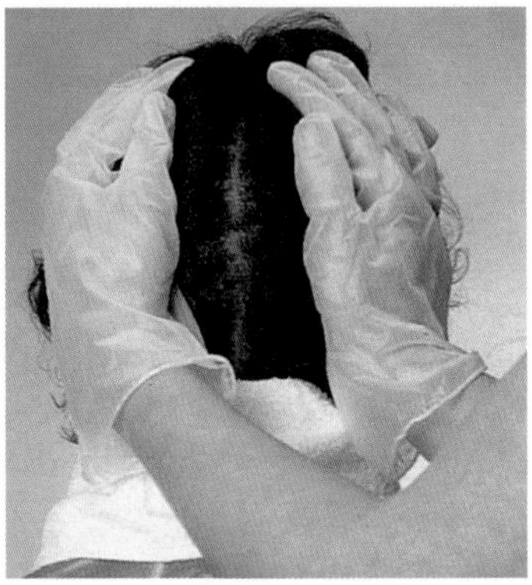

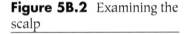

Figure 5B.2 Examining the scalp

Pull test

This test determines the degree of elasticity in the hair. Normally, dry, curly hair will stretch by about 20% of its normal length without breaking. Grasp half a dozen strands from the crown area and pull them gently. If the hair appears to stretch, it has elasticity and can withstand the relaxer. If not, conditioning treatments are recommended prior to a chemical relaxing treatment.

Relaxer test

Application of the relaxer to a hair strand will indicate the reaction of the relaxer on the hair. Take a small section of hair from the crown or another area where the hair is wiry and resistant. Pull it through a slit in a piece of aluminium foil placed as close to the scalp as possible. Apply relaxer to the strand in the same manner as you would apply it to the entire head. Process the strand until it is sufficiently relaxed, checking the strand every 3 to 5 minutes. Make careful notes of timing, the smoothing required, and the hair strength. Shampoo the relaxer from the strand only, towel dry, and cover with protective cream to avoid damage during the relaxing service. If breakage has occurred, you should do another strand test using a milder solution (see Figure 5B.3).

CHEMICAL HAIR RELAXING PROCESS (WITH SODIUM HYDROXIDE)

The procedure outlined below is based primarily on products containing sodium hydroxide. For this or any other kind of product, follow the manufacturer's directions.

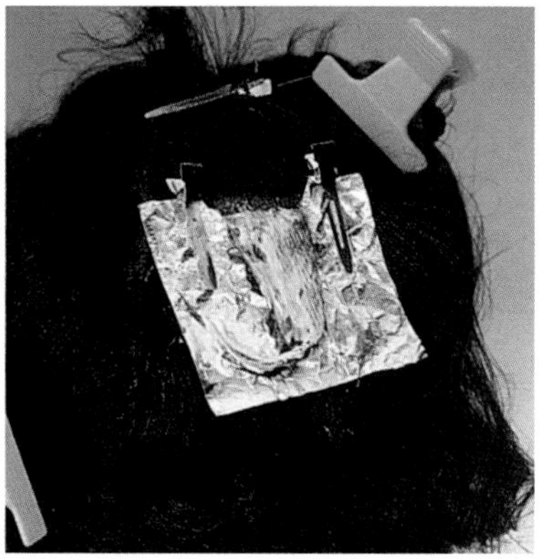

Figure 5B.3 Relaxer strand test

TABLE 5B.1 EQUIPMENT, IMPLEMENTS, AND MATERIALS		
Chemical relaxer	Protective gloves	Absorbent cotton wool
Conditioner	Neutraliser or neutralising shampoo	Towels
Rollers	Shampoo and cream rinse	Comb and brush
Spatula	Clips	End papers
Protective base	Timer	Setting lotion
Conditioner-filler	Record card	

Preparation

1. Select and arrange the required equipment, implements, and materials.
2. Wash and dry your hands.
3. Seat your client comfortably. Remove earrings and neck jewellery; adjust towel and shampoo cape.
4. Examine and evaluate the scalp and hair.
5. Give a strand test and check results.
6. Do not shampoo hair. (Hair ends may be trimmed after application of hair relaxer.)
7. Check the client's record card.

Procedure

1. Part hair into four or five sections (see Figures 5B.4 and 5B.5).
2. Dry the hair. If moisture or perspiration is present on the scalp because of excessive heat or humidity, place your client under a cool dryer for several minutes.

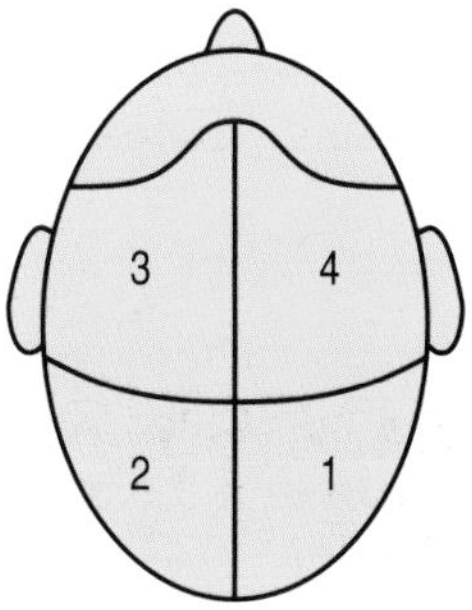

Figure 5B.4 Part hair into four sections

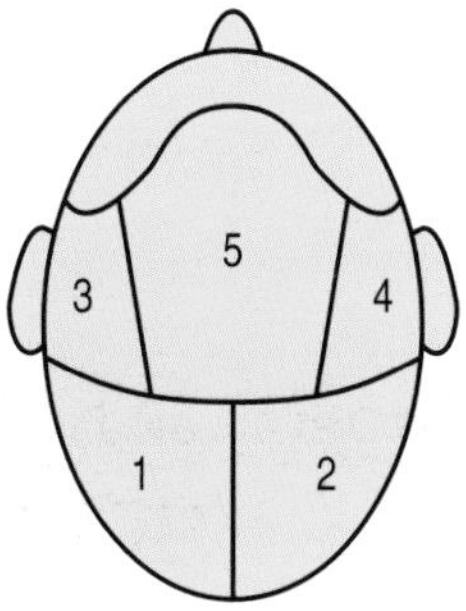

Figure 5B.5 Part hair into five sections; three sections in front area, two sections in back area

3. Apply protective base. Manufacturers recommend the use of a protective base to protect the scalp from the strong chemicals in the relaxer. To apply it properly, subdivide each of the four or five major sections into 1 to 2 cm partings, to permit thorough scalp coverage (see Figure 5B.6).

Apply the base freely to the entire scalp with your fingers. The hairline around the forehead, nape of the neck, and area over and around the ears must be completely covered. Complete coverage is important to protect the scalp and hairline from irritation.

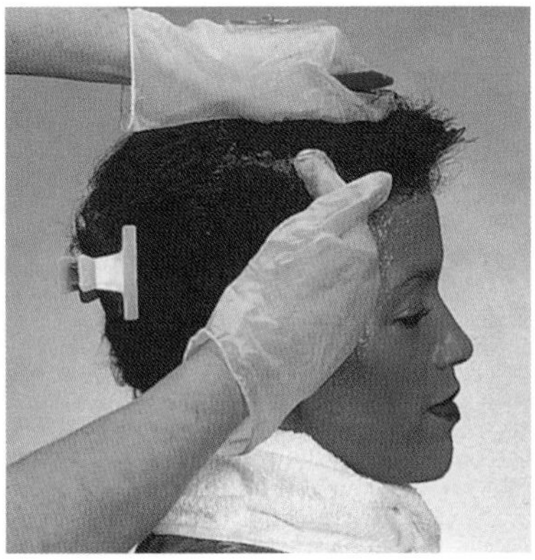

Figure 5B.6 Applying protective base

Applying the conditioner-filler

In many cases a conditioner-filler is required before the chemical relaxer can be used. The conditioner-filler, usually a protein polymer product, is applied to the entire head of hair when dry. It protects over-porous or slightly damaged hair from being over-processed on any part of the hair shaft. It evens out the porosity of the hair shaft, and permits uniform distribution and action of the chemical relaxer.

To give the full benefit of the conditioner-filler, rub it gently onto the hair from the scalp to the hair ends, using either the hands or a comb. Then towel dry the hair or use a cool dryer to completely dry the hair.

Applying the relaxer

Divide the head into four or five sections, in the same manner as for the application of the protective base.

The processing cream is applied last to the scalp area and hair ends. The body heat will speed up the processing action at the scalp. The hair is more porous at the ends and may be damaged. In both these areas, less processing time is required, and, therefore, the relaxer is applied last to these parts.

> ***TIP*** When using a 'no-base' relaxer, a protective base is not necessary. It is recommended that a protective cream be used on the hairline and around the ears.

There are three methods in general use for the application of the chemical hair relaxer: the comb method, the brush method, and the finger method.

Comb method

Remove a quantity of relaxing cream from the tub, using a spatula. Beginning in the back right section of the head, carefully part off 0.5 cm to 1 cm of hair, depending on its thickness and curliness. Apply the relaxer with the back of the comb, starting 0.5 cm to 1 cm from the scalp, and spread to within 1 cm of the hair ends. First apply the relaxer to the top side of the strand (see Figure 5B.7). Then, raise the subsection and apply the relaxer underneath. Gently lay the completed strand up, out of the way (see Figure 5B.8).

HEALTH AND SAFETY Avoid the use of heat, which will open the pores of the scalp and cause irritation or injury to the client's scalp. Protective gloves must be worn by the hairdresser to prevent damage to hands.

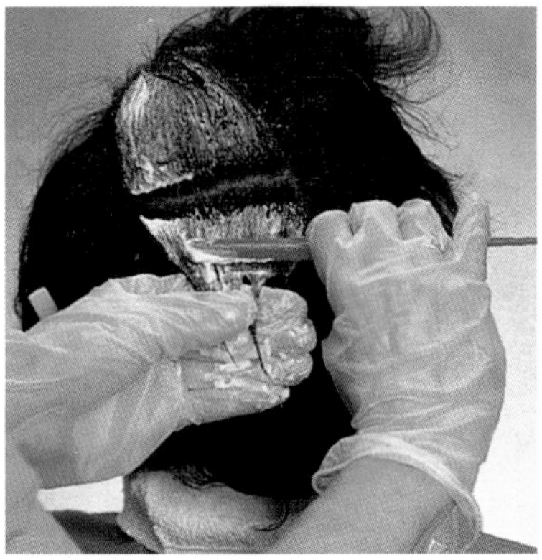

Figure 5B.7 Applying relaxer on top of strand

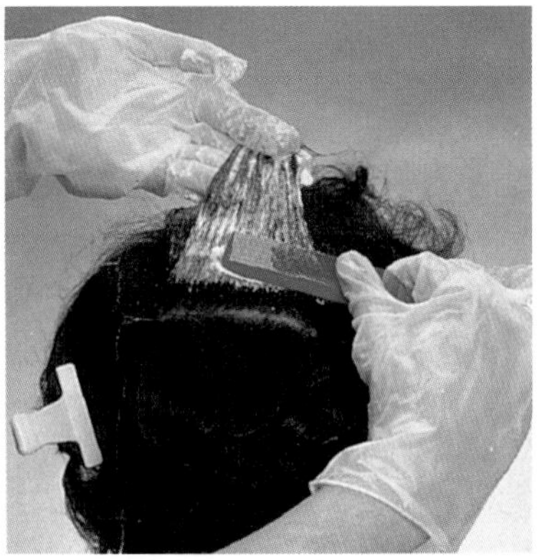

Figure 5B.8 Applying relaxer underneath strand

Complete the right back area and, moving in a clockwise direction, cover each section of the head in the same manner. Then, go back over the head in the same order, applying additional relaxing cream if necessary, and spreading the relaxer close to the scalp and up to the hair ends. Avoid excessive pressure or stretching of the hair.

Smoothing the cream through the hair not only spreads the cream, but also stretches the hair gently into a straight position.

An alternative technique is to begin application at the nape, approximately 2 cm from the hairline, and continue towards the crown. The last place to apply relaxer is at the hairline. Be guided by the manufacturer's instructions.

Brush or finger method

The brush or finger method of applying the relaxer to the hair is the same as the comb method, except that the brush or fingers and palms are used instead of the back of the comb.

HEALTH AND SAFETY Wear protective gloves.

Periodic strand testing

While spreading the relaxer, inspect its action by stretching the strands to see how fast the natural curls are being removed. Another method of testing is to press the strand to the scalp using the back of the comb or your finger. Examine the strand after your finger is removed. If it lies smoothly, the strand is sufficiently relaxed; if the strand revert or 'beads' back away from the scalp, continue processing.

Rinsing out the relaxer

When the hair has been sufficiently straightened, rinse the relaxer out rapidly and thoroughly. The water must be warm, not hot (see Figure 5B.9). If the water is too hot, it may burn the client and cause discomfort because of the very sensitive condition of the scalp. If the water is too cold, it will not stop the processing action. The direct force of the rinse water should be used to remove the relaxer and avoid tangling the hair. Part hair with fingers to make sure no traces of the relaxer remain. Unless the relaxer is completely removed, its chemical action continues on the hair. The stream of water should be directed from the scalp to the hair ends.

HEALTH AND SAFETY Do not get relaxer or rinse water into the eyes or on unprotected skin. If the relaxer or rinse water gets into the client's eyes, wash it out immediately and refer the client to a doctor without delay.

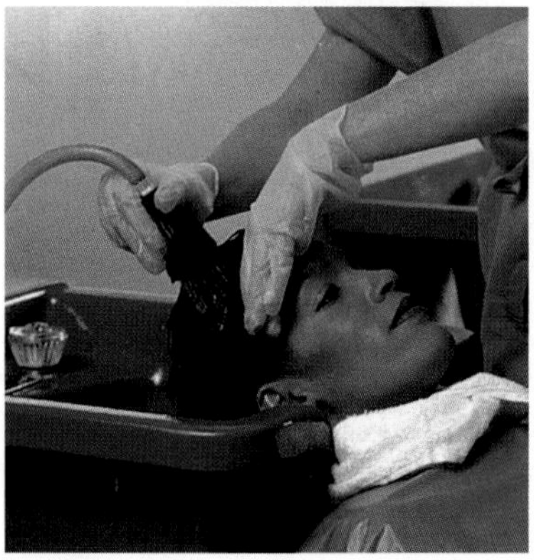

Figure 5B.9 Rinsing out relaxer

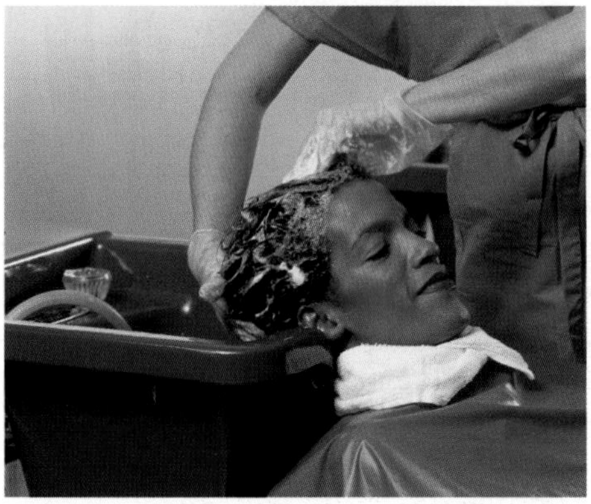

Figure 5B.10 Shampooing the hair

Shampooing/neutralising

When the hair is thoroughly rinsed, neutralise the hair as directed by the manufacturer's directions. Most manufacturers provide a neutralising shampoo that is applied to the hair after rinsing. Others prescribe the use of a non-alkaline or a cream shampoo followed by a neutraliser.

Gently work the shampoo into the hair. Use care to avoid tangling the hair or breaking any fragile ends. Manipulate the shampoo by working with the fingers underneath the hair, not on top. Rinse with warm water, making sure to keep the hair straight. Repeat the shampoo until the hair lathers well and all the relaxer is removed (see Figure 5B.10).

After shampooing, completely saturate the hair with the neutraliser if it is required by the manufacturer. Begin at the nape, and comb carefully with a wide-toothed comb, working upward towards the forehead. Use the comb to:

- keep the hair straight
- ensure complete saturation with the neutraliser
- remove any tangles without pulling.

Time the neutraliser as directed and rinse thoroughly. Towel blot gently. Condition hair as necessary and proceed with styling. Discard used materials. Clean and sterilise equipment. Wash and dry your hands. Complete the record of all timings and treatments during the service, and file the record card.

> ***NOTE*** Different products used for relaxing require different methods. Always follow the manufacturer's directions.

Applying the conditioner

Many manufacturers recommend that you apply a conditioner before setting the hair, to offset the harshness of the sodium hydroxide in the relaxer and to help some of the natural oils to the scalp and hair.

Two types of conditioners are available: cream-type and protein-type.

Cream-type conditioners

These are applied to the scalp and hair, then carefully rinsed out. The hair is then towel dried. Apply setting lotion; set the hair on rollers; dry and style the hair in the usual manner.

> ***TIP*** Because of the fragile condition of the hair, it is advisable to wind the hair on the roller without great tension.

Protein-type (liquid) conditioners

These are applied to the scalp and hair prior to hairsetting and allowed to remain in the hair to serve as a setting lotion. Set the hair on rollers, dry, and style in the usual manner.

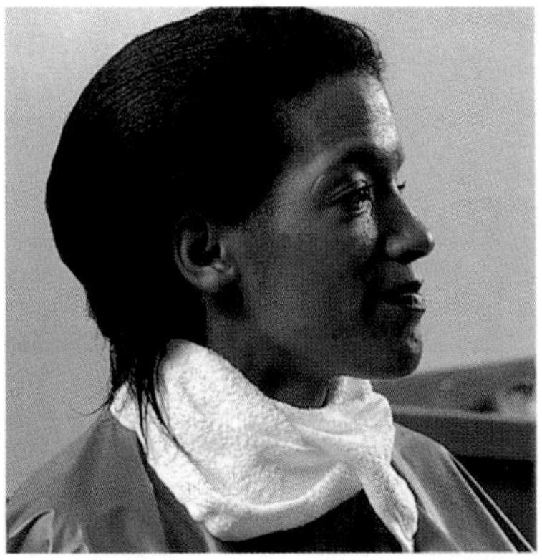

Figure 5B.11 Straightened hair

Hot thermal irons

To avoid hair breakage, excessive heat and excessive stretching should be avoided. Thermal curling with warm heat can be used to curl chemically relaxed hair. Conditioning treatments should be recommended and the hair dried completely before thermal curling.

> ***WHAT THE EXPERT SAYS*** Relaxing services are regular on-going processes that form a large proportion of the chemical work carried out on clients with over curly and/or Afro-Caribbean style hair. It is the essential skill of the hairstylist who wants to work on this type of hair.
>
> Due to the high alkalinity of the chemicals used in the process it is essential that the hairstylist is fully conversant with the process and observes the safety precautions.

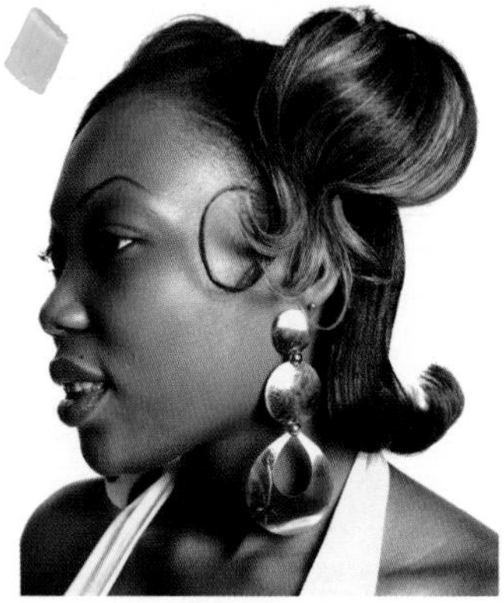

Figure 5B.12 Straightened fashion look

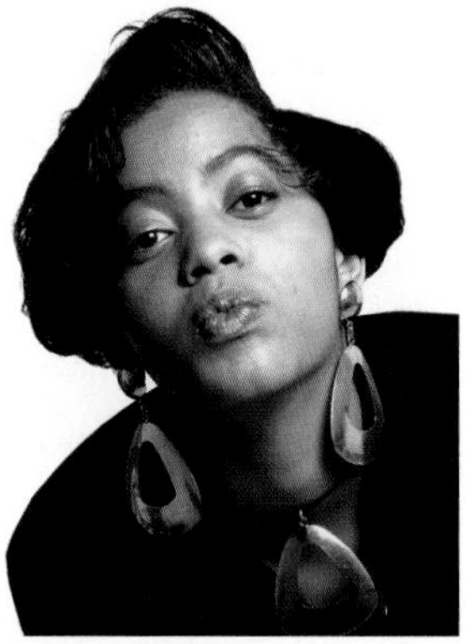

Figure 5B.13 Afro-Caribbean styling

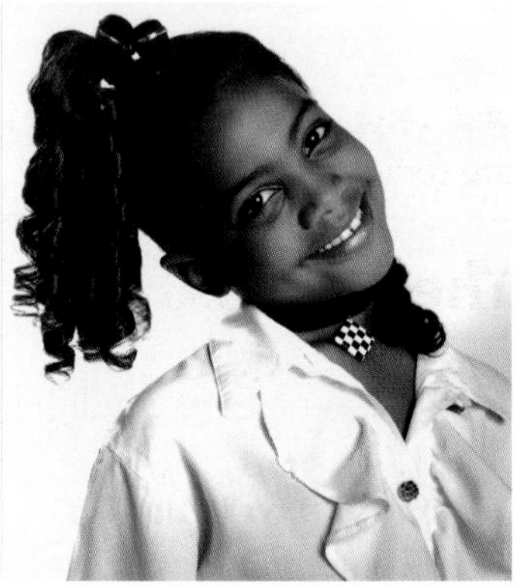

Figure 5B.14 Afro-Caribbean styling

HEALTH AND SAFETY

Always follow the manufacturer's instructions.

If you are unaware of how to proceed with the relaxing process ask your trainer/supervisor for guidance.

The Control of Substances Hazardous to Health Regulations 1988 requires your employer to arrange that all staff are informed, instructed and trained in the safe use of chemicals. You as an employee have responsibility, via the Health and Safety at Work Act, to comply with your employers' reasonable requirements in pursuance of the Act.

SODIUM HYDROXIDE RETOUCH

Hair grows about 0.5 to 1.25 cm per month. A retouch should probably be done every 6 weeks to 2 months, depending on how quickly your client's hair grows.

Follow all the steps for a regular chemical hair relaxing treatment, with one exception: apply the relaxer only to the new growth. In order to prevent previously treated hair from breaking, apply a cream conditioner over the hair that received the earlier treatment, thus avoiding overlapping and damage.

TWO-STEP PERMING

In order to produce a controlled curl on tight, curly hair the natural curl must first be relaxed and then the new curl pattern introduced onto this straightened hair. This process is known as two-step perming or curl rearrangement.

A solution (curl re-arranger) containing ammonium thioglycolate is applied to the tight curly hair. The hair is relaxed to a straight curl pattern. This solution is then rinsed from the hair.

A milder solution of ammonium thioglycolate is applied and the hair is wound onto large perm rods and processed, often under a pre-heated dryer. Once processed the hair is rinsed with water.

A neutraliser, usually containing sodium bromate (which will not lighten the hair in the way that a hydrogen peroxide based neutraliser can), is applied, processed and then the curlers are removed and the hair conditioned.

The method of perming

TIP Always read and follow the manufacturer's directions. These may vary slightly between manufacturers.

1. Only shampoo the hair if it is heavily oiled, as oil may create a barrier. If shampooing is required, do not use hot water or stimulate the scalp by rubbing. It is better if the hair is shampooed a few days earlier (see Figure 5B.15).
2. Hair that is fragile due to heat or chemical treatment should be treated with a protective polymer pre-treatment (conditioner/filler). This provides a protective coating of polymer to the hair This is usually dried onto the hair.
3. Apply protective cream to the complete hairline and divide the hair into four. Apply the re-arranger to small sections, to within 0.5 cm of the scalp, starting at the most resistant areas of the head (see Figure 5B.16).

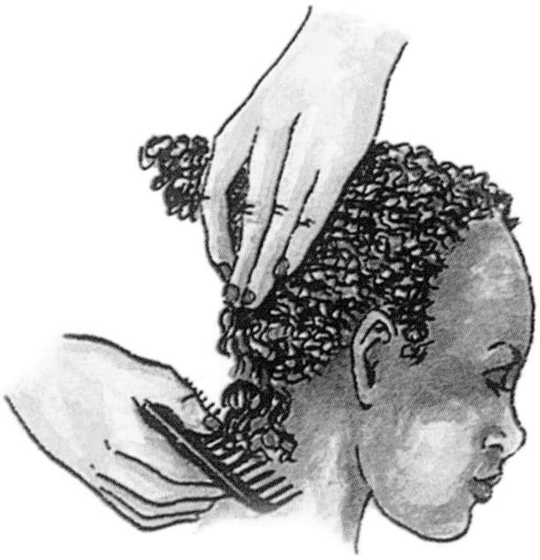

Figure 5B.15 Remove tangles from hair

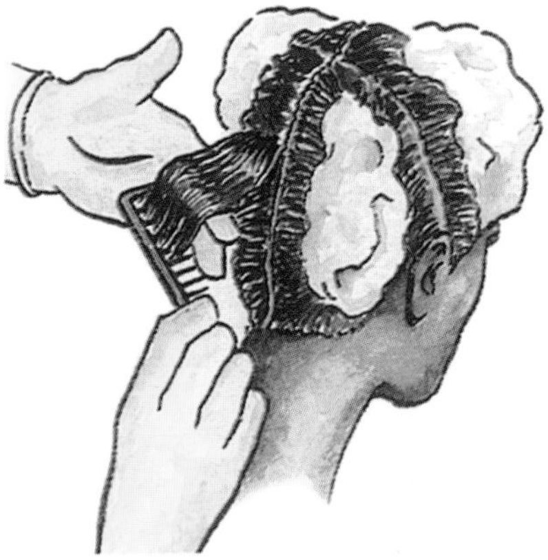

Figure 5B.16 Part hair into sections and coat with thiogel

4. Once the application is complete, cover with a plastic cap and a towel. Do not allow the product to dry out. Follow the manufacturer's guidance for timing. Process until the hair is straight, and take care not to over-process as this may result in hair breakage.
5. The re-arranger is then rinsed from the hair, taking care not to tangle the hair.
6. Section the hair, taking care as the hair will be fragile. The hair may be wound following the orthodox nine-section pattern or by brick winding.

TIP Hair that has already been relaxed should not be given a curly perm.

Permanent waving, pages 71–104

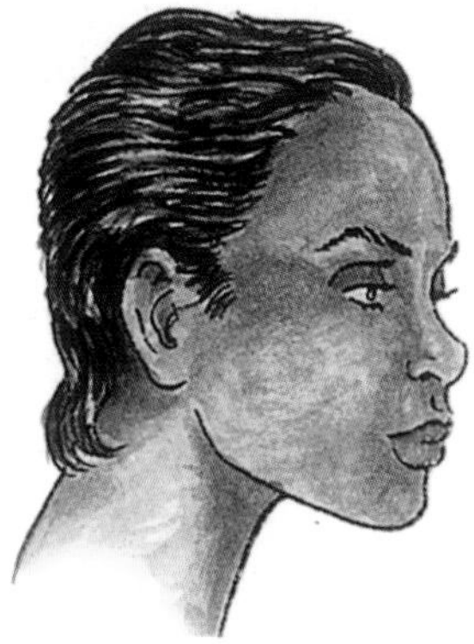

Figure 5B.17 Comb re-arranger from hair

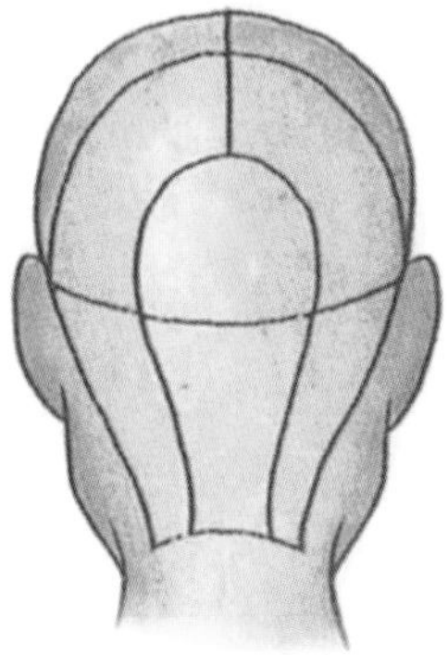

Figure 5B.18 Divide the hair into eight sections

7. Perm curler sections should be half the depth of the perm rods. The sections of hair should be overdirected, that is combed up and away from the direction of the wind. This will ensure controlled curl as close to the scalp as possible (see Figure 5B.18).
8. Wind evenly, without tension, using the width of the curler. The ends are protected using end tissues; fragile hair should be protected (see Figure 5B.19).
9. Protect your client by placing barrier cream around the hairline followed with a moist cotton wool strip. Then using the applicator, apply the curl booster, ensuring complete coverage of the wound hair (see Figure 5B.20).
10. Cover the head with a plastic cap and process under a pre-heated dryer, following the manufacturer's guidance for timing (see Figure 5B.21).

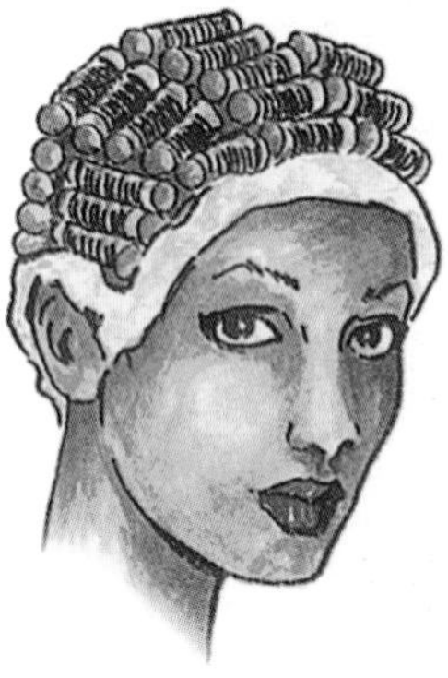

Figure 5B.19 Protect client's skin with cotton wool around hairline

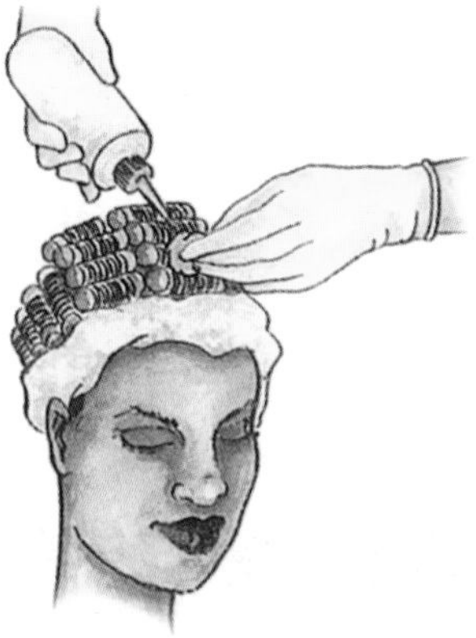

Figure 5B.20 Apply the gel to curls

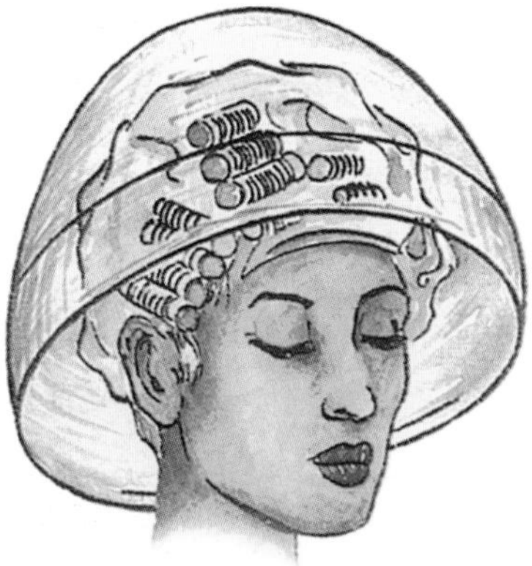

Figure 5B.21 Process under pre-heated drier

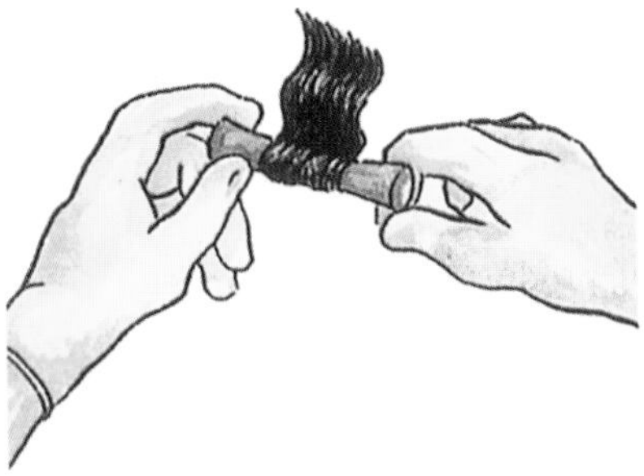

Figure 5B.22 Test a curl

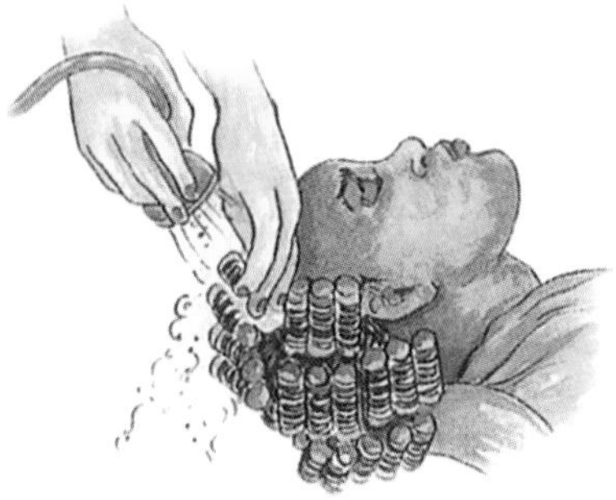

Figure 5B.23 Rinse the hair

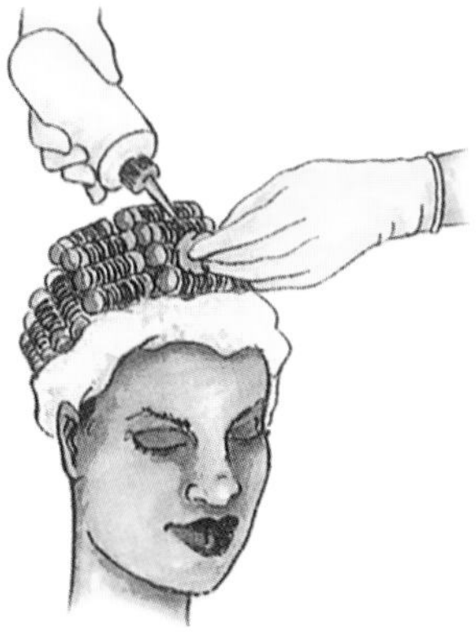

Figure 5B.24 Apply neutralizer

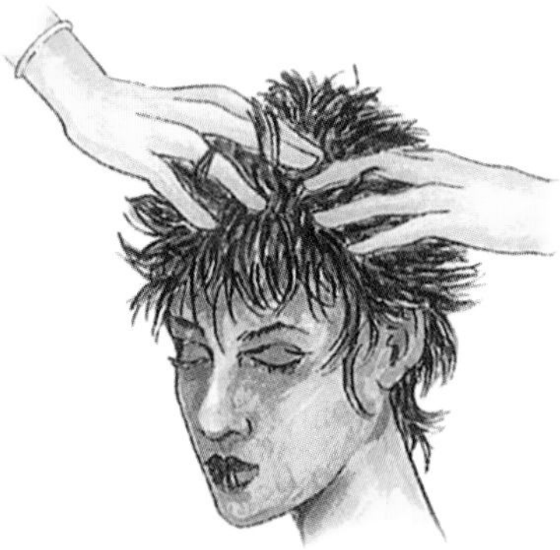

Figure 5B.25 Work neutralizer through hair

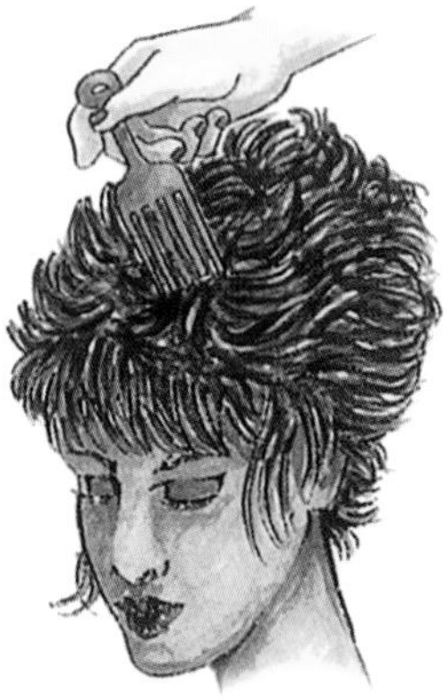

Figure 5B.26 Style hair

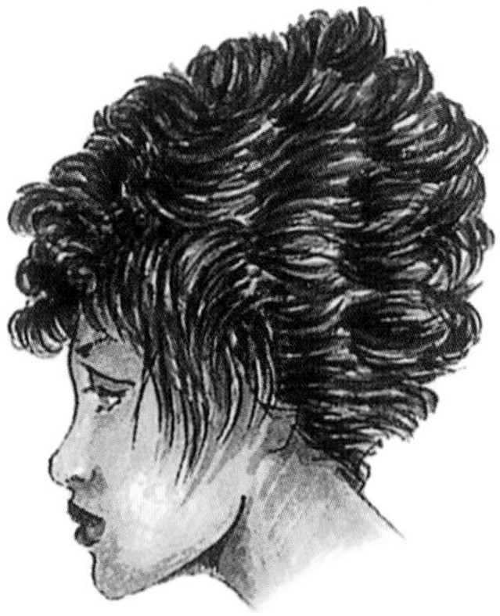

Figure 5B.27 Finished

11. Check the processing, taking samples from various areas of the head. Gently unwind the curler for half of its length and gently push the hair towards the scalp. A full 'S' shape indicates full development (see Figure 5B.22).
12. Once the hair is fully processed, rinse the wound curlers with tepid water, to remove the curl booster from the hair (see Figure 5B.23).
13. Blot the wound curlers, thoroughly.
14. Re-apply barrier cream and moist cotton wool to the client's hairline and then apply the neutraliser (see Figure 5B.24 and Figure 5B.25).
15. Rinse the neutraliser, thoroughly, from the hair, blot dry and then remove the perm rods, gently and without any tension.
16. Condition the hair, thoroughly. This should be followed by the application of a scalp conditioner to compensate for the drying effect.
17. The hair may now be styled (see Figure 5B.26 and Figure 5B.27).

TWO-STEP PERM RETOUCH

The main difference between the two-step perm and the two-step perm retouch is that the curl rearranger is applied only to the regrowth area. The protective polymer lotion will protect the previously treated hair when the curl booster is applied.

After-care

It should be remembered that the chemical processes described within this chapter cause damage to the hair, causing it to become dry and brittle. Excessive or incorrect use of strong chemicals on the hair can result in severe hair breakage.

Following straightening processes clients should be informed of how best to care for their hair. This becomes an opportunity to guide your client in the selection and purchase of suitable products to moisturise their hair. There are shampoos that will replace the oils lost and moisturise the hair, preventing further damage from atmospheric conditions. Deep penetrating conditioners, usually containing protein, should be recommended for use.

Styling lotions should be suggested to suit the method of styling, as well as setting lotions which contain protein and will strengthen the hair. For curly looks, curl activators may be used to maintain the level of moisture and oil in the hair.

FURTHER STUDY

- Look on the packages of straightening products to see the range of product strengths available for use in the salon and at home.
- Manufacturer's directions for use vary; look at a range of instruction leaflets to see the range of variations.
- Find out the range of after-care products available for the care of hair that has been straightened and relaxed.

REVIEW QUESTIONS

1. Name two chemicals often used in chemical hair relaxing products.
2. What does the term 'base' mean in relation to hair relaxation processes?
3. How may the client's hairline and face be protected during these chemical processes?
4. What are the three main stages of the chemical hair relaxation process?
5. What is a strand test used for?
6. How should hairdressers protect themselves when working with relaxing/straightening substances?
7. How close to the scalp should straightener products be applied?
8. What are the main stages of a two-step perm?
9. What is meant by 'over-directing' when curler winding?
10. What tension should be used when winding hair during a 'two-step perm'?

CHAPTER 6

Hair colouring

This chapter will give you the essential knowledge necessary for you to understand the hair colouring process. It will guide you in hair colour and product selection as well as in the application techniques available to the professional hair colourist and their suitability.

Level 1	
Unit 101	
Element 101.1	Maintain effective and safe methods of working when shampooing, conditioning and drying hair
Element 101.2	Shampoo and surface condition hair
Unit 102	
Element 102A.3 + 102B.3	Add temporary colour to hair
Element 102A.4 + 102B.4	Remove colouring and lightening products from hair
Unit 104	
Element 104.1	Develop effective working relationships with clients
Element 104.2	Develop effective working relationships with colleagues
Element 104.3	Develop self within the job role
Unit 105	
Element 105.2	Support health and safety at work

Level 2	
Unit 201	
Element 201.1	Consult with and maintain effective relationships with clients
Element 201.2	Advise clients on salon products and services
Element 201.3	Advise clients on after-care procedures
Unit 202	
Element 202.1	Maintain effective and safe methods of working when shampooing and conditioning hair
Element 202.2	Shampooing hair and scalp
Element 202.3	Condition hair and scalp
Unit 206	
Element 206.1	Maintain effective and safe methods of working when colouring hair
Element 206.2	Add colour to hair
Element 206.3	Permanently change hair colour
Element 206.4	Create highlight and lowlight effects in hair
Unit 208	
Element 208.1	Develop and maintain effective team work and relationships with colleagues
Element 208.2	Develop and improve personal effectiveness within the job role
Unit 209	
Element 209.2	Support health, safety and security at work

Contents

INTRODUCTION

Hairdressing is a career that offers you opportunities to develop your creative talents in many different ways. One of the most exciting and challenging areas of creativity in your career as a professional hair stylist will be colouring and lightening hair.

Hair colouring includes the processes of:

- adding artificial pigment to the natural hair colour
- adding artificial pigment to previously coloured hair
- adding artificial pigment to pre-lightened hair
- lightening natural pigment and adding artificial pigment in one step.

(The terms 'tinting' and 'colouring' are used interchangeably in this text.)

Hair lightening involves the diffusing of the natural pigment or artificial colour from the hair. Hair lightening involves the process of:

- lightening the natural pigment to prepare the hair for the final colour (pre-lightening)
- lightening the natural or artificial pigment to the desired colour (lightening)
- lightening the natural or artificial pigment for corrective colouring
- lightening the natural or artificial pigment in selected areas (highlighting).

WHAT THE EXPERT SAYS Hair colouring is one of those professional services that separate the enthusiastic amateur from the skilled professional. Hair colour products are increasingly available to the consumer via the high street retail outlets, but the vital ingredient of professional advice and technical service can only come from the experienced and skilled hairdresser. As a professional hairdresser you must capitalise on this skill. The chemical services are profitable sources of salon income and colouring represents repeat business. The client who has tinted or lightened hair usually returns for retouching at regular intervals. Satisfactory service and trust in their colourist encourage clients to remain loyal to the same salon and will in all probability mean that they use additional services that the salon offers.

Your success as a colourist depends only on the time and energy you are prepared to give to the continuous study and practice of your hair colouring skills. As you expand your skills and gain confidence, you may choose to specialise in hair colouring services, similar to medical professionals who practise in and develop one area of expertise. Colourists have a major role to play in the success of any hairdressing business. Their skill and expertise will enhance the work of the hair stylist and satisfy the client's need. There is the potential for the skilled colourist to establish a reputation for their own skills in guiding the client towards the most suitable colour choice and in using the most appropriate technique to apply the colouration to the hair. Colourists have the opportunity to develop their own formulations and techniques, using the product manufacturer's guidance and their own skill and experience to vary techniques to produce bespoke colouring for their clients.

The styling revolution

Thanks to the styling revolution in the 1960s and 1970s, there are many stylists who have mastered hair cutting or perming, and concentrate their energies solely on these frequently requested services. Add colour to a great haircut and perfect texture, and you have a powerful attention-getting combination. Specialist hair colourists are less numerous than cutters, and their skills are in increasingly high demand due to renewed publicity and popularity.

Keeping up to date

Colouring manufacturers are always willing to promote and inform the professional about their products. Use this facility to develop your skill and to maintain the currency of your product knowledge and your application technique skills. Manufacturers are generally very keen to inform and update the hairdresser.

Help and advice

Most hair colouring manufacturers have a telephone help line to offer professional advice and guidance in the use of their products. Should you experience problems in the use of their products make use of this facility.

As a professional hair colourist you should ensure that you constantly update your skills and make yourself aware of what is available so that you can advise both the business and your clientele of the most recent developments and technology.

HAIR COLOUR CONSULTATION

As with all facets of the hairdresser's role, consultation with the client is of crucial importance.

TIP Hair stylists willing to develop their colouring skills and expertise can serve the needs of a huge and growing market.

Reasons clients colour their hair

There are five main reasons why clients wish to colour their hair: to boost self-image, to keep up to date with fashion, for artistic reasons, in reaction to greying and to correct faults in their current colour. These may be sub-divided as follows.

Self-image boost

- To alleviate boredom or depression.
- To promote a more professional appearance.

Fashion

- To subtly enhance their existing hair colour.
- To create a fashion statement or follow a trend which expresses their personality.

Artistic

- To accentuate their hairstyle design, making it look more finished.
- To enhance or minimise their features, using colour to create illusions.

Greying

- To conceal premature greying.
- To keep and enhance their natural white or grey and eliminate yellow.

Corrective

- To eliminate the damaged look of sun-lightened hair ends.
- To remove the unsightly cast of chlorine or minerals caused by their water.
- To improve upon the results of previous colour experimentation.

Almost everyone at one time or another has considered doing something a little different with their hair. Our potential clients may have already done some experimentation at home or in another salon by changing their haircut or style, their hair texture by perming, or their hair's natural colour.

With the emergence and availability of non-professional products that your clients can purchase, why should they come to you, a professional colourist, for advice and service? And who are the 'typical' hair colouring clients today? (see Figure 6.1).

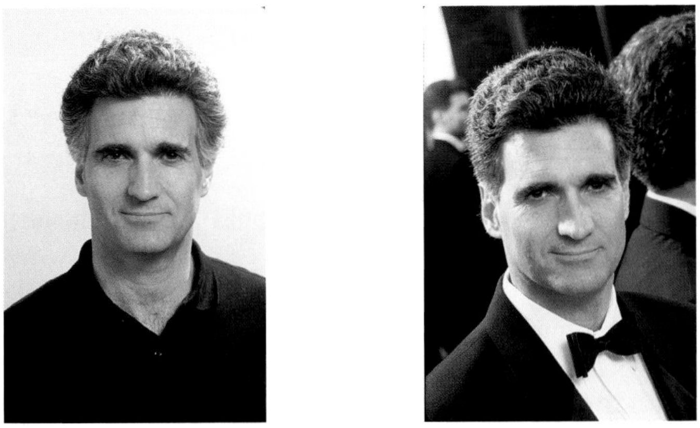

Figure 6.1 There are many reasons clients choose to colour their hair. To cover grey is one

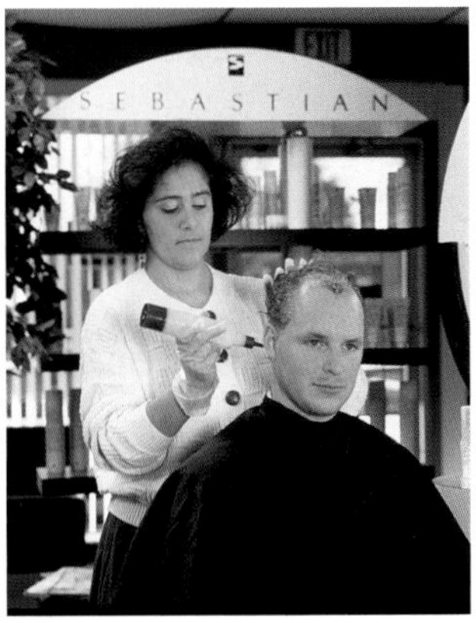

Figure 6.2 Hair colouring is a popular service for the male clientele today

Typical clients

Hair colouring offers a wide variety of choices and therefore attracts the attention and interest of anyone who wants to look good and feel better. Gone are the stereotypes of the obviously tinted client – the damaged hair, the flat or unnatural appearance. Typical clients may want to cover or enhance their grey; they may be teenagers, women, and men who enjoy frequent fashion changes; they are often clients currently unhappy with their natural colour or who want to improve the shine and texture of their hair; they may be current hair colouring clients who come in for their retouch applications and a little relaxation time to themselves. Even the male clientele for hair colour is growing rapidly and is expected to be the fastest growing category of hair colouring client this decade (see Figure 6.2).

As a trained professional hair colourist, you will have access to professional-only products that far surpass those your clients may purchase; in selection, performance, and stability. You will know the colour that will look best on your clients, which products and application techniques will best achieve the desired look, how to choose these products and customise them to fit hair conditions at different times of year, and how hair colouring and lightening products will react on clients' hair. The key to your success in hair colouring is communication.

With continuously developing technology and the latest advancements in hair colour education, hair colouring manufacturers are moving to standardise terminology in order to simplify learning and provide greater assistance to colourists.

The colourist's role in client communication

Observe

Simple observation gives you a chance to use your training and analyse client's needs. Your eyes are your primary information-gathering tools. The following is a list of factors about hair that influence colour choice. With time and practice, you will notice certain physical characteristics relevant to hair colour selection when you first see a client. These are items you will need to note when observing clients prior to hair colouring service:

- colour level
- colour tone
- eye colour
- skin tone
- length
- porosity
- density
- texture
- shape
- percentage of grey.

Each of these will be described in detail as we go through a typical hair colour consultation.

The consultation is a time when your greeting and appearance should be at their most impressive. The greeting establishes your credibility and trustworthiness.

You only have one chance to make a first impression on your clients, so make it a good one. You alone are responsible for the image you project. Make sure your clients and potential clients see you as you want them to. Establish and maintain eye contact, make clients comfortable, and listen.

> ***TIP*** Your professional appearance, confident manner and use of professional industry terminology will establish you as an authority in your client's eyes.

Listen

Listening allows you to find out how clients view their needs. The finest formulation combined with the most talented application will still result in colour failure if clients are dissatisfied.

Despite all the activity in a busy salon, your client's thoughts are centred mainly on their own concerns. So, naturally, all clients expect to be treated with courtesy and attention. The hair stylist who recognises this fact and gives clients respect, courtesy, and attention will win their confidence. And, when this hair stylist sincerely recommends a hair colour service, clients are likely to listen carefully and seriously consider the recommendation.

Make suggestions

To recommend a hair colour service with sincerity means to suggest a colour only when you honestly believe that your client would be happier and more attractive with the colour service. You must be attentive to your clients' needs by listening closely, by being genuinely interested, and by treating every client as you would like to be treated yourself in the same situation. In doing so, you can be confident that your choice will reflect and meet any client's needs, improve your client's appearance, and enhance your reputation as a colourist (see Figure 6.3).

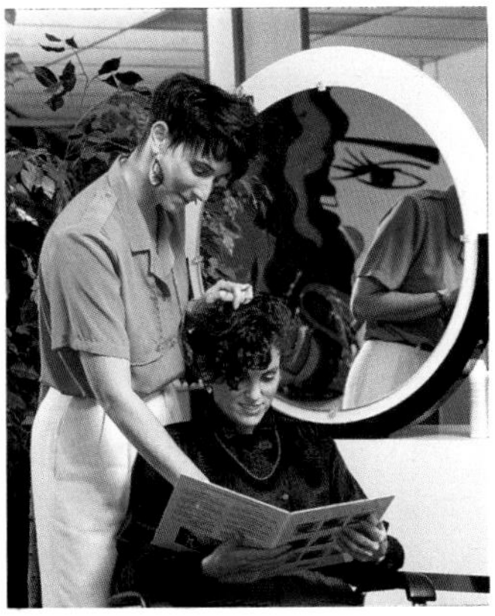

Figure 6.3 Good communication is essential when discussing a hair colouring service with a client

Explain time and monetary investment involved

At the completion of your consultation, you should have an agreement with your client as to what is needed, how long it will take, and how much it will cost.

Determine a solution to fulfil the client's needs

Hair colouring is a wonderful service, and can make a tremendous difference to your client. Whether you choose a subtle change or something quite dramatic, the opportunity to create is greatly enhanced by being able to offer a hair colour service.

In the following pages, you will learn how to analyse your client's needs and choose and perform a hair colour service. There are many choices and considerations. Hair colouring is an art, something to be learned over time, not simply by reading books. The people who walk into your salon to become your clients bring not only their hair, but their likes and dislikes, their hopes and dreams – a whole wealth of experiences in which you can share. Take your time, look carefully, listen well, and offer the gift of your art.

Hair colour consultation: the environment

The consultation is one of the most important steps in the hair colouring service. But first there are other important elements to consider that will allow you to 'set the stage' for your consultation success.

Setting the stage: the proper environment

Adequate lighting

Light, and how it plays with hair colour, is of prime importance to the hair colourist. Bright natural light makes hair colour appear different than does dim light. Electric lights of varying intensities and hues also alter the eye's perception of colour.

Perform the consultation in a well-lit room, preferably with natural lighting. If this is not possible, arrange the lighting so that there is incandescent light in front of the client (around the mirrors) and fluorescent behind the colourist (ceiling fixtures).

Incandescent lighting alone will make the hair and skin tones appear warmer than they truly are; fluorescent lighting alone has a cool cast and will give the skin and hair a pale and unnatural 'grey' appearance. Always remember to consider the lighting in which your clients will see themselves; a beautifully subtle highlight in natural sunlight may disappear under office lighting. Conversely, a strong, attractive colour in your salon lighting could become neon-looking in the sunlight.

The best mix of lighting for hair colour is to use full-spectrum white fluorescent tubes, or consider adding track lighting spot lights (incandescent) to existing fluorescent lighting in most buildings.

Colour of consultation area

Privacy and good lighting are important. Ideally, a separate room (or area) in the salon should be reserved specifically for consultations. If possible, the walls should be white or neutral, and neutral gowning should be used to conceal your client's street clothes, especially if they are strong colours that may influence your perception of the clients' hair and skin tonality.

Gathering and using colour consultation tools

In your consultation room or area, you will keep all of your professional hair colouring consultation tools – items that will make communication with your clients go smoothly. Keep a hair colour portfolio of your work or magazines and picture books with different hair colouring levels, tones, intensities, and application techniques, so clients can show you the general hair colour they have in mind. Ink colours on the page will not exactly match coloured pigments in hair, but if you tell your clients this you will both still be able to use these tools as a guide to understanding the desired colour.

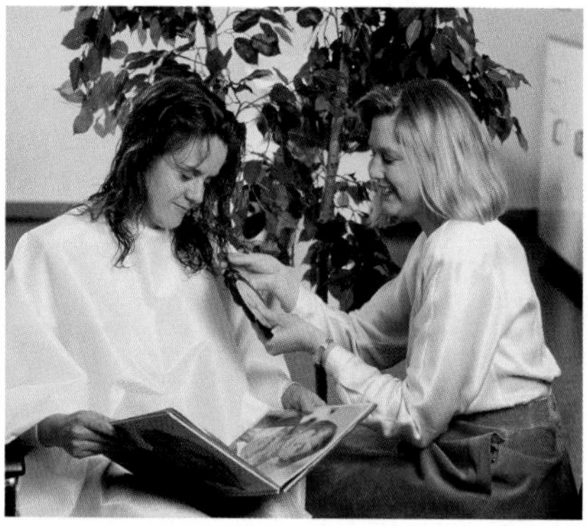

Figure 6.4 Hair colourist

Manufacturers' paper colour charts and hair colour swatches, although showing colour on white paper or on white hair, will at least give you an idea of the client's wishes. After all, your idea of red and a client's idea of red may be different – as different as strawberry blonde and burgundy. Manufacturers also make available to colourists their natural colour swatches, to help you judge the natural hair colour depth or level based on their colour product's system (see Figure 6.4). These are usually part of the product shade chart.

A client record card (see Figure 6.5) will be necessary to transfer your hair analysis, testing, and consultation information into a permanent file, whether paper based or computerised. You will also want to gather together your materials for strand and predisposition tests, which will be performed prior to each service in this chapter.

> ***TIP*** Computerised multi-media style selection systems may be used to illustrate to your client the effects of differing hair colour upon their hairstyle.

<table>
<tr><td colspan="2">Mr/Mrs/Ms
Surname

First names</td><td colspan="3">Address

Post Code
Tel. no.</td></tr>
<tr><td colspan="2">Date of skin test</td><td colspan="3">Result Hair type/colour/%grey</td></tr>
<tr><td>Date</td><td>Product</td><td>Oxidant</td><td>Notes</td><td>Cost</td></tr>
<tr><td></td><td></td><td></td><td></td><td></td></tr>
<tr><td></td><td></td><td></td><td></td><td></td></tr>
<tr><td></td><td></td><td></td><td></td><td></td></tr>
<tr><td></td><td></td><td></td><td></td><td></td></tr>
</table>

Figure 6.5 Client record card

Pre-colour testing

Strand test to confirm colour selection

Before applying a tint, conduct a preliminary strand test to confirm your selection. You will learn the following information:

- whether the proper colour selection was made
- timing needed to achieve the desired results
- whether further preconditioning treatments are needed
- whether it is necessary to apply a filler (pre-pigmentation).

Strand test procedure

1. Mix a small amount of the colour, intended for use, with peroxide according to the manufacturer's directions, using plastic measuring spoons to ensure accuracy of proportions (see Figure 6.6).
2. Apply mixture to a 0.125 cm section of hair, usually in the crown area of the head. (Remember to test each area where the hair colour varies. More than one formula may be necessary to achieve even results.)
3. Separate the strand from the rest of the hair using foil or plastic film. Process with or without heat according to the manufacturer's directions, keeping careful records of timing on the client's record card (see Figure 6.7).
4. Rinse the strand, shampoo, towel dry, and examine results (see Figure 6.8). Adjust the formula, timing, or preconditioning as necessary and proceed with tinting on the entire head.

> ***TIP*** It is important that the hair has received all pre-treatments necessary according to your analysis before the strand test is given, so that results will be accurate.

5. If results are unsatisfactory, adjust the formula and repeat the process on a new test strand.

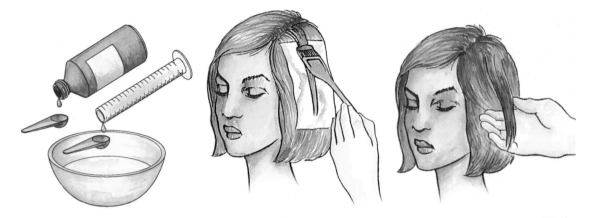

Figure 6.6 Mix colour with peroxide

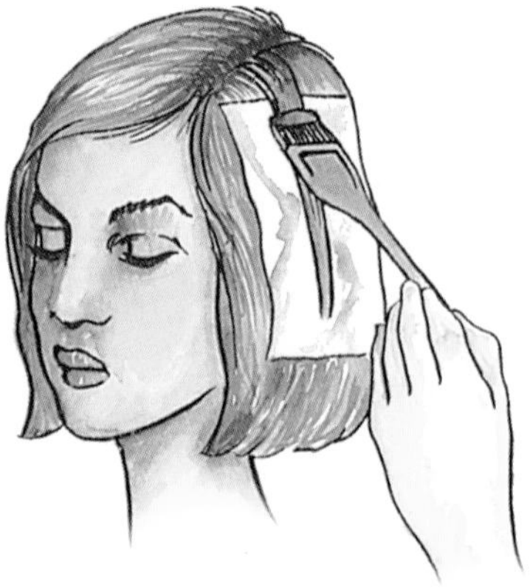

Figure 6.7 Apply mixture to strand

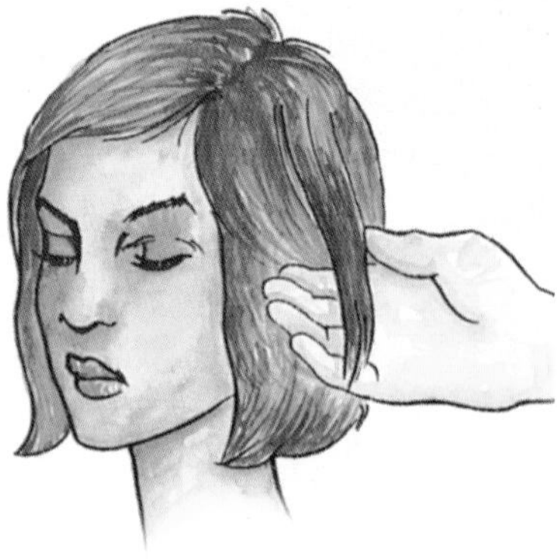

Figure 6.8 Examine results

Predisposition test to check for client sensitivity (skin test)

> ***HEALTH AND SAFETY*** A predisposition test must be given before colouring the hair with an aniline derivative product. Operator dermatitis, although rare, involves the same types of reactions as the client can experience. Since the colourist's hands are in water and contact chemical solutions repeatedly throughout an average day, it is important to take proper precautions. You should protect yourself from allergic reactions by wearing protective gloves until the product is completely removed from the client's hair.

Allergy to aniline derivative tints is unpredictable. Some clients may be sensitive, and others may develop a sensitivity after years of use. To identify an allergic client, a patch, or predisposition test should be given24 to 48 hours prior to each application of an aniline tint or toner. The tint used for the skin test must be the same formula as that used for the hair colouring service.

Predisposition test procedure

1. Select the test area – behind one ear extending into the hairline or at the inside bend of the elbow (near a pulse point).
2. Using a mild unperfumed soap, cleanse an area about the size of a one pence piece (see Figure 6.9).
3. Dry the area.
4. Prepare the test solution according to the manufacturer's directions (see Figure 6.10).
5. Apply to test area with a sterile cotton wool bud or the end of a clean tint brush. Tell your client what to do should a reaction occur. Your client should remove the patch test and, should the symptoms continue, should consult their medical practitioner. They should also inform you of this occurrence.
6. Leave the area undisturbed for 24 to 48 hours.
7. Examine the test area.
8. Note the results on the client's record card.

A *negative* skin reaction will show no sign of inflammation or skin irritation, and colour may safely be applied. If the skin test is *positive*, you will see any or a number of the following: redness, swelling, burning, itching, or blisters. A client with these symptoms is allergic, and

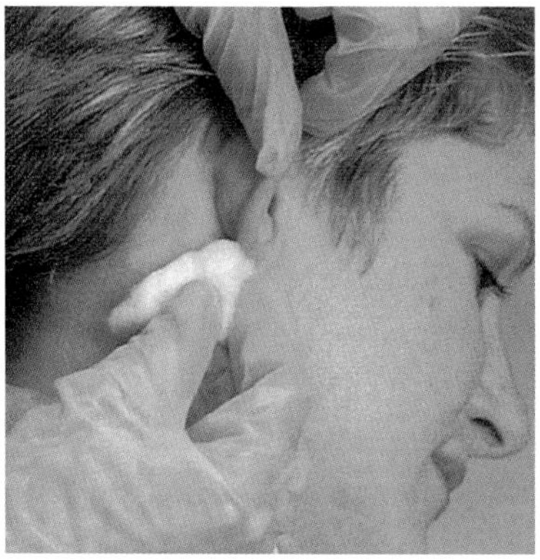

Figure 6.9 Clean patch test area

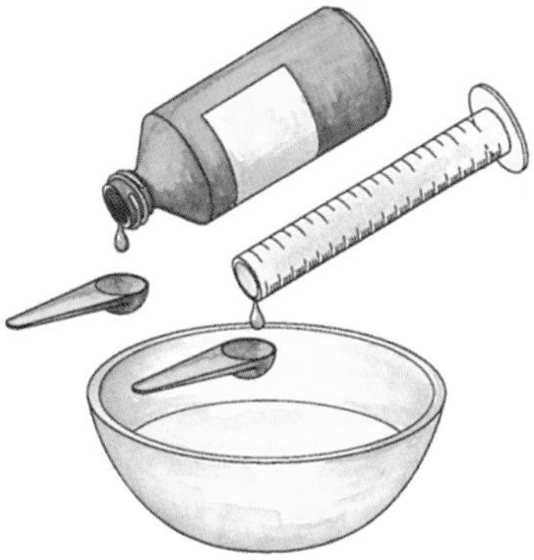

Figure 6.10 Mix tint and peroxide

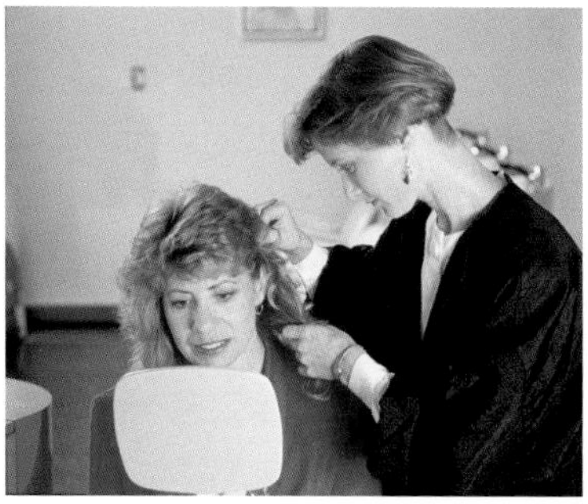

Figure 6.11 Analysing a client's hair physiology

should under no circumstance receive the colour service for which the test was performed. Application in this instance could result in a serious allergic reaction for the client, and a professional negligence claim for the hair colourist.

The skin test is also known as an allergy test, a patch test, a predisposition test or a Sabouraud-Rousseau test.

Client record card

Always record the consultation on the client's record card. It is important to keep an accurate record so that successful services can be repeated and any difficulties encountered in one service may be avoided in the next. A complete record should be kept, containing all analysis notes, strand test and whole head results, processing, timings, costs, and suggestions for the next service.

Analysing the client's hair physiology

No two people are exactly alike, and no two heads of hair are exactly the same. Even an individual client's hair will vary from season to season and from year to year. Every person has a natural hair colour that is either a dark, medium, or light colour, but no two people have exactly the same hair colour. Inside the hair shaft, where you cannot see, the factors that create or affect hair colour are always different from person to person. That is why the same hair colouring formula and procedure will produce a different result for every client (see Figure 6.11).

How hair structure relates to colouring

The hair is a remarkable and resilient fibre. Every hair colour service will affect or be affected by the structure of the hair. Some hair colour products cause a dramatic change in the hair's structure; others affect it very little. When a product significantly changes the hair structure, it usually creates a weaker strand of hair.

Knowing how products affect the structure will allow you to make choices. Your perceptions of what the hair can or cannot tolerate will allow you to be the best judge of what is most appropriate for each client.

Generally every hair on a person's head is composed of three parts: the *cuticle*, the *cortex*, and the *medulla*. The medulla is at the innermost layer, centre, of the hair shaft. The cuticle is the outermost layer of the hair. It is made up of overlapping bands of keratinised protein that is very similar to the protein that makes up our fingernails. It is translucent, allowing diffused light to pass through. The cuticle protects the interior cortex layer of the hair. The shiny appearance of the hair depends on this cuticle layer being smooth and intact. A healthy cuticle contributes 20% to the overall strength of the hair.

The cortex is the second layer of the hair. The natural colour we see in the hair is within this layer. The cortex structure is made up of elongated, fibrous cells bundled together. Melanin pigment granules are scattered between the cortex cells. These granules are embedded in the cortex layer like chips in a chocolate chip biscuit. The strength and elasticity of the hair depend on the cortex layer being intact. A healthy cortex contributes 80% to the overall strength of the hair.

Hair texture is described as the diameter of the individual hair strand. The terms coarse, medium, and fine are used to differentiate between large, medium, and small diameters. Texture has an effect on hair colour because the hair's natural melanin pigment is distributed differently in the different textures. Each diameter also has a different resistance to the changes hair colour chemicals make on the hair shaft (see Figure 6.12).

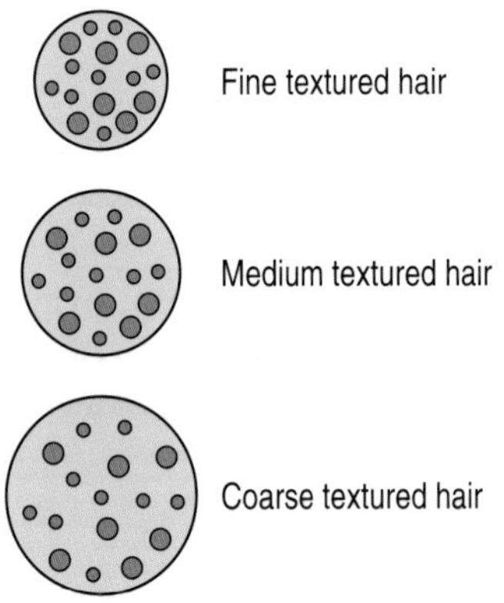

Figure 6.12 Diameters of various hair strands.

Fine-textured hair's pigment is grouped more tightly together. Because of this tighter grouping, when you deposit colour, you will have a darker result on fine hair. By the same token, fine hair is less resistant to lightening because there is less structure to resist the chemical. When lightening fine hair, a milder lightener can be used successfully.

> ***NOTE*** Due to the compact nature of fine hair, depositing colour molecules in the cortex may cause more damage to the structure than it would in coarser hair textures.

Medium-textured hair will have average responses to hair colour products. Note any variations in texture throughout the hair. The front hairline is usually finer in texture than hair further back on the head.

Coarse-textured hair has a more open grouping of hair pigment due the larger diameter hair shaft in which the pigment is located. Because of this open grouping, you will have a slightly lighter result when depositing colour. When lightening the hair, you will encounter greater resistance to the lightener, and a stronger lightening product may be needed.

Porosity is necessary for colour to take properly. Each product you put on the hair requires a different degree of porosity.

Porosity, in simple terms, is the ability of the hair to absorb moisture. Porous hair will accept liquid (hair colour for example) more readily than non-porous hair. Uneven porosity can create problems if even colour results are desired.

As hair grows longer, the ends are subject to frequent shampooing, drying, styling, and environmental influences. There will be visual and textural changes. The cuticle will be slightly abraded (worn away), and the rough hair fibre will loose some of its flexibility, body, and shine. There will also be some variation in colour from strand to strand and even from the scalp area to the mid-lengths. Hair may be lighter and more faded-out towards the ends.

This longer, older hair is described as over-porous, a condition in which hair reaches an undesirable level of porosity. This hair will respond differently to hair colour products from the newer hair closer to the scalp. Those different responses can only be determined by performing a strand test. As a general rule, overporous hair will look duller, flatter and will reflect cooler tones, while the healthier hair will reflect warmer tones.

Occasionally, a client's hair has a cuticle so smooth and compact that you will need to create the proper porosity for the success of your hair colouring service. The hair is considered resistant to the swelling effects of alkalis that allow hair colour to penetrate, and, if necessary, cover grey hair. Pre-softening of grey or resistant hair will be covered later (see Figure 6.13).

TIP The dense areas of your clients' hair will require more product and more careful application. Remember: for hair colour to work effectively, each hair shaft must be surrounded by product.

Hair density is the number of hairs per square centimetre on the scalp. Hair can be described as sparsely, moderately and thickly distributed on the head. It is important to notice that hair density varies, even on the same head. For some, the hair around the face line is more sparsely distributed, and the hair over the crown is more densely distributed. For others, the opposite is true (see Figure 6.14).

Hair length will be a factor in your hair colour choice. The hair on heads grows by an average of 1.25 cm per month. This translates to 15 cm per year. If your client's hair is 30 cm long, the hair furthest away from the scalp is two years old.

Longer hair has been exposed to the elements for a longer period of time and is referred to as older hair. Older hair will vary in porosity throughout the length of the hair shaft.

Unequal reactions to liquid and chemicals along the length of the hair shaft are due to variations in porosity. To observe variations in porosity, hold several strands of hair away from the scalp by their ends. Note any variations in colour or surface texture. Older, more porous hair will appear lighter in colour and rougher in texture.

Since the hair is longer, more hair colouring product may be needed for the application.

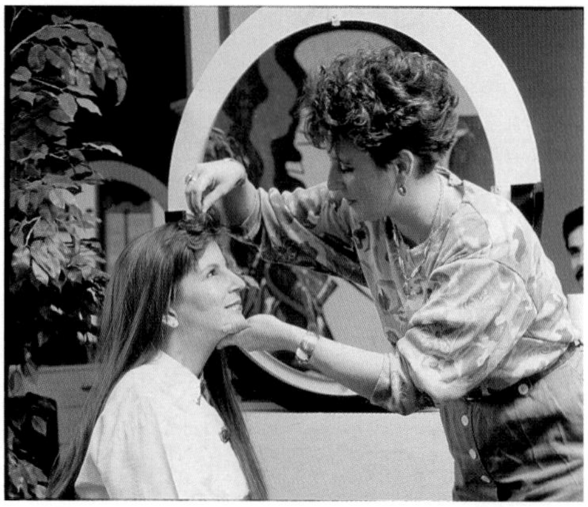

Figure 6.13 Checking the porosity of hair before a colouring service is given is important

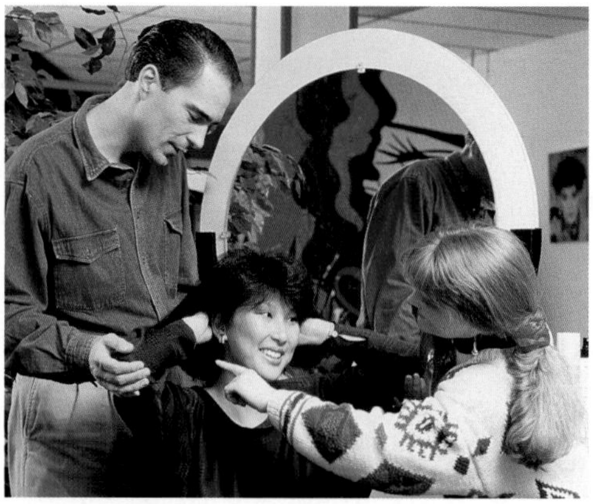

Figure 6.14 Note the variations in hair density prior to a colouring application

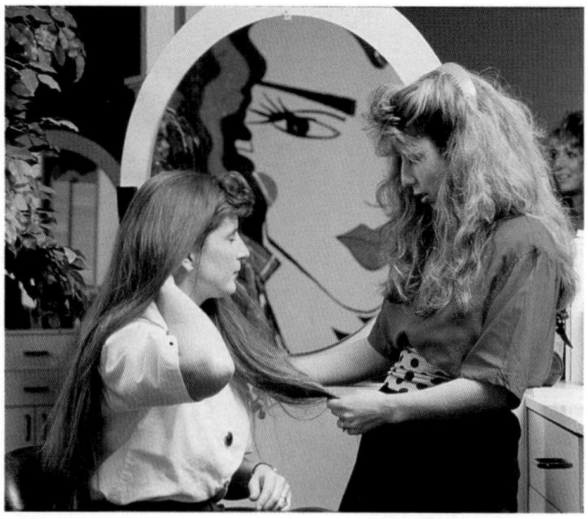

Figure 6.15 Hair length will be a factor in your choice of hair colour

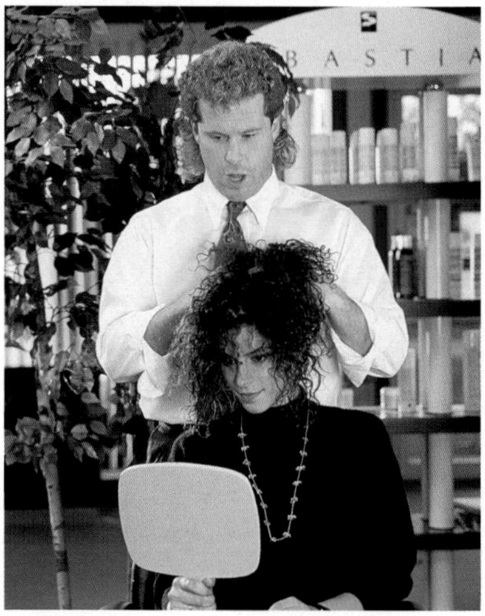

Figure 6.16 A curlier hair form may require a stronger tone

Pre-treatment conditioners may be necessary prior to a colour application to help equalise porosity and provide the foundation for even colour results. Many colourists accordingly charge more for colouring long hair (see Figure 6.15).

The shape of the hair as it grows from the follicle is a genetic trait and is described as being straight, wavy or curly. The smoother the hair shape, the more light reflection. The curlier shapes will refract, or bounce back light, and hair colour may not reflect as strongly as on straighter forms. Careful colour choice and application will create satisfactory colour results on any hair texture. To compensate for excessively curly hair, a more intense or stronger tone may be used, as determined by your strand test. Polymer hair colouring products or those that fill in, or smooth, the cuticle layer may also increase the perception of colour as well as shine (see Figure 6.16).

As a colourist, you should work with the hair's natural attributes, and use texture, shape, density, and porosity to your advantage. Follow the hair's natural pattern or style and insert highlights or lowlights to enhance a cut and give a more polished appearance.

Identifying the natural hair colour

Natural hair colour is the base of the colourist's work. Understanding the science of natural colour will help you develop informed hair colouring choices for each client. It is amazing to realise that nature creates an end-less variety of hair colours, with no two alike, using a single substance called melanin.

Natural pigments are classified as melanins. Melanin is made of molecules capable of reflecting colour. They are classified into two groups: black-brown or eumelanin and yellow-red or pheomelanin. Special cells called melanocytes receive the amino acid tyrosine from the blood vessels at the bottom of each hair follicle. Within the melanocytes, a chemical reaction occurs. An enzyme known as tyrosinase gives oxygen to the tyrosine, and the result is a change in its molecular structure. This oxi-dation of tyrosine produces the melanin that creates all the natural hair colour variations.

Once the melanin is developed, it is coated with melanoprotein to form a granule. While the hair is forming, these pigment granules called melanosomes are pushed up between the cells that are forming as cortex fibres and become a part of the hair structure. These melanin-filled granules are scattered through the cortex of the hair, in no set pattern or amount. This is how nature creates so many hair colour variations from only one natural substance.

The natural hair colour we see (black, brown, blonde, or red) will depend upon the type of melanin – eumelanin, pheomelanin, or a combination of both. The lightness or darkness (depth) of the hair will depend on the amount and distribution (whether closely packed or scattered) of melanin present in the hair.

The keratin protein of the hair is colourless. It is the melanin alone that gives hair its colour. When hair turns grey, it has the same basic structure as it has always had, except that it does not have pigmented melanin. The melanocytes don't necessarily stop producing pigment all at once. Sometimes they produce less and less until gradually the hair appears lighter. Some hairs have no colour and others do, producing the grey effect, sometimes known as 'salt and pepper'.

> ***TIP*** As our hair colour changes and becomes greyer, our skin colour changes as well. When advising the older client about hair colour suggest the lighter colours rather than the darker.

Often, clients will wish to colour their hair long before the grey hair is noticeable, because their colour lacks richness. When we lose all the pigment in a few of our hairs, we lose a little pigment in all our hair. This is a great motivation for colouring one's hair.

Understanding melanin is important to the professional colourist because melanin is a contributor to any new hair colour the colourist wants to create.

In hair colouring, hair stylists and hair colour manufacturers use a system to analyse the lightness and darkness of a colour. It is called the *Level System*. The materials you receive with your hair colour products will describe your particular manufacturer's system. Generally, in the majority of product labelling systems, a scale of 1 to 10 is used to describe the lightness or darkness. Level 1 colours are the darkest; level 10 colours are the lightest. Some manufacturers will elect to use a level system starting with zero; others extend their levels beyond 10 to 12. The scale works the same regardless of the starting and ending points – low numbers are darker; high numbers are lighter.

Hair colour manufacturers provide a chart depicting the colours in their product line. This colour chart shows the level and tone of the various colours. Natural hair colours can also be analysed with this tool. By comparing the manufacturer's colour chart with you client's hair, you can determine the hair colour level. You can then describe the lightness or darkness (depth) with a number from the level system.

> ***TIP*** The names for the natural hair colour levels may vary from manufacturer to manufacturer. It is important for you to identify the varying degrees of lightness to darkness that distinguish each level. Use the selected manufacturer's colour shade chart as your guide in identifying your client's natural colour level.

To determine your client's natural colour level, take a few strands of hair and hold them up and away from the head, allowing light to pass through. Holding the hair away from the scalp, take the manufacturer's chart and fan out the hair strands. Place the chart next to the hair closest to the scalp. Sometimes the hair will be a different level due to exposure to the elements or another chemical service. Be certain to identify the natural level at the base of the hair shaft, closer to the scalp. Also identify the level or levels of the middle lengths and ends so you can adjust your formula accordingly.

Do not part the hair or hold it flattened against the scalp: this produces an incorrect reading, as without light passing through the hair will appear darker. Hair that is wet or heavily soiled will also appear darker.

The natural hair colour levels are:

1. black
2. very dark brown
3. dark brown
4. medium brown
5. light brown
6. dark blonde
7. medium blonde
8. light blonde
9. very light blonde
10. lightest blonde (see Figure 6.17).

Levels 1, 2 and 3 are considered to be dark hair. Generally, people with dark hair want their hair to stay dark. This is usually the best choice, because their skin and eye colours are also usually strongly pigmented. The dark hair colour in combination with richly toned skin and eye colour creates an intense and exotic combination.

Levels 4, 5 and 6 are medium levels. You will note that the client's pigmentation in skin and eye colour is also in the medium range. There are certainly more options for someone with a medium level hair colour. Generally, you will select colours with richness or vibrancy for these clients.

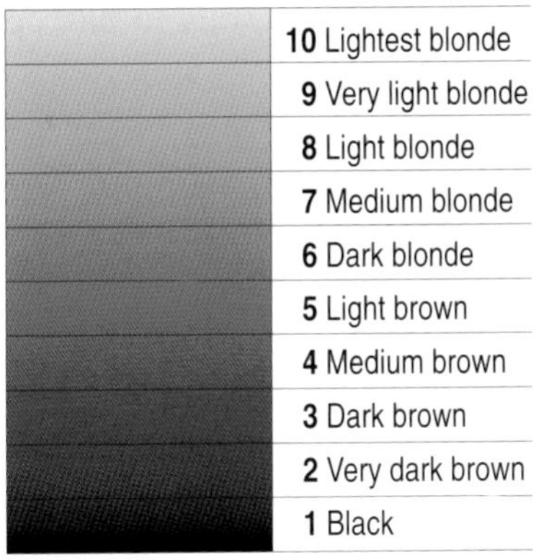
10 Lightest blonde
9 Very light blonde
8 Light blonde
7 Medium blonde
6 Dark blonde
5 Light brown
4 Medium brown
3 Dark brown
2 Very dark brown
1 Black

Figure 6.17 Natural hair colour levels

Levels 7 and 8 are the light levels. Again you will observe corresponding skin and eye pigmentation in this light range. Clients with light hair generally have most options regarding their choices. Darker or lighter hair works well.

Levels 9 and 10 are very light levels. We do not see many of these people as clients. Their hair colour is generally pleasing until it turns grey. We will discuss grey hair at a later point in this chapter.

The term *tone* is used to describe the warmth or coolness of a colour. The manufacturer's colour chart you used earlier to discover the colour level also describes the hair colours, indicating their tone.

The *warm tones* are red, orange, and yellow, although some hair colour labels use different names like auburn, copper, gold or bronze.

The *cool tones* are blue, green, and violet, often listed on labels as ash, drab, platinum, pearl, or smoky. Those words conjure up visual pictures of the properties or characteristics of the colour tone.

Intensity refers to the strength of the tonality in a colour. Intensity is described as being mild, medium, or strong. The difference in intensity can be as subtle as an auburn highlight or as strong as a traffic-stopping red. The strength of the warm or cool tone in a hair colour is indicated in Figure 6.18, with neutral (in the centre) representing an even balance of colour tones without showing obvious amounts of either warm or cool colours.

TIP Most hair colour manufacturers have their own training centres where you may learn how to select and use their own product lines. Some will also visit salons and training centres to give training in the use of their products.

Percentage and distribution of grey

Individuals in today's society are constantly being bombarded by advertisements and television commercials that emphasise youth. Because of this people often seek ways to look younger.

Grey hair can be a curse, or it can be a blessing. It is certainly most often the catalyst that convinces clients to colour their hair, which is a blessing to colourists. On the other hand, grey hair can also complicate the hair colour service because it does not respond to hair colouring in the same way as naturally pigmented hair.

Grey hair tends to be coarser, less elastic and occasionally curlier or straighter than other hair on the head. It also becomes more resistant to chemical services, and thus requires special consideration in hair colouring practice.

It is first necessary to determine the amount of grey hair (the actual percentage) on the head, relative to the naturally coloured hair. Then you must determine the distribution of those grey hairs (where they are located on the head). A person who is 50% grey could have their grey hair sprinkled equally throughout the head or located only in the front portion of the head. Each of these requires a different approach to formulating. Therefore, we must identify and note these factors regarding grey hair on the client's record card.

Determining the percentage of grey

Another consideration when formulating for grey hair is recognising the natural colour that has not yet turned grey. Most people retain some dark hair as they turn grey. The situation in which hair appears grey occurs when there is a mixture of white and dark hair. This blending, known as 'salt and pepper', creates different shades of grey depending on the ratio of pigmented to non-pigmented hair. This hair must be analysed for level and tone.

PERCENTAGE OF GREY	CHARACTERISTICS
10% – 30%	Mostly pigmented; difficult to see; generally most heavily located in the temples and sides with some blending of colours throughout the head.
30% – 50%	More pigment than grey hair: easy to see in dark colours but may blend in with lighter natural hair.
50% – 70%	More grey than pigmented; unnecessary to study hair to see grey.
70% – 90%	Mostly non-pigmented hair; generally majority of remaining pigmented hair is located in back with rest blended over head.
90% – 100%	Virtually no pigmented hair; tends to look white.

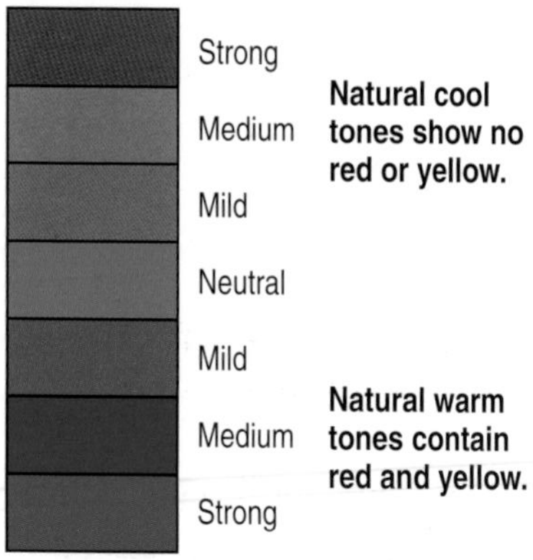

Figure 6.18 The strength or warmth of cool tones is called intensity

Be careful not to allow the reflection of the white or grey hair next to the pigmented hair to affect your judgement. In many instances, this will cause even the most experienced colourist to identify the naturally pigmented hair as darker than it really is, due to the contrast. By misjudging the depth of natural colour, you may not compensate adequately for the undertones present in the hair, which will create a warmer-than-expected end result when you begin to lift the natural hair colour.

What occurs during the greying process?

The melanin enters the hair shaft void of colour. The melanin pigment granule is still nestled in the cortex of the hair shaft and will still be evident as it is affected by the colouring process. When you lighten hair that is grey or white (non-pigmented hair), the melanin pigment diffuses in the same way as coloured melanin. The strand would become weakened, the cuticle would become lifted, and the hair would take on a yellow cast.

Another consideration when formulating for grey hair is what colour the client's hair was prior to turning grey. The hair colourist must recognise that when the hair starts to turn grey, the remaining natural colour changes as well. Grey hair does the masterful job of concealing the undertones that still remain in the hair. The undertones are there and are no less intensified than they were before the hair turned grey.

> ***TIP*** Each person is born with a particular combination of natural pigment. There is harmony between the hair, eye, and skin tones. At the point at which greying clients come to you for colour service, their hair has changed dramatically from the original birth colour. By knowing what colour their hair was when they were younger, you will be able to anticipate the changes that hair will undergo during treatment with an oxidative hair colour product. The answer to this question will indicate the intensity of pigmentation with which you will be dealing.

Selecting colour for desired result

Every hair colouring service must begin with a professional assessment of the client's current hair colour and what changes need to be made. Only then can the best procedure and formula be selected.

Basic rules for colour selection

- Make sure the client's hair is not over-greasy and is dry.
- Look through the hair. To see level as well as tone, raise the hair by pushing it up with the hands against the scalp.
- Analyse the level present in the hair. Does the client want to go lighter or darker?
- Analyse the level of the desired colour. Add or subtract from the form the natural colour to determine the level of colour necessary.
- What are the natural tones? What highlights does the client want? Select the colour within the level that will supply those tones, or determine which colour concentrate should be used.
- Know the properties of the product you are using. Consult the manufacturer's information on each colour and how it reacts on different hair colour levels (light, medium, or dark hair).
- Analyse the condition of the hair, especially its porosity. Does the hair need to be conditioned prior to the service to help the colour be true and prevent excessive fading?

Each manufacturer's colour product's directions will indicate their mixing formulas for adequate lift and/or deposit, and what hair colour classification and volume of developer (if any) is required to achieve the desired results, based on your thorough analysis of your client's hair and needs.

> ***REMEMBER*** The manufacturer's guidelines do require accurate analysis of your client's hair in order to direct you towards the correct colour product choice.

Examining the scalp

Carefully examine the scalp to determine the presence of any factors that would make it inadvisable to use a hair colouring product (these factors are called 'contra-indications'). An oxidation tint solution should not be used if the following conditions exist:

- positive skin test (predisposition or patch test)
- scalp abrasions, irritations, or eruptions
- contagious scalp disorders.

Examining the hair

Examine the hair to determine what, if any, pre-treatment may be necessary prior to your hair colour service. Elements to consider are:

Incompatibility test, page 158

- Evidence of prior chemical treatments (either colour, permanent wave or relaxer).
- Different degrees of porosity over the length of the hair shaft due to the effects of sun, harsh chemicals, or hair length.
- Variations in texture at the facial hairline, crown, or nape.

In some cases it may be advisable to postpone the hair colour service due to excessive damage or the presence of incompatible chemicals in the hair.

The results of such an examination may indicate the need for any of the following:

- reconditioning treatments
- colour removal
- removal of metallic colouring
- postponement of service due to breakage or some other problem.

All information about the condition of the client's hair should be recorded on the client's record card.

Discuss client's expectations and hair limitations

The difference between your client's current hair colour and what is desired will indicate the hair colour category and formula to use. Does your client want a temporary change or a more permanent one? Does your client want something close to their current colour or a dramatic colour change? Based on your thorough analysis, you can choose the appropriate product and technique to fulfil the client's expectations, but also respect the hair's limitations.

Be realistic in discussing colour selection with your client. It is best to select a general range of colour lightness and tone, rather than to promise an exact shade. Some clients will be able to change their colour in one process, creating the right level and tone at the same time. Others will need two separate products and processes to create the same effect. Be sure to consider carefully all the factors that will influence your client's decisions.

Consider the client's lifestyle

A colouring procedure that requires a great deal of care may be impractical for a very active person. Pale blonde may be the wrong choice for someone who swims regularly (pool chemicals can turn blonde hair green). Typically an iridescent aubergine colour would be inadvisable for someone who works in a conservative law firm. All of these factors must be considered.

An office job would dictate a more conservative colour choice than a freelance fashion photographer. A full-time mum might need a lower maintenance colour service. A businessman would wish for an undetect-able line of demarcation between the hair colour and his new regrowth.

Sun lovers will have different colour results from people who avoid exposure to the sun. Tennis, boating, and convertible cars all mean more sun. Pool swimmers have constant exposure to chlorine. which changes the texture and colour outcome. People who engage in heavy daily exercise need to shampoo their hair more often; this could cause their colour to fade.

Medicines can affect hair colour results. Sulphur-based drugs can add warmth to light blonde colours. High doses of vitamins and minerals can darken the natural hair colour level. Always ask your clients and note any medications they are taking on their record card.

Home care products are of great importance for hair colour clients. A shampoo for controlling dandruff or psoriasis may change your colour result. Rapid fading can occur due to highly alkaline, non-professional products. Some mousses, conditioners, and hair sprays can build up and coat the hair shaft. This will alter the porosity of hair, causing uneven colour results.

Educating your clients on how to care for their colour-treated hair will improve your results. Healthy, well-cared-for hair will be a positive reflection on your workmanship. Teaching your clients proper maintenance is the most professional approach to beautiful hair colour (see Figure 6.19).

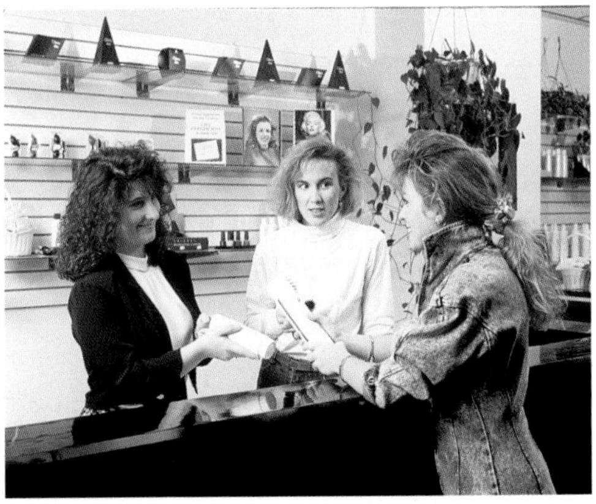

Figure 6.19 Discussing hair colour products

Time spent in the salon for services is a point of discussion. For some, looking good is a form of self indulgence; for others, it's pure torture. Frequency of maintenance must be presented during your consultation.

The time and money involved in committing to a colour service should be spelled out in advance.

This is a time to make direct eye contact with your client and wait for the answer. If the time or cost is objectionable, alter your suggestion. Continue this conversation until you and your client agree to the maintenance schedule you have presented. At this point, you will have an agreement with your client and can begin your service.

> ***TIP*** Your conversation should be something like: 'This colour (show a picture or swatch) can be achieved by (indicate the type of colour service i.e., weaving, single-process colour, etc.). The cost of this service will be (state cost). How do you feel about this?'

Choosing level, tone, and intensity

If necessary you will adjust the hair colour formula for each individual texture or condition. Remember the findings of your analysis, listed on your client's record card. Include the client's current colour in formulating for level, tone, and intensity. Generally speaking, a change of 1 to 2 levels will produce the most natural results. Any tone can be enhanced or subdued to the client's wishes by using the law of colour in selecting your formula. Adjust for grey, porosity, and length. Natural-looking hair colours are a balance between all three primary colours, including the client's contributing pigment and the artificial colour selected.

Selecting the appropriate application technique

After a thorough discussion with your client, you must then choose the method that will achieve the desired effect. Sometimes a combination of application techniques is necessary to first cover grey, then add carefully placed highlights, to make the transition from the lightness of grey to the contrasting darkness of a solid colour. Another example would be the use of a double-process, blending a pastel colour with a cool tone. Whatever you select, make sure the client understands each step of the procedure and the technique necessary to achieve your objective. This will avoid startled looks from clients when they see unexplained things happening to their hair during a procedure.

> ***TIP*** Remember that your client may not understand the jargon that you use. Explain the procedure that is about to be used on their hair, in terms that they will understand. This will help to gain their confidence in the process, so they will be more comfortable and therefore more likely to enjoy their visit to your salon.

Using colour keys to find the most flattering colour for the client

Analysing skin and eye colouring

The colour of client's eyes can be a clue as to what their hair colour could be. Eyes are rarely one colour. Usually they are combinations of two or even three colours. Basically there are brown, blue, and green eyes. Look more closely. Brown eyes with olive green, reddish brown, or gold flecks are quite common. Blue eyes may also have flecks of white, gold, or grey. Green eyes can range from grey-green to hazel (with brownish overtones) to yellow-green.

We can categorise eye colour as warm or cool. Warm eye colours contain red, orange, yellow, or gold flecks through the iris of brown, blue, or green.

Warm eye colours are:

- Brown with red, orange, yellow, or gold.
- Blue with yellow or gold.
- Green with reddish brown, orange, yellow, or gold.

People who have warm eye colours can wear warm hair colours. Cool eye colours contain black, grey-brown, grey-green, blue, violet, grey or white flecks through the iris of brown, blue, or green.

Cool eye colours are:

- Brown with black, grey-brown, grey-green, or grey.
- Blue with white, blue, grey, or violet.
- Green with blue or grey.

People with cool eye colours look most attractive with cool or neutral hair colours

The depth of eye colour is another factor in your colour choice. Lighter eyes reflect a lighter pigmentation throughout the client's colouring. A lighter intensity colour choice would be indicated. Medium eyes reflect stronger pigmentation, and more intense colour options are available. Dark eyes reflect the strongest pigmentation. A deeper colour choice is advisable. To choose a colour that will harmonise with the client's natural pigmentation, include the depth of eye colour (light, medium, or dark) in your colour equation.

> ***TIP*** Many clients choose coloured contact lenses to enhance their appearance. This can affect your colour choice. If you are not certain of the client's natural eye colour, always ask.

Skin tone can be broken down into four simple categories: olive, red, golden and neutral. It is easiest to observe the natural skin tone by looking at the skin on the neck, close to the clavicle. Skin on the face and arm is often affected by sun exposure, which masks the skin tone, making it difficult to determine.

Olive skin tones have an underlying tone of grey, green, or yellow. Olive-toned clients look best in cool or neutral colours. If a warm shade is desired, it should be in a darker level.

Red skin tones have an underlying tone of red-brown, red, or blue-red. Red-toned clients look best in cool or neutral colours. Warm colours are not recommended for these clients.

Golden skin tones have an underlying tone of golden brown, gold, or peach. Golden skin tones look best in warm colours. The level chosen would be affected by the client's natural level.

Neutral skin tones are a balance of warm and cool. Neutral skin can have an underlying tone of pink and yellow in combination. You will not observe one predominant underlying skin tone. Generally these skin tones are described as ivory, beige, or brown skin. Neutral skin tones look good in either warm or cool colours.

How does this information indicate a colour choice? The chart on pages 144–5 will help you in your selection. Remember that each person is unique, however, and consult with your trainer or product techician for advice. Gradually, as your skill develops, you will see these features automatically (see Figure 6.20).

Enhancing your client's natural colouring

When working with hair that has not been coloured, you will notice a natural harmony in the hair tone, skin tone, and eye colour tone. Maintaining that natural harmony will give you a pleasing, natural effect. A more avant-garde effect will be achieved by using complementary colour tones. The key to maintaining harmony in colour tone is understanding the *Law of Colour*.

Consider how tones change with maturity. Many clients initially want to return to the colour of their youth. They do not realise that the pigment of their skin is ageing in a process similar to that of the hair. To tint the hair back to the natural colour of their youth creates a

COLOUR KEY 1

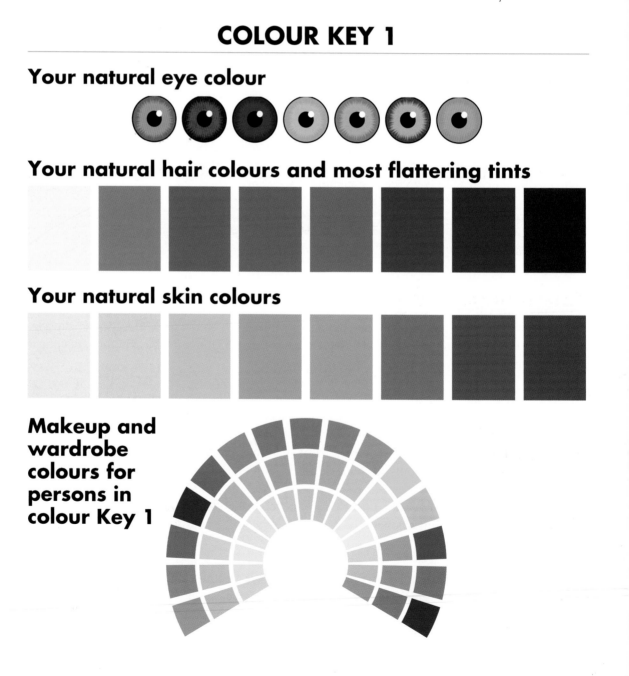

Your natural eye colour

Your natural hair colours and most flattering tints

Your natural skin colours

Makeup and wardrobe colours for persons in colour Key 1

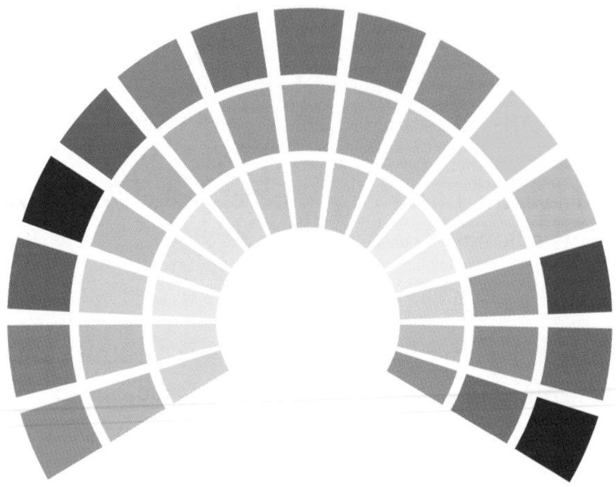

severe contrast that can be harsh. Generally, a colour of a similar tone but lighter level will be more flattering.

There will always be clients who break these rules. Many do so with great success. Attractiveness is a quality that incorporates the laws of art and balance, along with the client's personality and self-expression.

> ***TIP*** The level of your correction must be the same or slightly darker than the problem. For example, if you have a client whose hair is level 6 orange and she wants it to be more neutral looking, you would need to use a level 5 or 6 blue-toned hair colour to correct the warmth. A level 7 in a blue-toned hair colour will not have enough pigment to overcome the level 6 orange.

COLOUR KEY 2

Your natural eye colour

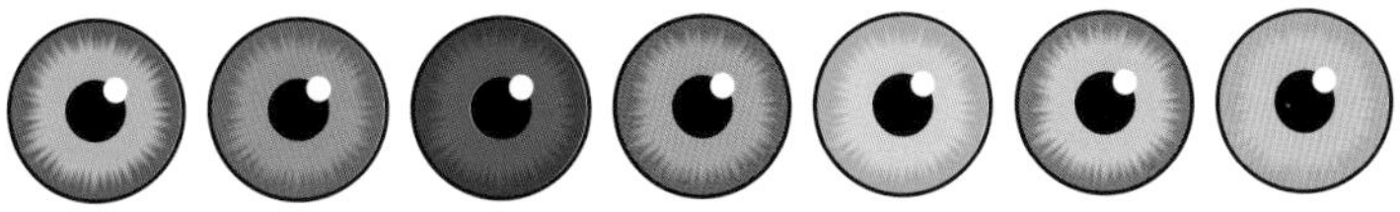

Your natural hair colours and most flattering tints

Your natural skin colours

Makeup and wardrobe colours for persons in colour Key 2

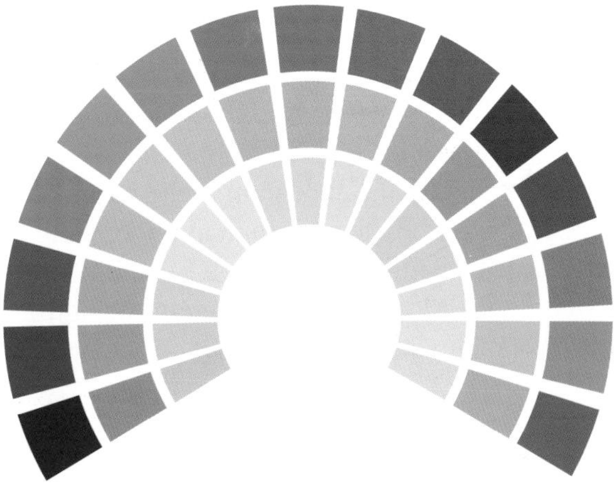

Creating natural-looking hair colour using artificial pigments

Most hair colours represent a balance of colours, which means that they generally contain a balance of each of the primary colours. However, colours will have a predominant base and a level of lightness or darkness that must be identified before formulating a tint for the hair.

Oxidation tints are identified by the predominant base and the level of colour formulated by the manufacturer. Most manufacturers provide literature that identifies the level and base colour for you. You may identify the level and base colour of the client's hair by comparing it to the manufacturer's colour or shade chart (as a guide, not as an absolute).

All colours – warm, cool, or neutral – can be formulated in tones that range from the lightest blonde to the darkest black, using the basic theory related to the Law of Colour.

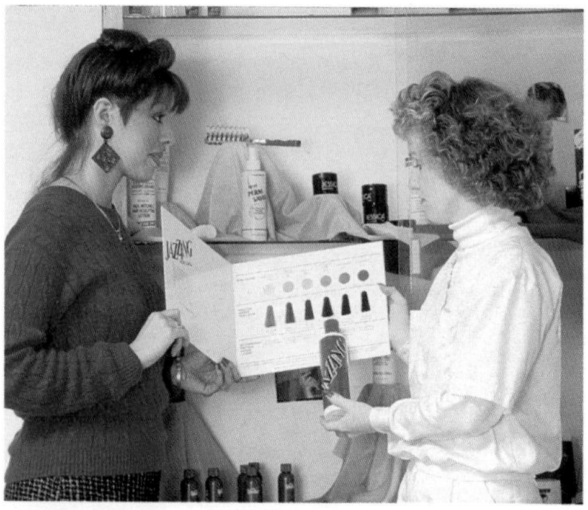

Figure 6.20 A hair colourist using a colour chart

Using level, tone, and intensity in selecting a colour

When you have decided on the hair colouring products to use, you must next find the correct level, tone, and intensity to achieve your desired result. In many manufacturer's product lines, you may find more than one colour choice at each level. However, each of these shades will create a different tonality.

Choose the one closest to what you need to achieve the desired result. To give the new hair colour the exact tonality and intensity desired, the basic shade can be adjusted or modified by adding a small quantity (2.5 – 5 ml) of a cooler or warmer shade on the same level, or by using a colour concentrate (usually added drop by drop (liquids) or centimetre by centimetre (cream)) to enrich or drab the final formula.

The four rules for natural-looking hair colour

In order to more easily mimic the characteristics of virgin hair colour, consider the following in determining your choice of colour and application technique:

- The hair should be lighter at the ends than at the base of the hair shaft
- The hair should be lighter on the surface than underneath
- Face-line hair should be lighter than the hair behind it (crown and nape)
- The darker hair should always be the dominant colour, i.e. in reverse highlighting, it should always have more dark hair than light on the head.

> ***TIP*** Manufacturers identify their hair colours by the use of number. The first number indicates the depth or level, the second number indicates the tone. If there is more than one tonal number, the first number indicates the stronger tone. Therefore a colour 6.43 indicates a colour of level *dark blonde* with a strong tone of *red* with a secondary tone of *yellow.*

CLASSIFICATIONS OF HAIR COLOUR

Hair colouring falls into three main categories: temporary, semi-permanent, and permanent. These classifications refer primarily to staying power (lasting ability), they also reflect their actions on the hair. These characteristics are determined by chemical composition and molecular weight, or size, of the pigments within the products found in each classification.

Temporary hair colouring

Temporary colours utilise pigments that have the largest molecules of all classifications of hair colour. The large size of the colour molecule prevents penetration of the cuticle layer of the hair shaft and allows only a coating action on the outside of the strand. The chemical composition of temporary colour is acidic and makes only a physical change rather than a chemical change in the hair shaft (see Figure 6.21).

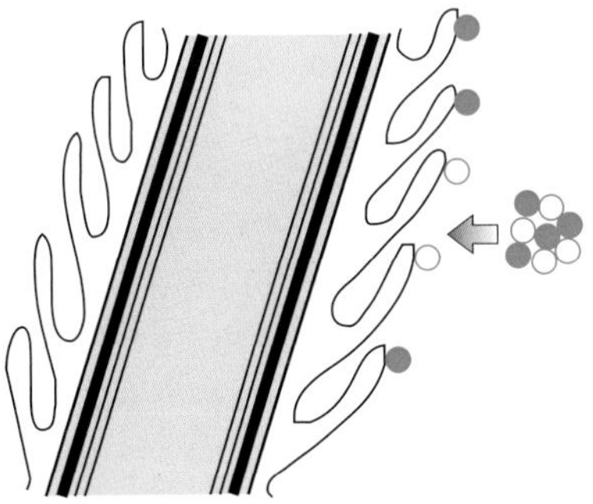

Figure 6.21 The action of temporary hair colour

Action of temporary colour on the hair

Since the colour remains on the cuticle and does not penetrate into the cortex, it lasts only from one shampoo to the next. However, excessive porosity can allow temporary colour to penetrate, 1
making it last much longer.

Temporary colours can be used for the following:

- to introduce your client to hair colouring
- to produce short term fashion colour effects on hair
- to temporarily restore faded hair to its natural colour
- to neutralise the yellowish tinge in white of grey hair
- to tone down over lightened hair without creating further chemical damage 1
- to temporarily add colour to the hair without changing its condition
- to add red colour when recolouring bleached hair (pre-pigmentation).

Temporary hair colours have several disadvantages:

- Colour is of short duration; it must be applied after every shampoo
- Coating is thin and may not cover hair evenly
- colour may rub off on pillows or collars and may run with perspiration or other moisture
- They can only add colour; they cannot lighten
- Staining may result if the hair is porous or if a dark colour is used on very light hair
- They have a limited ability to darken hair.

Temporary colours come in a wide array of shades from light to dark, warm to cool. They are easy to apply and are valuable as an introduction to hair colouring, or as a 'quick fix' in corrective colouring situations when the hair may not tolerate a stronger chemical.

An allergy or patch test is usually not necessary for this type of hair colour, except if your client has a history of hypersensitivity.

Types of temporary hair colouring

A wide variety of products are available within this classification: colour rinses; coloured setting lotions; coloured mousses; colour gels and creams; colour sprays; colour shampoos.

Colour rinses

The traditional temporary hair colourings. There are two forms of colour rinses, basic colour concentrates (water rinses) and prepared ready to use colour rinses. This form of hair colouring contains no setting or blowdry styling lotion.

Coloured setting lotions

HEALTH AND SAFETY Skin and hair are composed of similar types of keratin, with the soft keratin of the skin and scalp even more reactive than the hard keratin of the hair. This allows rinses to stain the scalp and the skin. Therefore, it is advisable to wear gloves to protect your hands even though the solution itself is relatively harmless.

Temporary hair colourings together with a setting lotion. The pigment is of mineral origin. These colours are applied direct from the bottle to pre-shampooed and towel-dried hair

Following consultation with your client, gown and shampoo the hair. Towel dry the hair and using a wide-toothed comb, comb the hair back off the face and locate a towel suitable for use when hair colouring. Shake the bottle and then remove the top. Apply to the hair by sprinkling the colour over the hair, gently massaging it onto the hair to distribute the colour throughout the hair as well as to prevent it running down the scalp onto your client's face and neck. Apply the bulk of the colour to the top area of the head and, depending upon the porosity, thickness and length of the hair, apply some to the sides and back. The bulk applied to the top area will comb down. Use a wide-toothed comb to distribute the product through the hair and along its length.

When applying coloured setting lotion to very porous hair, it may be necessary to use a tint brush style application to ensure an even colour coverage and to avoid a patchy result.

Strong red colours may stain the scalp, particularly if used on clients with dry scalps. In these cases a tint brush application, avoiding applying to the scalp, can help to avoid this. To apply the product close to your clients scalp, at the hairline or parting, slide a clean comb into the hair at the scalp and apply the coloration, using a brush, up to and onto the teeth of the comb, then draw the comb down the hair away from the scalp.

Remember to check your client's hairline for any skin staining before placing the client under the hair dryer and when removing the setting tools from the hair when dry. Skin staining may often be removed using cotton wool moistened with water. In extreme cases a proprietary skin stain remover may be used.

> ***TIP*** If your are unfamiliar with the product that you are using consult the manufacturer's directions or consult your line manager or trainer for guidance.

While this form of colour is not harmful to the skin, the hairdresser is well advised to wear protective gloves when applying these colours, in particular when applying strong vibrant shades.

Some coloured setting lotion ranges include a clear liquid version, called a lightener or brightener. It should be noted that while its affect on the hair colour may appear temporary, any lightening of the hair is not temporary and manufacturers will often recommend that no more that three consecutive applications of this be made, so as not to produce a noticeable regrowth.

Coloured styling mousses

Temporary hair colours within a styling mousse formulation. Most styling mousses are made for use when either blow drying the hair or when setting. They offer a wide array of colours that are fast and easy to apply. Colour mousses stay put on the hair shaft. They do not drip, run or blow off the hair when blow drying. Some mousses also have detangling and conditioning abilities as well as giving control during drying and style retention.

Prepare your client in the same manner as for coloured setting lotions. Shake the mousse can thoroughly and place a ball, the size of a golf ball, onto your hand. The exact amount to be used will be dependant upon the porosity, thickness and length of your client's hair. Using your hands, in a claw like action, distribute the colouration throughout the hair. Comb the hair with a wide-toothed comb to ensure distribution.

This colouration may stain both your client and yourself in the same manner as the coloured setting lotion. Any skin staining should be removed as soon as noticed in the same manner as for coloured setting lotion.

> ***TIP*** The metallic salts in some colour sprays can build up after repeated use and cause an adverse reaction with future chemical services. These products are also extremely flammable, so they cannot be used around clients who are smoking.

Coloured gels and creams

These are available in a variety of shades, some natural, others wild and vibrant. These colours are designed to shampoo completely out, but because they tend to be tones of great intensity, they may stain porous, bleached, or very dry hair (see Figure 6.22).

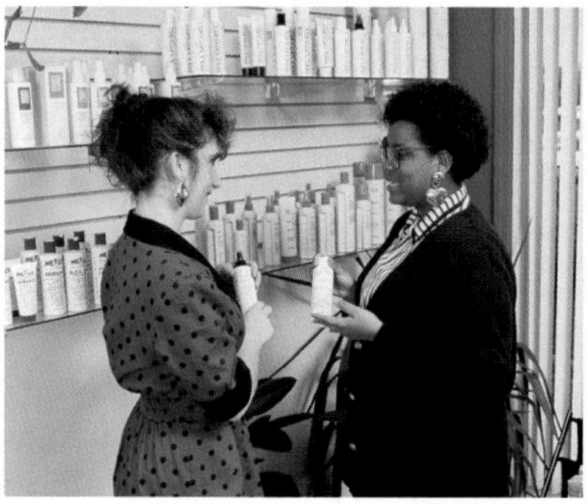

Figure 6.22 A variety of colour mousses and gels are available

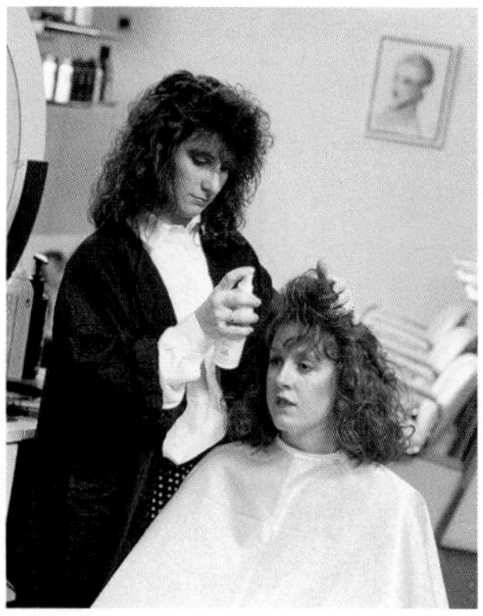

Figure 6.23 Spray-on hair colouring products are popular for creating special effects

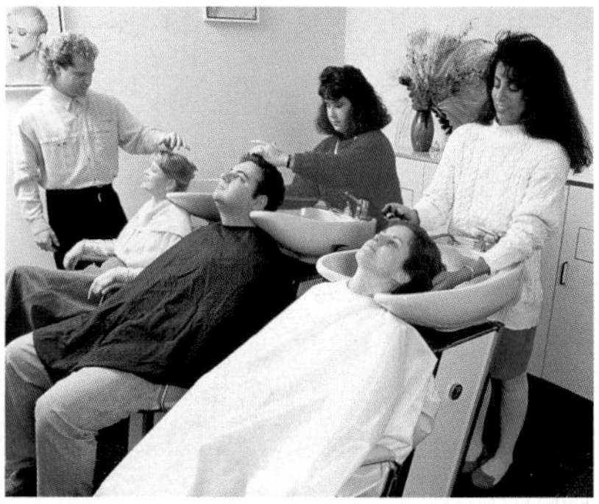

Figure 6.24 Colour enhancing shampoos combine the action of a colour rinse with that of a shampoo

Spray-on hair colouring

This is applied to dry hair from aerosol containers. These are generally used for special or party effects (see Figure 6.23).

Colour-enhancing shampoos

These combine the action of a colour rinse with that of a shampoo. These shampoos add colour tones to the hair (see Figure 6.24).

Semi-permanent hair colouring

Semi-permanent colour offers a form of hair colouring suitable for the client who is reluctant to have a permanent colour change. The semi-permanent colour is formulated to be more lasting than temporary colour techniques but milder than permanent ones (see Figure 6.25).

Semi-permanent colour may be excellent for clients who feel that their hair is dull, drab, or showing grey, but are not yet ready to begin permanent hair colouring. Semi-permanent colour can blend grey and deepen colour tones without altering the natural colour, since there is no lightening action on the hair.

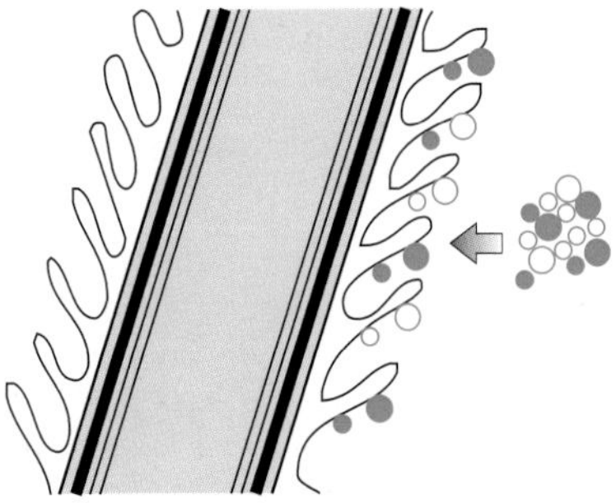

Figure 6.25 Action of semi-permanent hair colour formula

Semi-permanent colour is available in a wide range of shades. It can be purchased as a gel, cream, liquid or mousse. Such products are often chosen by younger clients to produce fashion trend looks. Semi-permanent colour products can deposit a dramatic colour, or can be used for special effects in bright colours. Providing the hair's porosity is normal, the colour will naturally fade without a regrowth, so the client can change the colour at any time or discontinue the effect.

Semi-permanent hair colour is formulated to last for between 4 to 12 shampoos. No developer is required. The colour molecules penetrate the cortex and stain the cuticle somewhat, so that the colour gradually fades with each shampoo. Due to this gradual fading of colour tone from the hair, there is no noticeable regrowth (depending upon the colour applied). If the hair is extremely porous, or if heat is used with some types of semi-permanent colour, the results can be more permanent. Results depend on the hair's original colour and porosity, processing time, and technique.

Semi-permanent colouring can have the following advantages:

- The colour is self-penetrating
- The colour is applied the same way each time
- Retouching is not necessary
- Colour does not rub off on a pillow or clothing
- Hair returns to its natural colour after approximately 4 to 12 shampoos
- This colour does not detract from the hair's condition; in fact these formulations will often condition while colouring the hair.

Semi-permanent hair colour uses

Semi permanent hair colour can be used in the following ways:

- to enhance hair's natural colour. Semi-permanent colours can be used to add golden or red highlights, and to deepen the colour of the hair. This type of colour is especially effective on Afro-Caribbean hair and natural hair colour that is too light or too drab to set off the client's complexion.
- to tone pre-lightened hair. Semi-permanent colours can serve as a non-peroxide toner for pre-lightened hair. Pre-lightened hair is porous and the toner will penetrate.
- to refresh faded tints. Excellent for between permanent colour services and for corrective work, when a non-peroxide alternative is desired.
- to add colour to grey/white hair. Most semi-permanent colours are designed to cover hair that is 25% or less grey or create a blending effect on higher percentages. They are also recommended for clients who want to keep and enhance their grey or white hair.
- as an alternative to oxidation tinting for hypersensitive clients. Clients who are allergic to oxidation tints may find semi-permanent colour, which is direct colour, a safe alternative. Clients with a history of sensitivity towards hair colour should be skin/patch tested before use.
- for pre-pigmentation. Semi-permanent colour may be used, when recolouring bleached hair, to pre-pigment hair.

Action on hair

Traditional semi-permanent colours are formulated with pigment molecules that are smaller than those of the temporary colours but larger than those of the permanent tints. They have a mild penetrating action that results in a gentle addition of colour in the cortex as well as some staining of the cuticle (see Figure 6.26).

The chemical composition of semi-permanent colours falls within the approximate pH range 8.0–9.0, thus causing an alkaline action on the hair. The alkali swells the cuticle, opening imbrications and allowing the molecules to enter the cortex. However, this solution is mildly

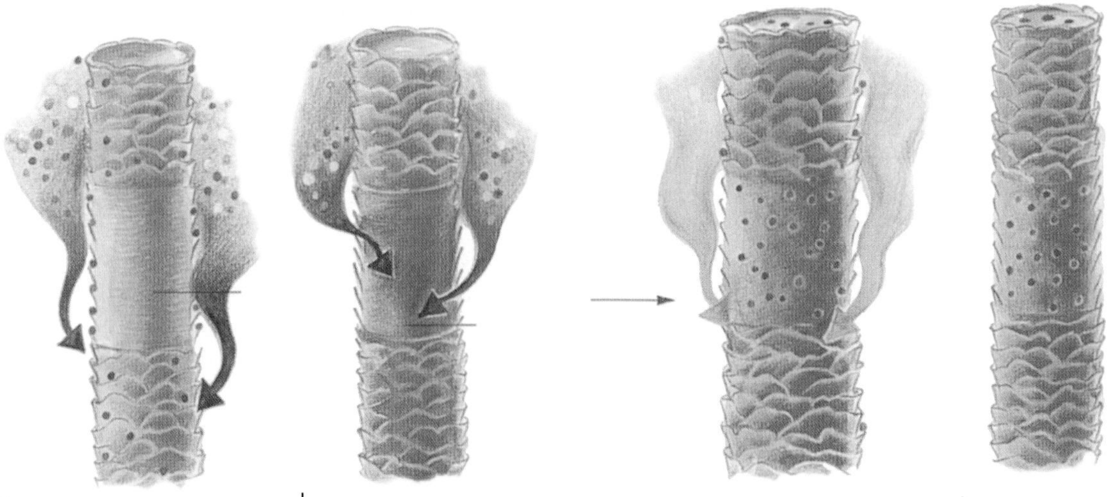

Figure 6.26 Action of semi-permanent hair colours

alkaline, which causes limited swelling and opening. Only a small number of these medium-sized molecules enter and remain in the cortex.

The pigment molecules are trapped within the cortical layer of the shaft as the hair shrinks back towards normal during the rinsing step of the service. A neutral or slightly acid after-rinse helps to close the imbrications and hold the pigment molecules within the cortex. However, even the mild swelling that occurs with shampooing allows some of the colour to fade.

Traditional semi-permanent colours have several distinct differences from temporary and permanent colours. They last longer than temporary colours and do not rub off. They are also easy to use, requiring no retouch application. Because semi-permanent colours make no significant permanent changes in the structure of the hair, they are less damaging. Many brands even give a conditioning effect. They are excellent for toning bleached hair that is too weak or porous to accept another peroxide treatment and for use on hair that is exceptionally fine or damaged from permanent wave or relaxer services.

Semi-permanent colour selection

The following steps, used in conjunction with the manufacturer's colour chart, offer a guide to selecting the correct colour with which to perform a strand test:

1. On solid hair (no grey) select a level of semi-permanent colour that is slightly lighter than the desired shade.
2. Due to the absorption of light, the use of an ash or cool shade will create a colour that the eye interprets as darker than if a warm shade is applied.
3. Due to the reflection of light, the warm colours will appear shinier.

The addition of artificial colour molecules to the natural pigment of the hair shaft will create a colour that is darker than the sample on the colour chart. Most colour charts show the approximate colour that will be achieved on white hair. This colour is to be used as a guide to estimate the colour results when it is applied to natural hair.

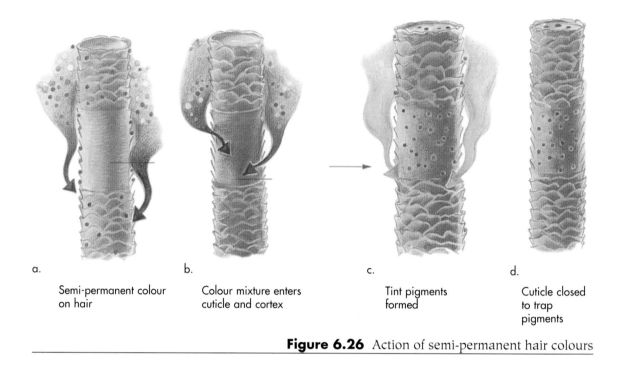

The natural hair colour must be considered as half the formula. Think of it as $\frac{1}{2}$ artificial colour and $\frac{1}{2}$ natural colour. Semi-permanent colours lack the strong oxidisers necessary to lift; therefore they deposit colour and do no substantial lifting. Think back to laws of intensity and remember that colour applied on top of colour makes a darker colour.

Since these products 'take' based on the hair's porosity, be cautious to avoid creating ends that are darker than the base of the hair. Semi-permanent colours, due to their depositing nature, may also build up on the hair's ends with subsequent applications. A strand test will determine your formula and timing before each service.

Many semi-permanent colours are used just as they pour from the bottle (i.e. they are direct colours), and the colour medium is the same colour as will be deposited in the hair. However, others require the mixing of an activator prior to their application. These are quasi-permanent hair colours. The activator is an oxidant that helps to swell the cortex and open the cuticle to allow colour penetration. This mild oxidiser also develops the colour pigments within the formula.

Some semi-permanent colours include a colour balancer in the packaging. This crystal need be added only if the semi-permanent colour is to be applied immediately following the removal of a lightening or bleaching product. It stops the residual oxidation that occurs on the hair shaft until the normal pH is completely restored.

Some semi-permanent colours come packaged with an 'after-rinse'. This rinse is acid-balanced to close the cuticle and trap the colour molecules within it. This helps prevent fading to a lighter colour as well as fading off-tone. The chemical composition of the after-rinse is designed to leave the hair soft, pliable and easy to comb. Whether or not the product you select is packaged in this way, it is always a good idea to finish your service with a mild conditioning rinse.

Application of semi-permanent hair colours

TOOLS AND MATERIALS		
Colouring towels	Applicator bottle or brush	Finishing rinse
Colouring cape	Plastic cap (optional)	Plastic clips
Protective gloves	Cotton wool	Barrier cream
Wide-toothed comb	Mild shampoo	Record card
Timer	Selected product	Colour chart
Measure		

Preliminary steps

1. Give a preliminary patch test if required. Proceed only if test result is negative. (This is not normally required for semi-permanent colours except when using them on clients with known hypersensitivity. A patch test is required prior to each quasi-permanent colour application.)
2. Thoroughly analyse the hair and scalp and select the appropriate colour product. Record your findings on the client's record card.
3. Assemble all necessary supplies.

TIP If you are in doubt about your salon's requirements for gowning the client, consult with your line manager or trainer.

4. Prepare your client. Protect their clothing using caps and towels: most salons have their own gowning procedure. Effective gowning must protect the client and their clothing from the risk of damage from the product to be used. Ask your client to remove jewellery and put it safely away.
5. Apply barrier cream around the hairline and over the ears, when pre-shampooing this would be applied following the shampoo.
6. If in doubt about suitability of the product or its outcome on a particular head, carry out a strand test.

TIP When applying strong colours or semi-permanent colours to hair where the scalp is dry and scaly, avoid allowing the product onto the scalp, as scalp staining often occurs. This may be visible through the finished hairstyle.

Procedure

1. Shampoo the hair using a mild shampoo, if required.
2. Towel dry the hair.
3. Put on protective gloves and apply barrier cream to the client.
4. Apply semi-permanent colour to the entire hair shaft (see Figure 6.27).

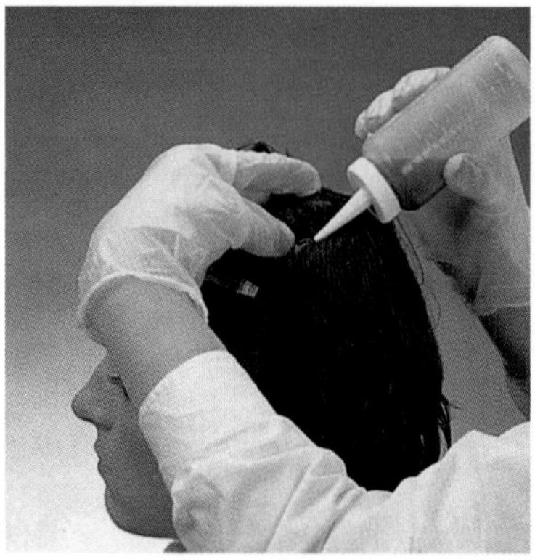

Figure 6.27 Applying semi-permanent colour

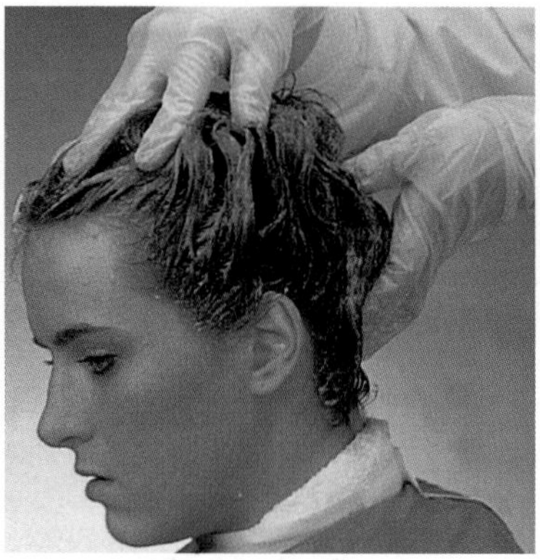

Figure 6.28 Gently work colour through hair

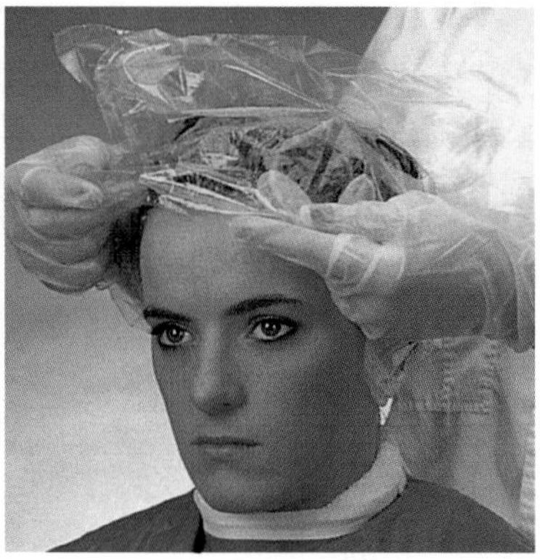

Figure 6.29 Use a plastic cap if required

5. Pile hair loosely on top of the head.
6. Follow the manufacturer's directions about using a plastic cap or heat (see Figure 6.29).
7. Process according to strand test results or manufacturer's guidelines.
8. According to the timing instructions provided by the manufacturer, when the colour has developed, wet the hair with warm water and lather.
9. Rinse and (subject to manufacturer's directions) then shampoo, then rinse again with warm water until the water runs clear.

10. Use a finishing rinse to close the cuticle and set the colour.
11. Rinse and towel-blot the hair. Style as required.
12. Complete the record card and file.

Clean up

1. Discard all disposable supplies and materials.
2. Close containers, wipe them off, and store safely.
3. Clean implements, tint cape, work area, and hands.

Deposit-only (quasi-permanent) hair colour

When semi-permanent colours were first introduced some years ago, clients generally shampooed their hair weekly, making the lasting ability of the semi-permanent colour of the time a satisfactory 4 to 6 weeks. Today, however, with more clients shampooing daily, a colour that lasts 4 to 6 shampoos may be unsatisfactory. For a colour that will act similarly in nature to the semi-permanent colours but will produce a longer-lasting effect, manufacturers have introduced a new category of hair colours called *Deposit-only* or *Quasi-permanent colours*.

Composition and action

The effect of a deposit-only hair colour lies between those of semi-permanent and permanent colour classifications. Deposit-only colours use a form of a catalyst, such as low-volume developers, to gently swell and open the cuticle layer and drive the colour into the cortex. Deposit-only hair colours have small- and medium-sized dye molecules. The small-sized molecules slightly penetrate into the cortex, and the medium-sized dye molecules penetrate the cuticle layers, resulting in a colour that has the gentleness of a semi-permanent colour with the longevity of a permanent hair colour. Deposit-only colours last 4 to 6 weeks, gradually fading from the hair and producing a diffused line of demarcation (see Figure 6.30).

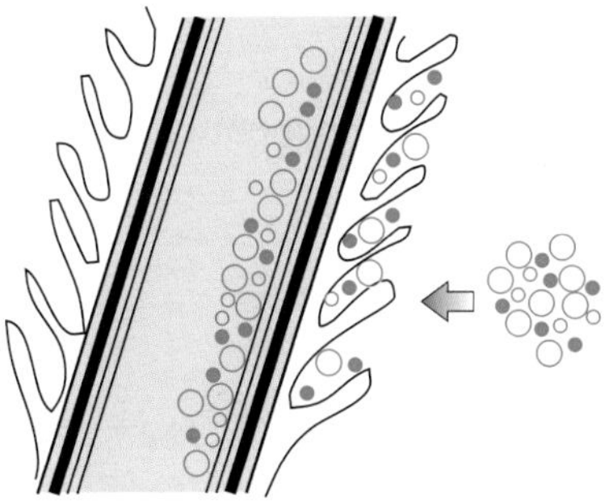

Figure 6.30 Action of deposit-only hair colour

Selecting and formulating a deposit-only (quasi-permanent) colour

Deposit-only hair colours are ideal for grey coverage, to refresh permanent tints, for corrective colouring, lowlighting and for creating quick fashion effects.

By its very nature, a deposit-only hair colour will darken the natural hair colour when applied. Remember, when formulating, that half of your formula will be the client's natural hair colour and half will be the depositing colour you have selected. Since colour on top of colour always appears darker, select a deposit-only colour lighter than the client's natural level if you intend to keep the same amount of depth but add tone.

Since grey hair has no pigment and appears lighter, it is important to consider the grey hair in your formulation of a deposit-only hair colour. As there is no lift, the resulting depth of colour when covering grey may appear too extreme unless you allow for some brightness in your formulation. It is often inadvisable to make grey hair one even shade when colouring with any product, since natural hair colour has different depths and tonalities that give the hair the added life that grey hair is lacking.

> ***TIP*** When selecting the formulation for the use of these colours on high percentages of white hair, to avoid over strong or bright results, add base tone to any fashion tone selected.

It is always better when taking a client from lighter to darker to err on the side of lightness, because a darker tone can easily be used to deepen the colour if necessary. A result that is too dark, on the other hand, will involve corrective procedures to lighten or remove the artificial pigment before re-applying to achieve the desired colour.

Hair previously treated with another colour service will have a greater degree of porosity, which must be considered carefully when formulating and applying a deposit-only hair colour.

Application procedure for deposit-only (quasi-permanent) colours

The application procedure for a deposit-only hair colour is similar to that of a semi-permanent colour, since neither type of colour alters the hair's natural melanin or produces lift. Follow the manufacturer's application and timing guidelines for the product that you have selected.

For successful hair colouring services, the colourist must follow a definite procedure. A system makes for the greatest efficiency, and the most satisfactory results. Without such a plan, the work will take longer, results will be uneven, and mistakes will be made.

> ***TIP*** Remember that while these colours fall within the semi-permanent hair colour section, most do require a skin test before each application.

Permanent hair colouring

Permanent hair colours are prepared from a variety of materials: vegetables, flowers, herbs, salts of heavy metals, organic and synthetic chemicals. All of these permanent colours fall into one of four classifications: vegetable tints, metallic dyes, compound dyestuffs, or oxidation tints. Practically all permanent hair colouring is done with the use of oxidising penetrating tints that contain aniline derivatives.

These tints penetrate the cuticle of the hair and enter the cortical layer. Here, they are oxidised by the peroxide added into colour pigments. These pigments are distributed throughout the hair shaft much like natural pigment.

Vegetable tints

In the past, before technology brought us the hairdressing industry as we now know it, many vegetable materials such as camomile and henna were used as hair colouring ingredients.

Camomile

Camomile flowers can be ground into a powder and used as a paste. It gives a lighter brighter effect to blonde hair. Shampoos and rinses containing powdered flowers are intended to add a bright yellow colour in the hair. However, camomile's effectiveness is limited to a minimal colour change.

Henna

Henna is the most noteworthy and popular of the vegetable colours and comes from plants grown in moist climates throughout Africa, Arabia, Iran, and the East Indies. The henna leaves are removed before the flowering cycle, dried, and ground into a fine powder. Hot water is added to create a paste that is applied to the hair.

> ***TIP*** Vegetable colours can form an alternative for clients who show an allergy to oxidation colouring.

Henna is a natural product that appeals to the young client and consumers who prefer organic products and avoid synthetics. Its 'natural' qualities appeal to many.

Current technology has brought to the market henna in black, chestnut, and auburn, plus a lightener. These hennas are made of concentrated herbal extracts that have both a cumulative and a semi-permanent effect. The dye coats the hair and is partially removed by shampooing.

The coating action of henna creates a hair strand that becomes thicker, and thus helps to give body to fine, limp hair. Because it makes no structural changes in the hair, it can be used on weak hair without damaging it. Henna fills in a roughened cuticle and holds together split ends to provide a slick, light-reflective surface. This, coupled with the additional warmth, creates hair that shines.

> ***NOTE*** The coating effect of Henna can make the hair resistant to permanent waving.

Metallic hair dyes

Metallic hair colours can be recognised by the descriptive terms used by manufacturers in their packaging even before reading the ingredients list. Metallic dyes are known as 'progressive hair colours' and 'colour restorers'. They are referred to as 'progressive' because hair progressively turns darker and darker upon each subsequent application. The term 'colour restorer' is used because the natural hair colour *appears* to be gradually restored. When the desired colour is reached, the consumer needs to reduce the frequency of application to maintain the colour.

Metallic hair dyes comprise a minor portion of the home hair-colouring market and currently are very rarely used professionally. Nevertheless, it is crucial for the professional colourist to be informed of the chemical composition, characteristics, and methods of removal, because metals react adversely with oxidation tints.

> ***TIP*** During your consultation with the client, if you see a progressive darkening of the hair towards the hair ends without a definite line of demarcation, and with a somewhat drab, lacklustre colour, it can often mean that metallic salts are present.

Clients occasionally request chemical services without knowing the incompatibility of metallic colour with professional oxidation products. Consumers generally do not even realise that they used a product containing metal. The colourist must be able to analyse and prescribe safe, professional treatments to avoid hair damage and discolouration.

The metallic coating builds up on the surface of the hair shaft. Repeated treatments leave the hair brittle and conflict with future chemical services that include in their formulation hydrogen peroxide, thioglycolate, ammonia, and/or most other oxidisers.

Resulting damage might be discolouration, breakage, poor permanent waving results, and even destruction to the point of a melted hair shaft due to the heat created in this adverse chemical reaction.

Compound dyes

Compound dyes are a combination of metallic salts or mineral dyes with a vegetable tint. The metallic salts are added to give the product more staying power and to create a wider range of colours. Like metallic dyes, compound dyes are not often used professionally.

Many clients use hair colouring products at home. Therefore, you must be able to recognise and understand their effects. Such colouring agents must be removed and the hair reconditioned prior to any other chemical service.

Hair treated with metallic or any other coating dye looks dry and dull. It is generally harsh and brittle to touch. These colourings usually fade to unnatural tones. Silver dyes have a greenish cast, lead dyes leave a purple colour, and those containing copper turn red.

Test for metallic salts (incompatibility test)

1. In a glass container, mix 30 ml of 20 volume (6%) peroxide and 20 drops of 28% ammonia water.
2. Cut a strand of the client's hair, bind it with tape, and immerse in the solution for 30 minutes.
3. Remove, towel dry, and observe the strand.

Hair dyed with lead will lighten immediately. Hair treated with silver will show no reaction at all. This indicates that other chemicals will not be successful because they will not be able to penetrate the coating.

Hair treated with copper will start to boil and will pull apart easily. This hair would be severely damaged or destroyed if other chemicals such as those found in permanent oxidation colours or perm solutions were applied to it.

Hair treated with a coating dye either will not change or will lighten in spots. This hair will not receive chemical services easily, and the length of time necessary for penetration may very well damage the hair.

Preparations designed to remove metallics and non-peroxide dye solvents may assist in the removal of metallic and coating dyes from the hair. Performing a strand test will indicate whether the metallic deposits have been removed.

> ***TIP*** The most effective guarantee of future successful chemical services is to cut the tinted hair off.

Oxidation hair colour

Permanent oxidation hair colours can lighten and deposit colour in one application, a feat performed by no other classification. This ability to create an infinite array of levels, tones, and intensities has made permanent colours irreplaceable in the industry. These tints penetrate the cuticle of the hair and enter the cortical layer (see Figure 6.31). Here, they are oxidised by the peroxide added into colour pigments. These pigments are distributed throughout the hair shaft much like natural pigment (see Figure 6.32).

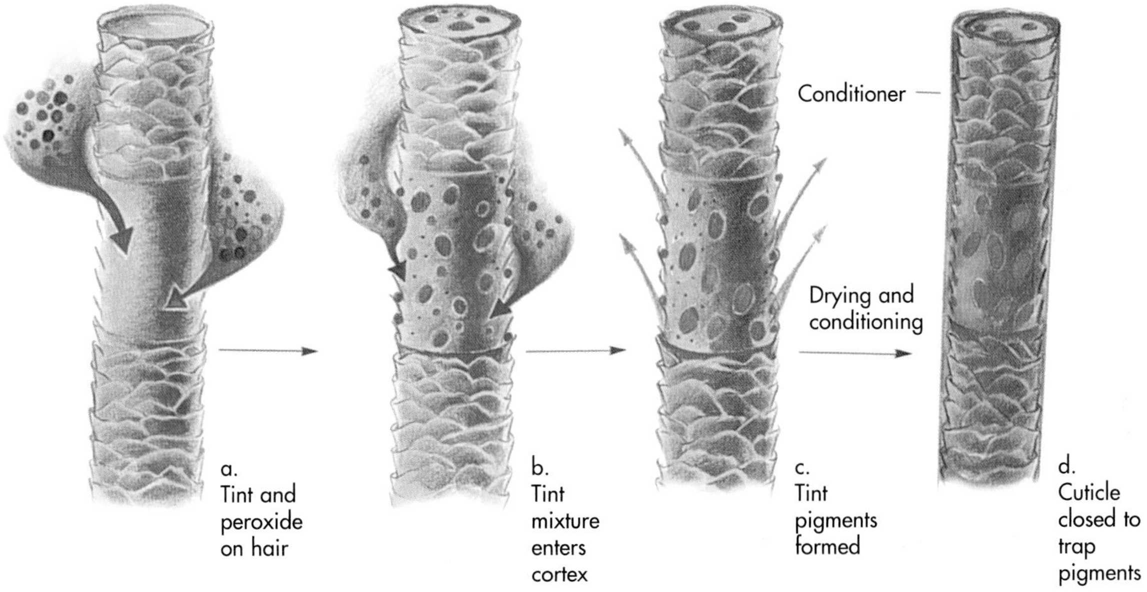

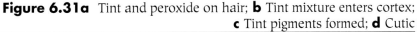

Figure 6.31a Tint and peroxide on hair; **b** Tint mixture enters cortex; **c** Tint pigments formed; **d** Cutic

Application classifications

Permanent hair colour applications are classified as either single-process colouring or double-process colouring.

Single-process colouring achieves the desired colour with one application. Although the application itself may have several different steps, the desired colour is achieved with a single application. Lightening of the hair's natural pigment and deposit of the artificial pigment in the cortex is done simultaneously as the hair colouring product processes. Some examples of single-process colouring are virgin tint applications and tint retouch applications.

Double-process colouring achieves the desired colour upon completion of two separate product applications. It is also known as double-application tinting and two-step colouring. Two

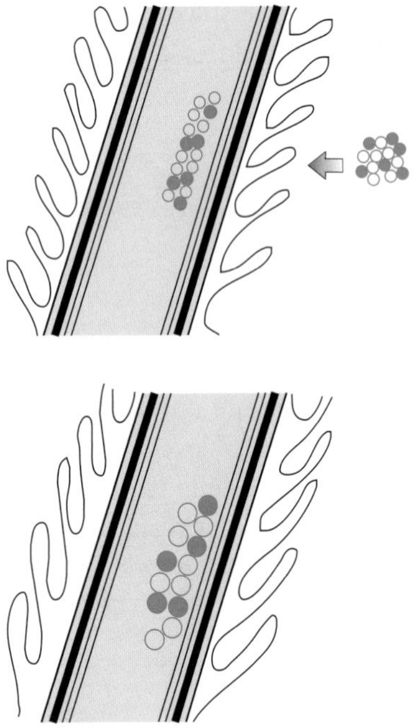

Figure 6.32 Action of permanent hair colour

examples are bleaching followed by a toner application and pre-softening followed by a tint application. Because the lightening action and the colour deposit are independently controlled, a wider range of hair colour possibilities is opened up for each client.

Hydrogen peroxide

This is available both as a cream and a liquid, and is the most widely-used provider of oxygen for the oxidation process that takes place when oxidation tints and bleaches are applied to hair.

In the case of oxidation tints, the oxygen provided by the hydrogen peroxide causes the development of the colour combining with the dye material within the cortex to form a colour molecule too large to exit the hair shaft.

When bleaching, oxygen also changes the natural pigment of the hair, changing the melanin molecule from a coloured to a colourless compound. Those pigments most easily affected are ash tones and brown shades, then reds and finally yellow.

Peroxide strength

The strength of hydrogen peroxide is desrcibed in two ways:

- volume
- percentage strength.

Volume describes the amount of oxygen released by the product during decomposition. Therefore one litre of 20 volume hydrogen peroxide will release 20 litres of oxygen leaving 1 litre of spent product. One litre of 60 volume will release 60 litres of oxygen. 5 – 10 – 20 volume hydrogen peroxide is mixed with oxidation tint when adding depth to the natural hair colour (darkening) and 30 – 40 – 60 is used when lightening. Always follow the manufacturer's directions when selecting the strength of peroxide to use.

> ***REMEMBER*** A predisposition test must be given before colouring the hair with an oxidation tint. You should protect yourself from allergic reactions and dermatitis by wearing protective gloves until the product is completely removed from the client's hair.

Forms of hydrogen peroxide

Cream peroxide contains additives such as thickeners, drabbers and an acid for stabilisation. The thickeners help to create a product that is easy to control. This thicker mix is less likely to bleed when producing woven highlights. The creamy formula also tends to stay moist on the hair longer than liquid peroxide.

Liquid peroxide, H_2O_2 appears similar to water, a clear liquid to which a stabiliser, usually an acid, is added. The acid reduces oxidation (oxygen loss) until mixed with a product containing an alkali, which neutralises this action and speeds up oxygen release. Once the available oxygen has been released, water is left behind with no dangerous residue.

> ***HEALTH AND SAFETY*** Hydrogen peroxide is an irritant to skin and eyes, rinse affected area with sterile water, if irritation perists seek medical advice immediately.

Oxidation tint application

> ***HEALTH AND SAFETY*** The Control of Substances Hazardous to Health Regulations (1988) require employers to:
>
> - identify substances in the workplace that are potentially hazardous.
> - assess the risk to health from exposure to the hazardous substances and record the results.
> - make an assessment as to which members of staff are at risk.
> - look for alternative less hazardous substances and substitute if possible.
> - decide what precautions are required, noting that the use of Personal Protective Equipment should always be the last resort.
> - introduce effective measures to prevent or control the exposure.
> - inform, instruct and train all members of staff.
> - review the assessment on a regular basis.

Materials preparation

All materials to be used should be in prime condition. Tint product may come in bottles, tubes or cans. Check that no oxidation has already taken place in the product; this may be indicated by a darkening of the product. Ensure that the developer or hydrogen peroxide is in good condition and is of the correct volume (percentage) strength. Materials required are:

- selected tint
- hydrogen peroxide
- cotton wool
- mild shampoo
- after colour conditioner/colour fixer
- protective cream.

All tools used should be in good repair, clean and dry prior to use. You will need:

- non-metallic bowl
- measuring cylinder/jug
- tinting brush/applicator
- timer
- record card
- tinting cape and towels
- protective gloves
- plastic clips.

Client preparation

1. Give a patch test 24 to 48 hours before the colouring service and record the outcome. Proceed only if the test result is negative.
2. Thoroughly analyse the scalp and hair. Consult and discuss with your client the colour and product to be used.
3. Check the scalp for any cuts, abrasions and contagious disorders. The presence of any of these will contraindicate the colouring process.
4. Gown your client, following your salon's procedures. This will normally include the use of a client gown, colouring towels and impenetrable tinting cape. Gowning should protect your client and their clothing from contamination from the tinting product about to be used. Jewellery should be removed.
5. Brush the hair, taking care not to scratch the surface of the scalp.
6. Assemble all tools that will be required during the colouring process (see section on *Materials preparation*).
7. Perform any necessary preconditioning treatments.
8. Carry out a strand test, if required.

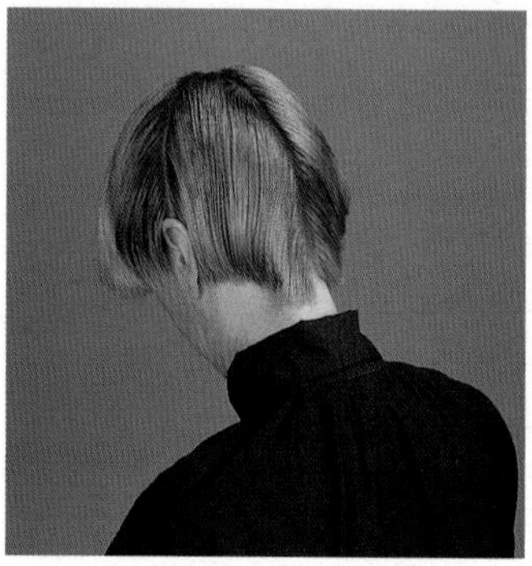

Figure 6.33 Hair sectioned for tinting

9. Divide the hair into four quarters (see Figure 6.33). Apply barrier cream to the hairline and ears when applying dark levels of colour or when the skin is very dry.
10. Prepare the product, mixing the formulation following the manufacturer's directions. Do this at the dispensary, not in front of your client, in case you spill product on the client. Ensure that all products that you use are in prime condition and are mixed in clean non-metallic utensils.

HEALTH AND SAFETY When mixing tint, an amount of ammonia is given of to the atmosphere, avoid inhaling this. Always prepare the product in a well-ventilated area.

Always follow the manufacturer's directions. Accurately measure the quantities of tint product into a non-metallic bowl. If using cream tint, cream the tint as this will aid mixing with the hydrogen peroxide. If preparing colours that are a combination of shades mix the tint product together before adding any peroxide.

TIP Accurate measurement of product is essential to ensure predictable and consistent results.

Accurately measure the hydrogen peroxide and then mix with the tint product. When mixing products of differing thickness, add only small quantities of peroxide at a time to the tint mixing the two together well. In some cases shakers and applicator bottles are used for the mixing process. Once mixed the oxidation process begins, so mix only quantities that you need to use immediately.

Procedure for first time application (virgin hair)

TIP Manufacturers often provide suggested methods of application. If in doubt, read their directions.

1. Put on protective gloves.
2. Begin in the section where the colour change will be the greatest or the hair is most resistant, and consult the record card for indication of any particular areas of resistance. If there is no specified area it is usual to start at the back of the head.

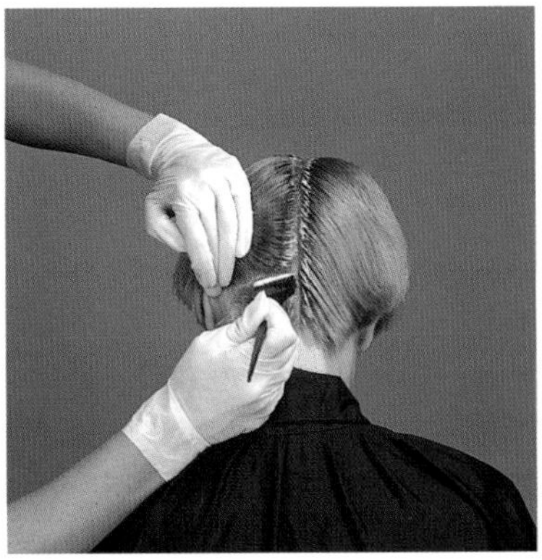

Figure 6.34 Applying tint to root area starting at the back of the head

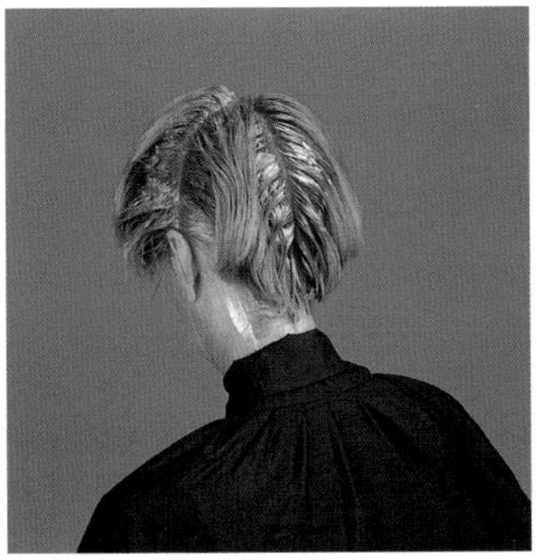

Figure 6.35 Back sections, regrowth application

3. Part off a section of hair 0.5 cm in depth, using the tail of the application brush.
4. Apply the product to the middle lengths and ends of the hair, to within 1 cm of the scalp. Scalp heat will aid and speed-up colour development at the root area. Application to the middle lengths and ends first will give this area a greater length of time to develop and therefore result in an overall even result.
5. Ensure that all the hair within each mesh of hair is covered by the tint product. Take care not to apply too much product, as this may result in product dripping onto your client, as well as product wastage.

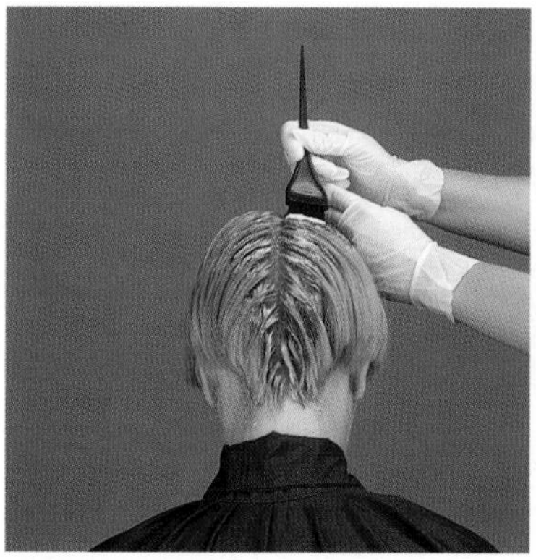

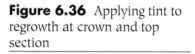

Figure 6.36 Applying tint to regrowth at crown and top section

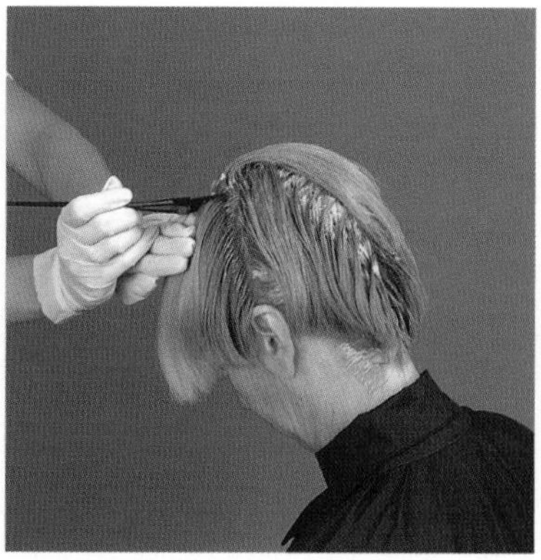

Figure 6.37 Applying tint to front regrowth sections

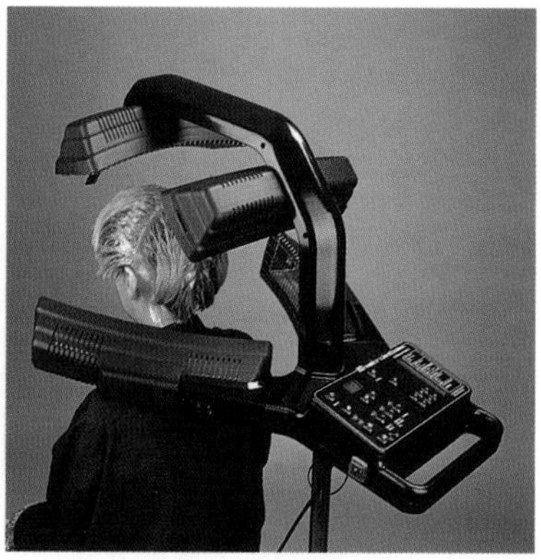

Figure 6.38 Using the accelerator to assist colour development

6. From the nape area progress up one side of the back of the head to the crown area. Take care not to press the tinted mesh of hair onto the untinted root areas of other meshes, as this will bring about an uneven result and overprocessing in certain areas.

> ***NOTE*** Some manufacturers recommend a one-step application when darkening hair in a first-time application. This means applying the product from the roots to the points in one application. Check the manufacturer's directions.

7. Once the crown area is reached, start at the nape on the other side of the back and progress up this side of the back to the crown area.
8. Apply the product to the two front sections, taking care not to allow the product to drip onto your client's face or ears.
9. Cross-check your application to ensure that all the hair's middle length is covered by the product.
10. Allow the product to develop, usually for 10 to 15 minutes (check manufacturer's recommendation). Heat may be applied to aid development (subject to manufacturer's directions). This may be applied in the form of a scalp steamer, the method of using which is described on page 34. An accelerator/radiant heater may also be used, methods of use described on page 35. Take care not to allow the product to dry out on the hair.

> ***HEALTH AND SAFETY*** Always unplug electrical appliances, using dry hands, once their use is no longer required.

11. Check the colour development by wiping a strand free of product, using moist cotton wool, and checking the colour against the required outcome, using the shade guide.
12. Once sufficient development has been identified, prepare a fresh supply of the product and apply this to the root area, up to the product already on the middle lengths. This is carried out by taking similar sized sections in the same order as for the first application.

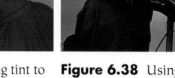

TIP Avoid sitting your client where draughts of hot or cold air may affect the hair, producing an uneven colour development. A cold room will slow down the development.

13. Check that all the hair has been coated with the product. Allow to develop, in the same manner as previous. A full processing period will be required for this fresh application of product to the hair.
14. Check the development of the colour by wiping a strand of hair free of tint using moist cotton wool. Check the resulting colour for evenness and for its match to the desired finished colour.
15. If the development is incomplete, re-apply product to the test strand and leave to develop further. If the development is complete move your client to the basin area.

Your client should view their new hair colour in natural daylight. They should be made fully aware of how their colour will appear once they leave the salon. The hair will be damaged by the chemicals during the colouring process. Most modern colour products reduce hair damage to a minimum, and contain buffers to reduce this effect and have conditioners to compensate. Your client may not be accustomed to handling their hair in its new condition and therefore will require guidance in its after-care. Home care products should be recommended and guidance in their correct use be given to your client, to enable them to maintain their new colour and condition, as well as reduce fade.

Guidance will be required in when to make follow-up visits to the salon.

Procedure for retouch application

The fresh growth of hair will require colouring at intervals of approximately one month. This is the job of the professional hair colourist.

Always consult with your client before undertaking a retouch colour. Check if the colour required is the same as the previous colour service given.

1. Put on protective gloves.
2. Begin in the section where the colour change will be the greatest or the hair is most resistant, consult the record card for indication of any particular areas of resistance. If there is no specified area it is usual to start at the back of the head (see Figures 6.39–6.41).
3. Part off a section of hair 0.5 cm in depth, using the tail of the application brush.

TIP Ensure accurate measurement of product to maintain continuity of hair colour.

4. Apply the product to the regrowth area. If the regrowth is longer than 1.5 cm it should be treated as if it were a first time application. This is because body heat from the scalp may not affect the hair past this point.
5. Ensure that all the regrowth hair within each mesh of hair is covered by the tint product. Take care not to apply too much product, as this may result in product running down the hair, as well as product wastage.

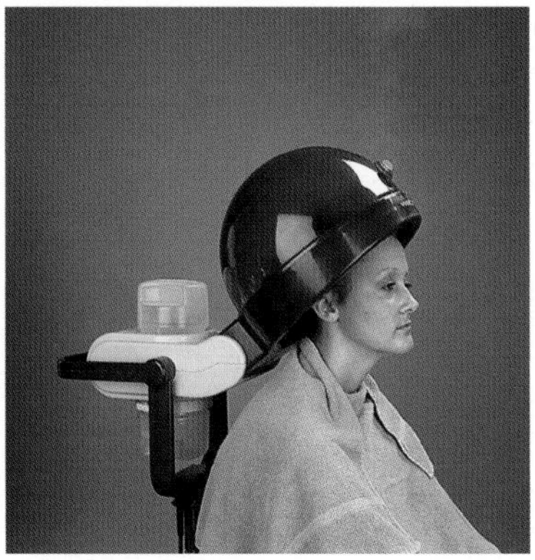

Figure 6.39 Scalp steamer

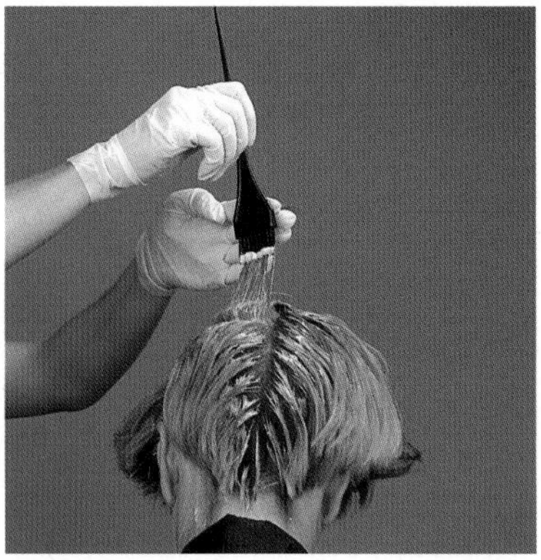

Figure 6.40 Applying tint to middle lengths and ends of hair

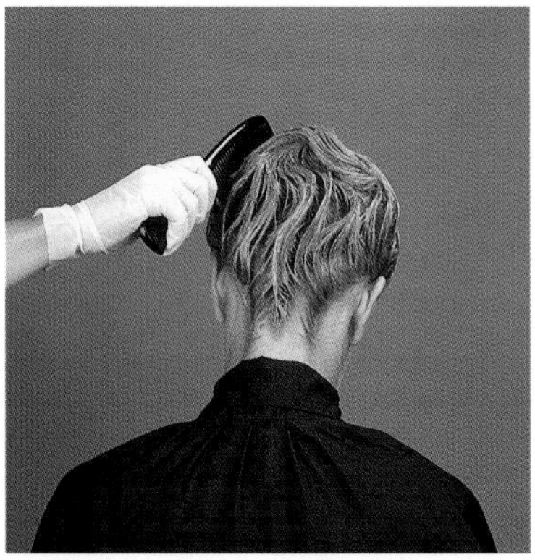

Figure 6.41 Tint applied to all the hair

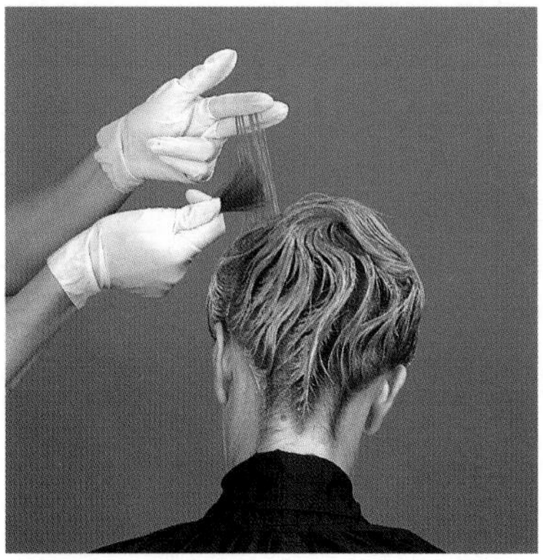

Figure 6.42 Checking hair colour development

TIP Overlapping colour onto previously coloured hair may result in banding of colour, damage to the hair, and even hair breakage.

6. From the nape area progress up one side of the back of the head to the crown area. Take care not to press the ends of the hair onto the tinted root areas of other meshes, as this will result in an uneven result and overprocessing in certain areas.
7. Once the crown area is reached, start at the nape on the other side of the back and progress up this side of the back to the crown area (see Figure 6.42).
8. Apply the product to the two front sections, taking care not to allow the product to drip onto your client's face or ears (see Figure 6.43).
9. Cross-check your application to ensure that all the regrowth is covered by the product.
10. Allow the product to develop, usually for 20 to 35 minutes. Check the manufacturer's recommendation. Heat may be applied to aid development (subject to manufacturer's directions). This may be applied in the form of a scalp steamer: method of use is described on page 34. An accelerator/radiant heater may also be used, its method of use is also described on page 37. Take care not to allow the product to dry out on the hair (see Figures 6.38 and 6.39).
11. Check the colour development by wiping a strand free of product, using moist cotton wool and checking the colour against the required outcome, using the shade guide.

12. Once sufficient development has been identified, consider if the colour of the middle lengths and ends require refreshing. Do not unnecessarily apply colour to the middle lengths and ends as this may result in damage to the hair and a progressive darkening (colour build-up). Fresh tint, diluted tint, or semi-permanent colour may be used to refresh the colour in these areas. The choice may depend upon the degree or amount of colour fade (see Figure 6.40).
13. Check that all the hair has been coated with the product. Allow to develop, in the same manner as previously. A full processing period will be required for this fresh application of product to the hair (see Figure 6.41).
14. Check the development of the colour by wiping a strand of hair free of tint using moist cotton wool. Check the resulting colour for evenness and for its match to the desired finished colour (see Figure 6.42).
15. If the development is incomplete, re-apply product to the test strand and leave to develop further. If the development is complete move your client to the basin area.

Removing the product from the hair

TIP At this time the scalp may be a little sensitive, so take care to control the water temperature applied to the scalp, and avoid the warmer temperatures.

1. Massage the product on the hair and scalp, paying particular attention to the hairline, where this process will help to lift any skin staining (moist tint will remove skin staining at this time). This massage will also help to emulsify the product and aid its easier removal from the hair. 1
2. Follow the manufacturer's directions in product removal. If you are in doubt about the correct process consult with your line manager, stylist or trainer. In most cases this will include adding a small quantity of warm water to the product on the hair. Massage this to emulsify, add more warm water, massage and then rinse away.
3. Thoroughly rinse the product from the hair.
4. Shampoo the hair thoroughly, using a mild (acid-balanced) shampoo. The acid-balanced shampoo will help to flatten the hair cuticle, prevent any creeping oxidation (continued oxidation action in the hair), and help to return the hair to its normal pH.
5. Apply an anti-oxidation, fixing, finishing rinse to the hair. The exact product to be used may depend on salon procedures and manufacturer's directions.
6. Style the hair.
7. Complete the record card and file or enter onto the computerised data base.

Clean-up

1. Dispose of all disposable supplies and materials. 1
2. Close containers firmly, wipe them clean and put them in their proper place. Never return unused products to their containers as they may be contaminated and will subsequently contaminate all of the product in the container.
3. Wash and dry all equipment, and place soiled linen in the laundry basket.
4. Clean the working area.
5. Wash and dry your hands.

HIGHLIGHT AND LOWLIGHT EFFECTS IN HAIR COLOURING

Highlighting and lowlighting techniques for hair colouring use lighter or darker shades of hair colour to enhance and accentuate your client's hair colour and hair style (see Figure 6.43). A combination of lighter and darker shades may be used to give depth and dimensions to the hair-style. A single additional shade may be used to accentuate natural tone in the hair or to define movement in the hairstyle. There are a number of techniques available, some of which produce effects throughout the entire head of hair and others which are designed specifically for small areas of the hairstyle.

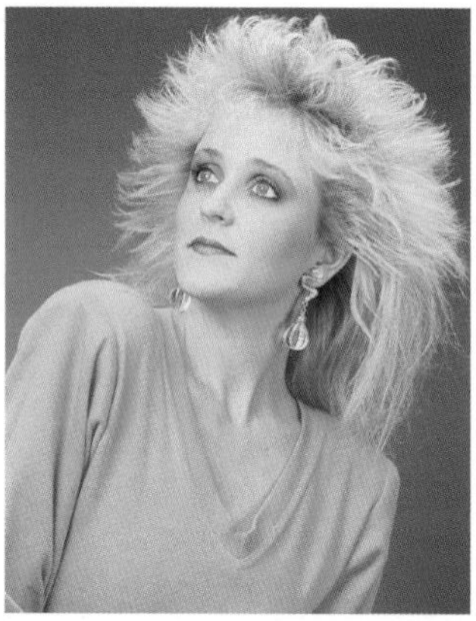

Figure 6.43 Special effects hair lightening

Techniques of highlighting and lowlighting

Weaving techniques

There are a number of techniques used to weave small strands of hair from the bulk that may then either be coloured or lightened, or a combination of both. There are a variety of specialist tools to produce this effect, but in most cases the point end of a pin-tail comb is used to weave out the strands of hair. These strands are subsequently separated from the bulk of the hair using aluminium foil, fine film wrap, proprietary brand sachets or tissue.

> ***TIP*** A predisposition test is not normally required prior to the application of a bleach product. However if your client has a history of hypersensitivity a skin test may be advisable.

Client preparation

1. Discuss and negotiate the required result with your client. This will include details of the required overall hairstyle, the required colour effect, the density of the woven sections and the cost of the service. Check any colour record cards available for your client.
2. Carry our predisposition test, 24 – 48 hours beforehand, if a permanent oxidation tint is to be used.
3. Gown your client as for a permanent form of hair colouring.
4. Section the hair, according to the required hairstyle, to give control over the hair when weaving.

Product preparation

1. Prepare the sachets that will be used in the process. When using aluminium foil these may be available in prepared batches, already cut to specified lengths. Others come on a continuous roll which must then be cut to slightly more than twice the length of the hair to be coloured. Fold one end of the foil over at approximately 5 mm deep to produce a more rigid band to hold against the root area at the scalp. When using fine film wrap this is cut as it is required, and is used at its full width. Proprietary brands of sachets consist of a plastic-based sachet with a transparent cover and a mild adhesive strip. If working without assistance a number of these should be opened ready for use. When working on very long hair it may be necessary to join two of these together. Sachets usually come in a variety of lengths. Tissue may be used to separate strands of coloured hair from the rest. The colour product must be of a thick consistency. For this technique, a spatula is required. The strands to be coloured are placed on the spatula and the colour product applied. The spatula is withdrawn and the coloured hair allowed to fall onto the tissue.
2. Prepare a small quantity of the colouring product. As this process can be quite lengthy, small measured quantities of product prepared when required are better than preparing a large quantity at the outset which then deteriorates before it is used on the hair.
3. You will require protective rubber gloves.

> ***TIP*** Remember that once mixed the colouring/bleaching product begins to oxidise and if too long a period elapses before its use it may have fully oxidised before it touches the hair. It will therefore have little or no effect on the hair.

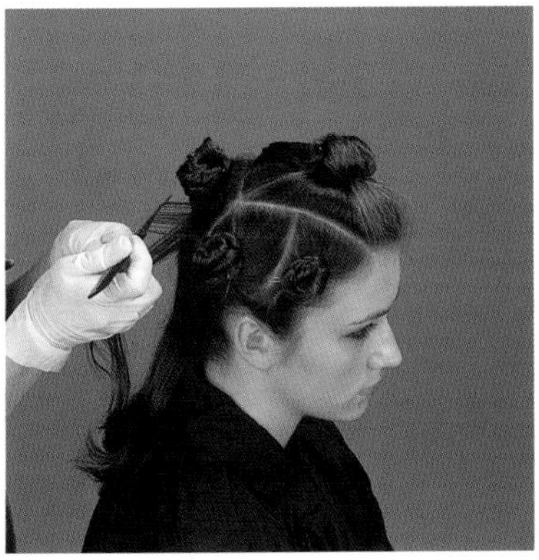

Figure 6.44 Weaving subsection with tail comb.

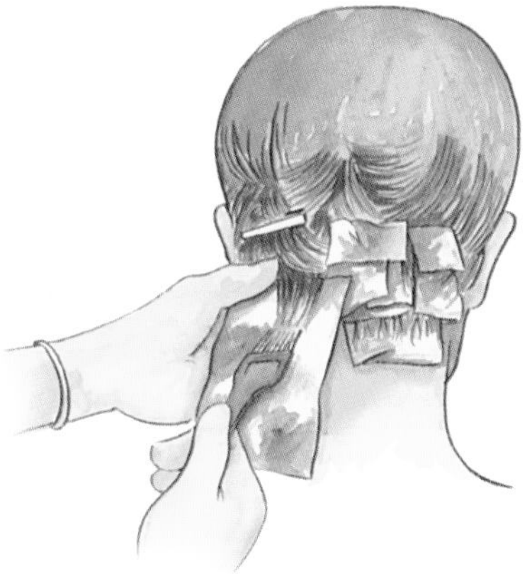

Figure 6.45 Place hair in foil packets

Weaving the highlights

1. It is usual to start at the bottom of the hair section, as the woven meshes will hang down and should not be disturbed. Start at that area of the head where the highest degree of colour change is required, or where the hair is most resistant, if the degree of resistance is known.
2. Using the pin tail of the comb, draw off a mesh which is 1 cm deep and then slice off the top 3 mm of this mesh (see Figure 6.44). Allow the larger section to fall and retain the smaller, held firmly outwards from the head, tangle-free.

3. Weave out fine strands to be coloured, by pushing the point of the pin tail (held parallel to the mesh) across the mesh, pressing down at those points when the strand to be coloured is required. When you begin to practise this skill it will be a slow process, however with much practice not only will your speed develop but also your ability to draw off consistent sizes of meshes (see Figure 6.44).
4. Now hold out the woven-off strands from the head while the remainder of the hair is allowed to fall. Place the sachet close to the roots of these strands at the scalp, and then lay the strands onto the foil and apply the colour (see Figure 6.45). Do not apply the colour product all the way to the scalp, as this may result in seepage onto the rest of the hair. Apply to within 5 mm of the scalp: the product will be drawn along the hair to the scalp.

TIP To assist in holding aluminium foil in place when laying the hair onto it, apply a small amount of the colouring mix to the foil before locating it in place. Once the hair is laid onto this the adhesion will help to hold the foil and hair together.

5. Once the colour/bleach mix has been applied to the strands of hair, fold the sachet to secure it on the hair and to retain the product within it. Avoid pressing on the bulk of the sachet as this may cause the product to ooze from the sachet and then contaminate the other hair.
6. Continue to do this throughout the head in a systematic manner. As this can be a lengthy process, check the colour development of those sachets placed earlier as you progress around the head.
7. When making a section at the front hairline, take a parting at a slight angle to the hairline, this will avoid obvious lines of colour appearing. Avoid locating strands of colour on the parting or on the very edge of the hairline, as the regrowth will be very apparent as the hair grows.
8. Allow the hair to process without additional heat as this can cause the product within the sachet to either become more liquid (if it is an oil-based product) or to expand (all oxidation products do this) and therefore ooze onto adjacent hair and cause unsightly patches of colour.
9. When using permanent hair colours allow the product to process for the full development period following the application of the final sachet. When using bleach you must check the degree of lift from the earlier made sachets, as these may have fully processed before the later ones. If this is the case remove these sachets and using moist cotton wool remove the bleach from the hair.

TIP Too much colour product within the sachet may result in seepage onto the rest of the hair.

10. Once the colour has fully processed take your client to the basin area. Recline them to the basin and then begin rinsing the hair using lukewarm water. As the water floods the hair the sachets may be removed by sliding them from the hair.
11. Rinse the colour from the hair, shampoo using a post-colour shampoo and follow with a pH balance/anti-oxidation conditioner. This will help to prevent creeping oxidation and to close the cuticle flat.
12. Complete your client's record card, noting the products used, the techniques applied and the results.

Clean-up

All used materials should be disposed off. Those highlighting sachets made for repeat use should be washed, dried and stored for future use. Used linen should be disposed of in the laundry bin, and all containers returned to their storage area.

Cap technique

The cap technique involves pulling clean strands of hair through a perforated cap using a hook (see Figure 6.46). This technique is best suited to use on short hair, though there are brands of highlight cap specifically designed for use on long hair. Due to the translucent nature of many brands of highlight cap, it can be difficult to determine the exact position of the highlights in relation to the hairstyle.

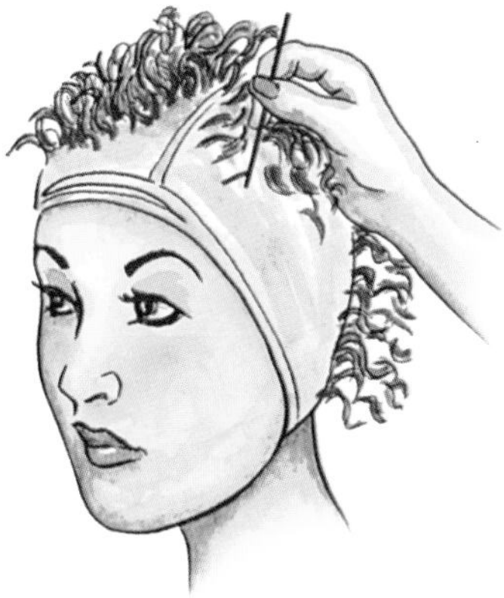

Figure 6.46 Draw strands through holes in cap

Preparation of the materials

1. Select the type of cap or material to create the cap, the selection of which will often be personal preference. Proprietary brands of highlight cap can usually be used for several applications. For its first use the holes in the cap will need breaking open, using the hook. Take care not to press the hook hard onto the scalp. The areas for the perforations are usually strengthened to avoid tearing and seepage of the colouring product from the outside surface. The interior of the cap should be lightly coated with talc, as this will enable it to slide into position on dry hair. Polythene sheet or fine film wrap may be used in place of the pre-formed cap. The scalp area is enclosed within the wrap and then secured around the hairline using clear adhesive tape. These styles of caps can be susceptible to tearing for those inexperienced with the technique.Other brands of cap may require the application of heat to tighten them to the head shape.
2. Select the hook size relative to the texture of the hair and the thickness of the strands of hair required. The larger the hook size the greater the size of strand drawn through.
3. Select the colouring products, **do not** mix the product until all of the strands of hair have been drawn through the cap.

> ***TIP*** Check that your client's ears are not trapped or folded under the latex cap.

Client preparation

This is the same as for woven highlights.

Drawing through the highlights

1. Brush the client's hair into the direction of the hairstyle and then ease the highlight

cap into place. You will need to locate the *latex* cap by placing your hands on the inside, palms open, and easing the cap into place. Ensure that the cap is tight to the scalp, particularly at the crown area.

2. Plastic caps are rather like bonnets which are located firmly over the hair and then held in place by a tie under the client's chin. Polythene sheet and fine film wrap is located onto the scalp area as firmly as possible and while it is held in place clear adhesive tape is bound around the hairline. Excess sheet or wrap is then trimmed off, taking care not to cut the hair beneath.
3. Lengths of hair which hang from beneath the cap should be gathered together in the nape and protected from colouring product.
4. Draw the strands of hair through the cap starting at the top of the hairstyle. Gently but firmly push the hook through the cap. As you collect hair in the hook, to ensure that the full length of the hair is coloured, gather hair at the root area. Ease this hair through the cap. The closeness and thickness of the strands depends on the thickness of your client's hair and the required outcome. When a subtle effect is required more fine strands may be drawn through. For a more obvious result fewer thicker strands are drawn through.

TIP Avoid using colour mixes which are too thin as these may seep through the holes in the cap and therefore result in a blotchy result.

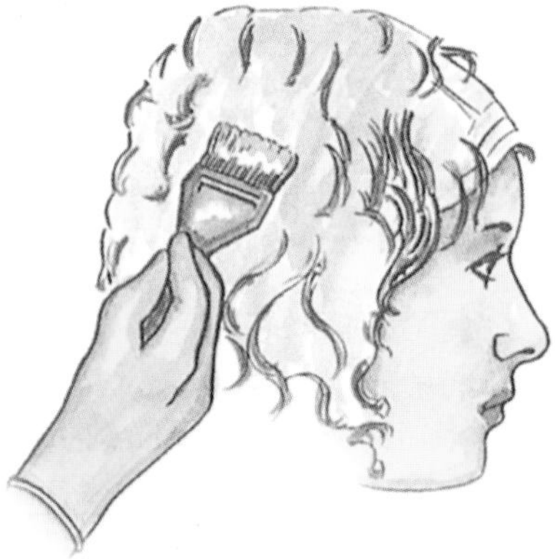

Figure 6.47 Apply lightener to selected strands

5. When all the strands are drawn through, check to ensure that the cap is still firmly against the scalp. Gently grasp the strands between the fingers and pull to ensure that they are fully through the cap, and using the fine teeth of a comb, gently comb the hair to ensure that there are no tangles or partly pulled through strands.
6. Mix the colouring/bleach product and apply this to the hair strands which have been drawn through the cap (see Figure 6.47). Start the application of the product to the top of the head, and section by section paste the product onto the hair in an upward direction. In this manner the product-coated hair will lay on the cap instead of hanging down on your client's face and neck.
7. Process as for other forms of permanent hair colouring. Take care: heat applied may cause oil-based colouring products to become more fluid and these may drip onto the client or seep through the hole in the cap.
8. Check the colour development as for other forms of permanent hair colouring. Once the processing is complete at the basin, rinse the product from the hair and cap. The use of high water pressure may result in wetting your client.

9. Apply a conditioning cream to the strands of hair if no subsequent colouring is required, and ease the cap off the head. The cream acts as a lubricant, preventing drag on the hair that might otherwise cause discomfort and hair damage due to over-stretching.
10. Continue as for the removal of other forms of permanent hair colour.

Clean-up

Dispose of all disposable items in a covered bin. Reusable highlight caps should be rinsed clean, dried and then a fine film of talc applied. Place used linen in the laundry basket and return part-used containers to the storage area.

OUTCOME	CAUSE	ACTION
Scalp irritation immediately	high strength of peroxide; allergy to product	remove product and rinse with cold water: seek medical advice
Hair breakage	over processing; overlapping onto previously coloured hair; too early comb through of product; incompatible chemicals	remove immediately; use restructurant; use penetrating conditioner
Uneven result	poor application; uneven application; uneven mixing of product; too large hair sections; seepage of product during highlight process – too much product – incorrect product – incorrect use of applied heat to product – product applied to scalp	spot colour to produce even result
Poor coverage	hair resistant; tint underprocessed; poor quality product; lack of red (white/blond hair)	pre-soften hair; re-colour; spot colour; pre-pigment
Incorrect tone	under processed; base too dark (yellow cast); base to light (green cast); incorrect H_2O_2 use	re-colour/bleach if hair tests confirm tensile strength; pre-pigment and re-colour

FURTHER STUDY

- Collect a portfolio of manufacturer's directions that you may use as a reference when using hair colouring products.
- Build a portfolio of your hair colouring achievements, which you may use as evidence of your skill as well as forming a tool for communicating your range of skill to your client.
- This chapter introduces you to the basic skills of hair colouring. Find out more about alternative colouring techniques and techniques of corrective colouring.
- Artificial pigment requires specialist techniques to remove it from hair. Consult with your supplier on the products available to do this and then find out how they may be used and what their features and limitations are.
- Recolouring lightened hair can result in the production of unwanted green tones. Pre-pigmentation is the technique use to prevent this. Find out the variety of techniques that may be used for this.
- Many clients seek quick, cost-effective ways of using hair colour to accentuate their hairstyle. Watch the trade press for ideas in these areas.

REVIEW QUESTIONS

1. Give three reasons why clients colour their hair.
2. State five factors about your client that may affect their choice of hair colour.
3. What form of artificial lighting is best suited for hair-colour analysis?
4. What is the name of the test used on hair to determine the result of using a particular colour formulation on the hair?
5. On what area of the client is the predisposition test carried out?
6. For permanent hair colouring, how often should a skin test be given?
7. Name the substance that produces the natural pigment of hair.
8. What is the term that describes hair's ability to absorb moisture?
9. What is meant by 'level' when hair colouring? What is meant by the term 'level 7'?
10. Provide another term to describe a green tone in hair.
11. List the three categories of artificial hair colour.
12. How does coloured mousse colour the hair?
13. How do oxidation tints act on the hair?
14. Why is a two-step application required when applying lightening oxidation colour to virgin hair?
15. During hair colouring, how may tint staining be removed from the skin?
16. What is meant by the term 'creeping oxidation', and how may it be prevented?

CHAPTER 7

Customer reception

This chapter will provide the essential knowledge you need to understand the process of effective client reception and the phasing of client appointments.

Level 1	
Unit 103	
Element 103.1	Attend to clients, visitors and enquiries
Element 103.2	Contribute to making appointments for salon services
Unit 104	
Element 104.1	Develop effective working relationships with clients
Level 2	
Unit 201	
Element 201.1	Consult with and maintain effective relationships with clients
Element 201.2	Advise clients on salon products and services
Unit 207	
Element 207.1	Attend to clients and enquiries
Element 207.2	Make appointments for salon services
Element 207.3	Handle payments from clients for the purchase of services and retail products
Unit 208	
Element 208.1	Develop and maintain effective team work and relationships with colleagues
Unit 209	
Element 209.2	Support health, safety and security at work

Contents

INTRODUCTION

The customer reception is usually one of the first points of contact that your client has with the salon. This contact may be either by their visit to the salon or by the telephone contact made when your client makes contact to make an appointment. It is therefore at this stage that the initial image of the salon and its customer orientation is perceived by your client. 1

When your client first visits the salon, their first impression may well be of the facade of the salon and the display provided by the salon window. The new client must make the conscious decision to enter the salon and the way they are greeted and their enquiry handled will shape the view that they have of the salon. The receptionist has a crucial role in this phase of the process, putting the client at ease and ensuring that their needs are identified and fulfilled.

When a new client makes contact by telephone, the response received will be all that influences the client and is therefore a crucial part of the process.

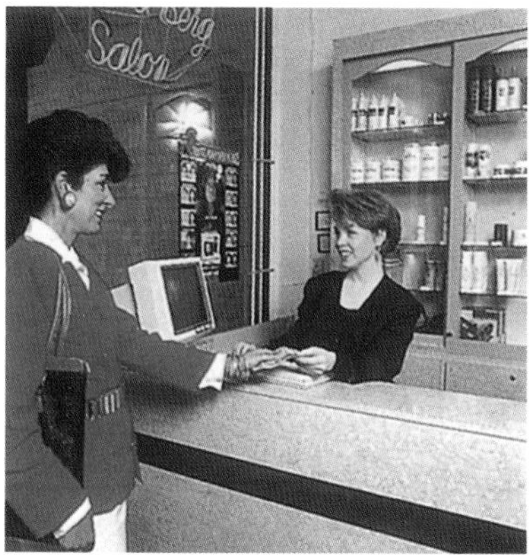

Figure 7.1 The hairdresser as sales person

THE ROLE OF THE RECEPTIONIST

The reception function is carried out in a variety of ways from salon to salon. At some the role is carried out by a reception specialist, in others it is carried out by the hair stylists as part of their overall duties. Whoever carries out the function and in whatever way this is done, the objective of the function is the same throughout: to attend to enquiries and to phase appointments effectively, to manage the allocation of work and satisfy the client's expectations. This will contribute to the success of the business. 1

> ***TIP*** When taking messages for others make a written note of the caller's name, date and time of call, the nature of the message and a contact telephone/fax number, email address or postal address if a response is required. This should be promptly passed to the person concerned. Remember messages taken that are not passed on may result in ineffective service to your clients.

The receptionist's duties

1 These duties include:

- responding to clients' enquiries, either by telephone or when they visit
- phasing appointments to ensure allocation of work in a way that is manageable by the hairstylist
- informing hairstylists of their client's arrival
- ensuring the comfort of the clients while they wait
- referring clients to the relevant person to fulfil their needs
- calculating client bills and collecting payments
- 1 receiving sales representatives and directing them to appropriate personnel
- providing a point of sale for retail goods (see Figure 7.1).

Qualities of a receptionist

1 This person should be organised, as they will be organising others and their workloads. They will project the salon's image and will therefore be expected to appear appropriately. Clear speech, together with the ability to communicate effectively, are essential features of a good receptionist.

ATTENDING TO VISITORS TO THE SALON

The clients

1 All clients who step over the threshold of the salon should be greeted courteously, with a smile and with body language which reflects pleasure in helping them. Greet the client, introducing yourself and asking how you may help them. You will require patience, as clients may be uncertain of their needs. They may require guidance and advice. Establish the client's requirements, which may range from purchasing retail products to seeking advice on their hair care, making an appointment for a hairdressing service to keeping an appointment or even to meeting a business associate in the salon. The receptionist may be able to handle many enquiries, but the client who requires advice and guidance over and above the scope of the receptionist should be invited to wait while a suitable person is informed or a consultation is arranged.

> ***TIP*** When clients visit the salon for the first time, they may feel vulnerable. Ensure that you guide these clients in the procedures of the salon and the location of cloakrooms, toilets and other client facilities. A client who is made aware of what to expect will feel more relaxed and more likely to enjoy their visit.

When a client arrives to keep an appointment they should, if possible, be greeted by name, their appointment details checked and the relevant member of staff promptly informed of their arrival.

Advice given to clients, about suitable services or retail products should be accurate and given in a clear manner. If in any doubt the receptionist should seek advice from a specialist within the salon. A knowledge of the features and benefits of services as well as of retail products is an essential aspect of the receptionist's skill. The cost of these should also be readily available.

Things to avoid

1 Do not:

- keep the client waiting for service while you carry on a conversation about a non-work related issue with a colleague. In all events the client's presence should be acknowledged even if you are unable to attend to them straight away due to a prior commitment

- allow any displeasure or harassment to be reflected in your greeting to the client. The client should be the centre of your attention
- keep a client waiting without informing them of possible delays and reasons for these. In the case of lengthy delays, consider options which the client may prefer, a revised appointment or alternative stylist. Effective phasing of appointments should avoid this occurrence
- eat, drink or smoke at reception. Responding to a client while you are eating or drinking is not a pleasant experience for them. Smoking can be anti-social and odours from this can be unpleasant for your clients.

Sales representatives

The receptionist will be the first point of contact for the visiting sales representative. Clients of the salon must take precedence over the representative. Check the credentials of the representative: most will carry a business card, which will indicate their name and the company that they represent. Having established their identity, ask them to take a seat in the waiting area and then inform the person with the responsibility for liaising with them. Some salons have a policy that sales representatives may only be seen by appointment with the relevant person and others will meet representatives if they are available. The receptionist must ensure that they are aware of the salon's policy in these matters. 1

Deliveries of product are usually made to the reception area of the salon. Salons may have policies regarding where goods should be delivered and who is eligible to sign the carrier's dockets, confirming receipt of goods in good order, and the procedure to be adopted.

Stock control, page 203

Other visitors

Any visitor to the salon should report to the reception. The salon may have policies on how visitors other than clients should be greeted. If in doubt, you should check the visitor's identity and, having seated them in the waiting area, seek advice from the salon management. 1

These visitors may include local authority representatives, training advisors and awarding body verifiers, business consultants, personal friends and acquaintances. The salon may have policies about members of staff receiving unofficial visits from acquaintances, except in emergencies. 1

If messages are taken for members of staff or management these should be recorded and passed to the relevant person. When taking messages, the salon may have its own procedures or pro-forma message pads. The detail usually required includes the name of the intended recipient, the name of the message leaver, the date and time of the message, the actual detail of the message and any action or response that is required. The salon may have a procedure for passing messages to ensure that they are passed promptly and that follow-up action is taken.

> ***TIP*** Details about the level of salon business should be considered as confidential to the business and should not be discussed with others either within or outside of business, without approval from the salon management.

USE OF THE TELEPHONE

The telephone forms a link between the salon and its clientele, enabling them to make contact without the need to actually visit the salon. With this in mind it is important that this service is available for as much time throughout the working day as possible. Personal telephone conversations should be avoided, and in many cases are prohibited, except in emergency. Conversations with clients should be clear and effective but at the same time as brief as possible without making the client feel rushed. When the telephone is in use other clients cannot make contact with you.

The telephone may also be used in a proactive manner in order to generate business, a method of checking on clients who have perhaps not visited the salon for some time and a way of reminding them of the services that you offer.

In cases of emergency, perhaps due to a member of staff's unplanned absence due to ill health, the telephone provides a method of contacting clients and rescheduling them.

Responding to the call

TIP The telephone can easily reflect, to the listener, the attitude of the speaker. Take care to always speak 'with a smile' and not to reflect annoyance or irritation.

The telephone should be answered promptly. Your salon may have a policy in always responding to the telephone within three rings. This should be considered good practice (see Figure 7.2). The caller should be informed of the name of the salon, who is responding to the call, and an invitation or offer of service, for example: 'This is Salon Hair, Paula speaking, how may I help you?'

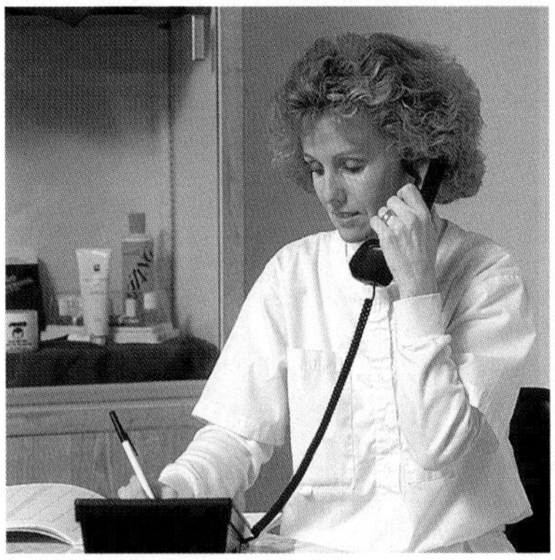

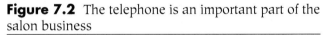

Figure 7.2 The telephone is an important part of the salon business

Speak clearly to the caller who is making an appointment, repeat the detail of the date, time, the service to be offered and if relevant the name of the stylist who will be undertaking the task. If in doubt about the spelling of a client's name ask the client to spell this out for you. This is not usually considered impolite. When you book clients who are visiting the salon for the first time, check that they are aware of the average cost of treatments. Your salon may have specific requirements when making appointments, particularly if a computerised appointment system is used, as details of the client will be 'called up' for checking when the appointment is entered. Remember to thank the caller for calling at the end of the conversation.

TIP Remember that information about clients is confidential. Receptionists should not release any information about a client to any one not normally authorised to ask without first consulting the salon management.

When responding to a telephone call where a message is taken, read this back to the caller to check the accuracy of the message taken.

When speaking to a telephone caller, remember that background noise from the reception area may be heard. Confidential conversations may be overheard, if you must keep the client waiting while you source information use the 'mute' button on the telephone, if available, so that comments not intended to be heard by the client do not become communicated.

Should a client telephone while the receptionist is busy dealing with another client, the 1
telephone should be answered and the caller asked if they can 'hold' while the current client's transaction is dealt with. If the client states that they cannot hold, then a return telephone number may be requested with an undertaking for the receptionist to return the call at the earliest instant. It is important that this undertaking is subsequently not neglected.

THE APPOINTMENT SYSTEM

Every salon requires a record of planned appointments for its clients. The record not only serves 1
to ensure that the hairdresser has a planned rota of clients with which to work and will assist the stylist in planning their working day, it will also serve as a reconciliation document, a check of takings by the stylist against the anticipated income from a number of clients.

The manual appointment book

The appointment schedule usually takes the form of a written appointment book, with a page per 1
day, containing columns allocated to particular hairstylists and specialists which is divided into time slots, usually in fifteen-minute intervals. The client's name, contact telephone number and the nature of the service required are then entered in the relevant stylist's column at the appropriate time of the day.

The receptionist must be aware of the stylist's competencies and the length of time that they require to complete services. This will enable them to realistically phase clients to ensure maximum efficiency without delay to the client.

The computerised reception system

More and more hairdressing salons are using computerised systems to retain their customer 1
information and to phase their appointments. In most systems the computer software will have built in to them the range of services available from the salon and the timings which are required for each stylist to undertake these tasks. This is usually linked to an automatic billing system that not only calculates the client's bill but is also often capable of re-booking appointments and generating reminders of these appointments for clients.

General guidance

The same guidance would be given as for when confirming appointments with clients via the telephone. Ensure that you communicate effectively, ensuring that the client is aware of the time and date of the next appointment, together with details of the service to be provided and the stylist who will provide this. Always confirm the appointment by completing an appointment card. This card will remind the client of the date and time of their next appointment as well as being a reminder to your client of the business, enabling them to recommend and direct new clients to you easily.

> ***TIP*** If you are dealing with a telephone request for an appointment which cannot be met, do not say 'no'. Always offer alternatives. 'No' can terminate the conversation leaving no area for negotiation.

Should someone request an appointment with a particular hairstylist for a particular day and time when that stylist is not available, there are several ways to handle the situation:

- If the client regularly uses that one hairstylist, suggest other times when the stylist is available.
- If the client cannot come in at any of those times, suggest an alternative stylist.
- If the client is unwilling to try another hairstylist, offer to call the client if there is a cancellation at or near the desired time.

When clients pay their bill at the end of the service, always offer to make further appointments for them. This will help to ensure repeat visits by clients and maintains the relationship between the salon and client.

RECEIVING CUSTOMER PAYMENTS

Part of the role of the receptionist is that of handling client payments. This requires the skills of numeracy and tact.

Following the treatment the client's total bill must be calculated. Salons may have differing ways of doing this. In some cases the hairstylist informs the receptionist of the various services and items that are to be added to the bill. In other salons each individual who contributes to the client's treatments reports this to the receptionist who then maintains a record of the service given and subsequently calculates the bill based upon this information.

Provided that all details of all services are correctly 'keyed' in, a computerised client reservation and recording system will then calculate the client's bill and will record all treatments. Many electronic tills will calculate the amount of change to be given to the client, if required. Some may also record the stylist's name so that commissions and performance figures can be established. Each day a cash 'float' is required so that change may be given to clients. This consists of an agreed amount of cash in small denominations. The receptionist should check the level of the float and record it, so that it may be accurately deducted when the takings are reconciled (actual takings are compared to recorded takings). The receptionist should operate the cash flow to avoid running out of a range of cash for change. A reserve may be kept in a safe and the receptionist should be aware of how to easily obtain this and should forecast when it may be required so as to save shortages at crucial times.

> ***TIP*** A client may request to make payment using travellers' cheques. Consult with a responsible person before undertaking this.

Unless otherwise stated on the price list, prices charged are assumed, if appropriate, to include Value Added Tax (VAT) at the current rate.

The salon receptionist must make themselves aware of acceptable forms of payment within the salon. These may include:

- cash
- cheques
- credit cards
- cash equivalents
- vouchers.

Cash payments

The most often used form of payment for services, coinage of the realm, is accepted in all salons. When receiving cash as payment note the following:

- Always count and agree the actual payment before the cash is placed in the cash drawer.
- When change is required, retain the original payment outside the cash drawer while change is calculated. This can help to avoid disagreements about the amount of the initial payment.
- Always follow the salon's policy in checking the validity of bank notes used for payments.
- It is not usual to open a cash drawer just to obtain change for a client; the opening of the till should normally coincide with a transaction.

Payment by cheque

Most salons accept payment from clients by cheque. Some do, however, set a minimum level above which the cheque payment should be, usually to offset the bank charges levied against the business for handling the cheque. When receiving a cheque, note the following procedures:

- The cheque should be signed in the presence of the receiver. The remainder of the detail may have been printed for the client by a computerised till or may have been written by the client.
- Check that the days date is correct, with the correct year, that it is made payable to the correct company name and that the amount payable is correct both in writing and in figures.

> ***TIP*** Remember, the checking of the validity of a cheque guarantee card or credit card can cause some clients embarrassment, therefore this process should be carried out with discretion and the utmost courtesy to the client.

- Most businesses require that a cheque payment be supported by a cheque guarantee card. If this is the case, the client should be asked to write the card number on the reverse side of the cheque. The receptionist should check the accuracy of the number, that the card will guarantee the cheque to the required level – this amount (usually £50 or £100) is indicated on the card – that the signature on the cheque is the same as that on the card, and that it is tendered within the card's start and expiry dates (you may be required to note this detail on the reverse of the cheque).
- If there is doubt about the validity of the card it should be retained by the receptionist while checks are made. If you are in any doubt about the salon procedures for doing this consult with your line manager.

It is not normal practice to cash cheques for clients without the agreement of the salon management, or to give cash change for cheques made out to greater amounts than that of the bill. It is unwise to accept cheques that are not made payable to a specific name, or where any detail is incomplete.

Credit card payments

Payment by this method is accepted by many but not all businesses. Agreement between the business and the particular credit card company is required. The business pays a percentage of each card transaction to the card company. Always follow your salon's policy in receiving these cards. These transaction may be completed via an electronic point of sale, which links direct with the card company and validates and records the transaction direct. The use of sales vouchers either printed via a computerised till or by hand may also be used. Some general notes of guidance are:

- Always check that the card is valid and within the start and expiry dates.
- If completing a sales voucher by hand, use a ballpoint pen, ensuring that the writing can be seen on all copies. The details from the card may be transferred to the sales voucher using an imprinter. Pass the top copy of the voucher to the client, for their record. All others to be placed in the cash drawer.
- Check that the card is not the subject of a warning notice. From time to time card companies will circulate a listing of card numbers that should not be accepted, and if used should be retained by the salon who should inform the card company.
- Do not accept damaged or torn cards, particularly if the signature strip has been partially or completely removed.
- Each business will have been set a 'floor limit', the level of payment above which authorisation must be obtained from the card company if the payment is to be guaranteed. This may be done by a simple telephone call and a 'transaction number' recorded on the sales voucher; you will need to have at hand your 'merchant number' when making this call.

If you are in doubt whether a particular card is accepted by your salon, consult with the manager. Do not accept payment via this method if you are not fully aware of the process, as errors may invalidate payment. If in doubt seek advice and help.

Cash equivalents

Some clients may offer payment via traveller's cheques, either in sterling or in a foreign currency. Sterling cheques may be received very much like an ordinary cheque. Ensure that the customer signs the traveller's cheque in your presence and that this signature is the same as that on the traveller's cheque folder or passport. If accepting traveller's cheques in non-sterling currency the bank will give a valuation for the exchange.

If you are in any doubt about the procedures for receiving traveller's cheques then consult your manager.

Vouchers

The salon may offer vouchers for sale, which may then in turn be used as gifts that are in turn used by clients to purchase goods or services from the salon. These may be used to the equivalent value of the stated cash figure. Salons' policies with regard to giving cash as change on these occasions may differ; if in doubt consult with your manager.

- Remember always to follow the salon's policies in receiving payments from clients.

- If you are in doubt about the validity of the payment being made, follow the salon procedure or consult with your manager.
- A receipt for payment should be given. This is your client's proof of payment, particularly for unrecorded treatments or retail sales, and will be required should a refund be necessary.
- Do not give refunds to clients unless you have the authority to do so, or you have consulted with and have permission from the authorised person.
- Do not leave the cash drawer open when not in use. When the reception is unattended the cash drawer should be locked.
- Large amounts of cash, or notes of high denomination should be removed from the cash drawer and placed in a safe. This will help to reduce any security risk.

THE DATA PROTECTION ACT 1998

Data held on computer can easily be processed and transmitted to others, there are issues about the rights of people to be aware of what personal information is held about them, its accuracy and the use to which it is put. The law requires that people and organisations who retain information about living people on computer, to register this with the Data Protection Registrar. This also applies to certain paper-based manual data retention systems.

To register it must be indicated that data will:

- be processed fairly and lawfully
- not be used for a purpose other than for which it is collected
- be adequate, relevant and not excessive for the purpose
- be accurate and up to date
- not kept longer than necessary
- be processed in accordance with the data subject's rights
- be kept secure and protected from unauthorised processing, loss or destruction
- be transferred only to those countries outside of the European Economic Area that provide adequate protection for personal information.

If your salon keeps personal information about you and your clients it may be registered with the Data Protection Registrar. You may wish to find out what your salon regulations are regarding access to this information, who has access to data, provisions for data security. You may be required to comply with your salon's regulations.

FURTHER STUDY

- Ensure that you are aware of whom to go to for advice and guidance when making appointments for clients and when receiving payments.
- Familiarise yourself with the range of services offered within your salon, their duration and cost.
- Find out if your salon has a policy for:
  - the manner in which the telephone is answered;
  - who makes client appointments;
  - how the client's bill is calculated and who gives information on the services provided;
  - who is empowered to receive payments or to authorise particular methods of payment;
  - the process of making refunds.

1

REVIEW QUESTIONS

1. May information about clients be given to whoever asks?
2. How should the client be greeted when they visit the salon?
3. List three functions of the salon's receptionist.
4. When booking a client what detail is normally required to be listed in the salon's appointment book?
5. How should a telephone appointment booking be confirmed with a client?
6. What two purposes may the appointment cards serve?
7. What is meant by 'phasing' of appointments?
8. What action should be taken following receipt of a message for someone within the salon?
9. What detail must be checked when receiving a cheque guarantee card in support of a cheque payment?
10. What is the purpose of a cash float?
11. What is the 'floor limit' in relation to credit card usage?

CHAPTER 8

Working with others

This chapter provides the essential knowledge to help you understand the principles and practices involved in working as a hairdresser. The information in this chapter will affect all other areas in the book.

Level 1	
Unit 103	
Element 103.1	Attend to clients, visitors and enquiries
Unit 104	
Element 104.1	Develop effective working relationships with clients
Element 104.2	Develop effective working relationships with colleagues
Element 104.3	Develop yourself within the job role
Unit 105	
Element 105.2	Support health and safety at work

Level 2	
Unit 201	
Element 201.1	Consult with and maintain effective working relationships with clients
Unit 208	
Element 208.1	Develop and maintain effective team work and relationships with colleagues
Element 208.2	Develop and improve personal effectiveness within the job-role
Unit 209	
Element 209.2	Support health, safety and security at work

Contents

INTRODUCTION

As a professional hairdresser you will project an image that is manifold, both as a professional hair artist and as a socially conscious person, aware of current fashion trends who may be both caring and objective when advising clients (see Figure 8.1). Your development in the profession of hairdressing is integral with all of the other tasks that you carry out. It is impossible to separate your development from the day to day work that you perform. As a novice hairdresser you will always be learning, either from formal training sessions or by watching and being involved with the effective running of the business. Every experience that you have in this profession must be viewed as a learning process that enables you to develop your skills further.

Always reflect upon your performance of a task. Consider what you did well and build on this; for those areas where you feel that you did not perform so well, be objective and consider what changes you should make in your future actions which will improve yourself. Be aware of who you may approach for advice and guidance in these matters and at what time this may be most appropriate.

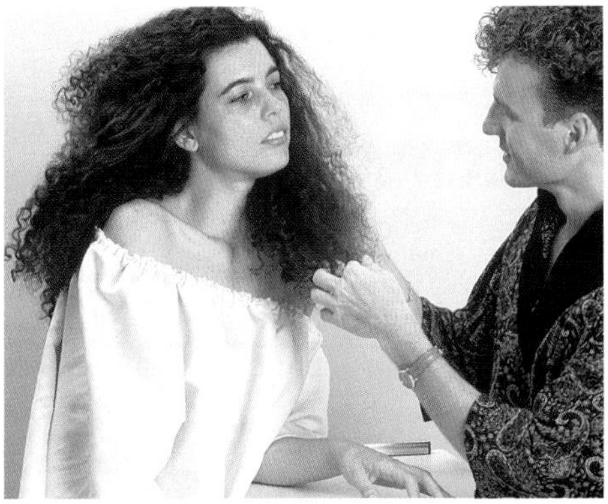

Figure 8.1 Be caring and objective

As a hairstylist the learning and development process never ends. In the early stages it may be that you have basic skills to acquire and you must develop a work ethos that ensures that you approach your work with enthusiasm, remembering that in a service industry your performance with your client is what ensures their return and therefore your ongoing success. Not only will you be developing your practical skills but also your social skills. Very rarely will you work in isolation. At all levels you will need to be able to interact with colleagues, supporting each other in your workplace, and this will be seen by your clientele. You must therefore develop skills of working together as part of a team, as well as relating with your client on a 'one to one' basis.

Fashion does not stand still, so neither will the requirements of your clients or your employer. As a commercial hair stylist you must keep abreast of both current and emerging fashion trends. This may be achieved in a variety of ways that are mentioned elsewhere in this book. Your role within the hairdressing salon will also develop. You will be expected, at certain stages, to accept responsibilities. These may appear quite minor – preparing work stations, for example – or they may take the form of supervisory skills, allocation and checking of work being carried out by others, or making judgements on other people's performance. All are important and may be essential to the running of the business. They all require different skills, which must be developed and do not normally happen without a level of planning.

As an employee in a business, you will interact with your line manager. You must take on the skills of negotiation and interaction not only with your colleagues, but with those for whom you have responsibility, and with your line managers.

PROFESSIONAL IMAGE

Image is the pivotal focus for hairdressing. Each hair stylist and salon will seek to project an image that will relate to a particular type of client. This will usually be shown by the appearance and manner of the hair stylist together with the style of hairdressing produced. Some salons will have an image that will focus on a specific segment of the market and will be quite clearly defined, whether by the salon decor, the salon facade, the atmosphere generated or a combination of all three. Other salons will have a professional image that will be attractive to a wider market segment in terms of gender, age and socio-economic grouping.

> ***TIP*** Potential clients will often form opinions about you as a hair stylist by your appearance.

PHYSICAL DEVELOPMENT

As a hairdresser, the main tool that you use is your body. Take care of this machine to ensure that it serves you throughout your career. Your service to your client is achieved partly through the skills that you have developed, and partly through the atmosphere of relaxation and pleasure that you create. You must be physically able to provide this service throughout the working week, and this means taking care of your health.

Personal health and hygiene

For your client to feel at ease and relaxed while in your company, you must be pleasant to be with, and this means attending to your personal hygiene. Open sores or cuts on exposed areas of the skin should be covered with a waterproof dressing, helping to prevent the spread of any infection. This is often a requirement of the local bye-laws affecting the registration of hairdressing salons with local authority regions.

As a hairdresser, you will work in very close proximity to your client, so you must be aware of their discomfort if you have body odour or bad breath. Smoking will leave an odour on your breath and clothes that can be most unpleasant, particularly for non-smoking clients. Your client may also find odours from strongly flavoured foods unpleasant, and these may linger for some considerable time. Put yourself in your client's position and consider how you would react to these situations. Remember that your client has a choice of which salon they visit.

As a member of a team, remember that these same factors may affect your working relationships with your colleagues.

You must consider your salon's policy with regard to working with clients when your are suffering with colds or disorders which may be contagious, and you should make yourself aware of legislative regulations that may have an effect.

> ***TIP*** You may be able to insure against loss of use of certain parts of your body, your hands for example, which may prevent you from carrying out your hairdressing role.

Care of your feet

For more information about this see Chapter 10, pages 207–214

As a hairdresser you will spend a great deal of time on your feet. Proper foot care will help you maintain a good posture and a cheerful attitude. Sore feet or poorly-fitting shoes can cause great discomfort (see Figure 8.2).

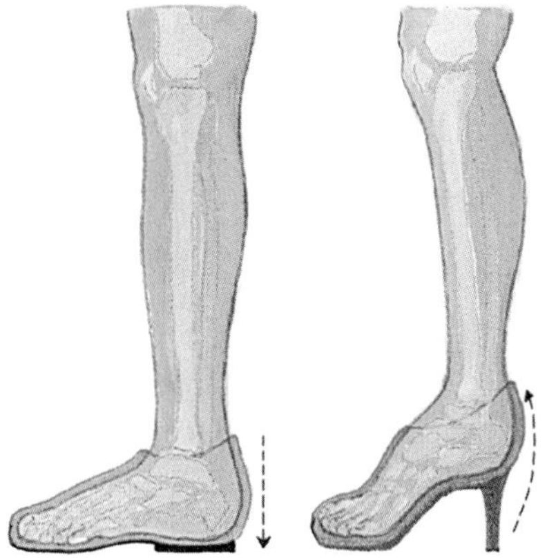

Figure 8.2 For comfort and to maintain good posture, wear well-fitted, low-heeled shoes

Shoes

Wear shoes with low, broad heels and cushioned insoles. They give you support and balance, and help to maintain good posture, offsetting the fatigue that can result from hours of standing. It also helps if you can stand on a carpeted or cushioned surface.

Daily foot care

After bathing, apply cream or oil and massage each foot for 5 minutes. Remove the cream or oil and apply an antiseptic foot lotion. Regular pedicures that include cleansing, removal of callused skin, massage, and toenail trims will keep your feet at their best. When your feet ache, chiropodists recommend that you soak your feet alternately in warm and cool water. See a chiropodist if you suffer from corns, bunions, ingrown toenails, or other foot disorders.

Healthy lifestyle

You should practise stress management through relaxation, rest, and exercise. Avoid substances that can negatively affect your good health, such as cigarettes, alcohol, and drugs.

PHYSICAL PRESENTATION

Your posture, walk, and movements all make up your physical presentation. People form opinions about you by the way you present yourself. Do you stand straight or slouch; do you walk confidently or do you drag your feet? Your physical presentation is part of your professional image and can help to reduce fatigue.

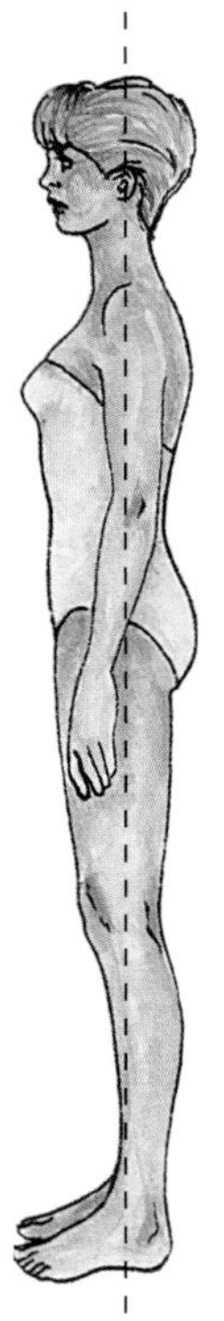

Figure 8.3 Good posture

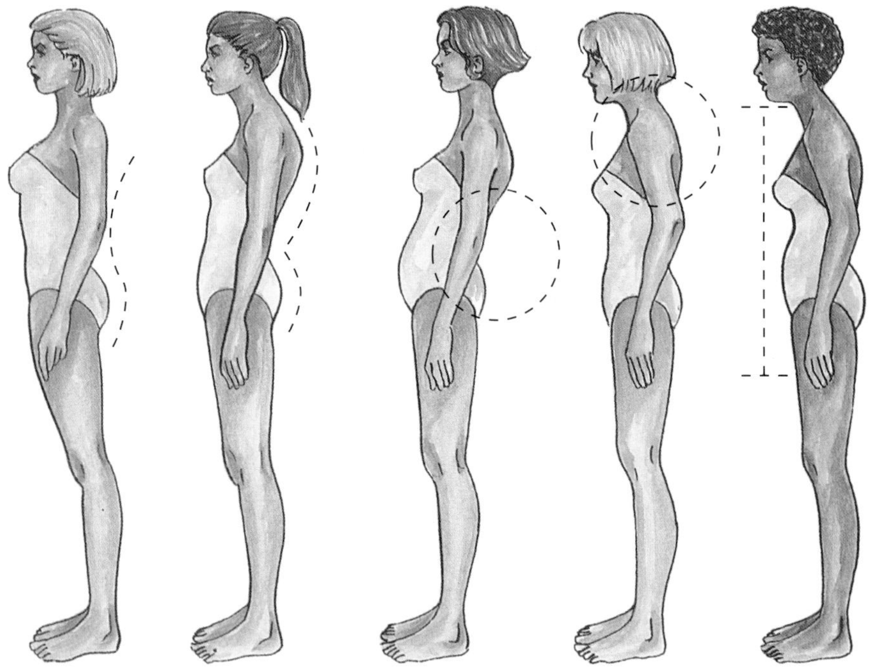

Figure 8.4 Five defective body postures

Good posture

Good posture not only improves your personal appearance by presenting your stature to advantage and creating an image of confidence, it also prevents fatigue and many other physical problems (see Figures 8.3 and 8.4). As a hairdresser you spend most of your working time on your feet, so you should develop good posture as early as possible through regular exercise and self-discipline.

Physical presentation on the job

To prevent muscle aches, back strain, discomfort, fatigue, and other problems, and to maintain an attractive image, it is very important to practise good physical presentation while performing work activities (see Figures 8.5 to 8.6).

Checkpoints of good posture

- Crown of head reaching upward while chin is kept level with the floor.
- Neck is elongated and balanced directly above the shoulders.
- Chest up; body is lifted from the breastbone.
- Shoulders are level, held back and down, yet relaxed.
- Spine is straight, not curved laterally or swayed from front to back.
- Abdomen is flat.
- Hips are level (horizontally) and protrude neither forward nor back.
- Knees are slightly flexed and positioned directly over the feet with the ankles firm.

Basic stance for women

- Place most of your weight on your right foot and point your toes straight ahead in a straight line.

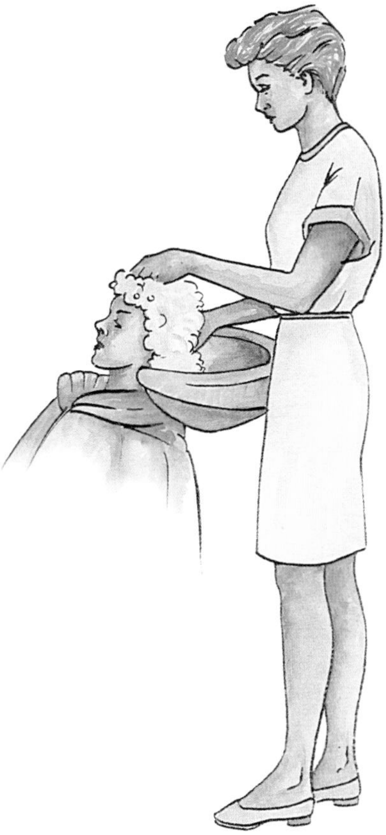

Figure 8.5 To avoid back strain, maintain good posture when giving a shampoo

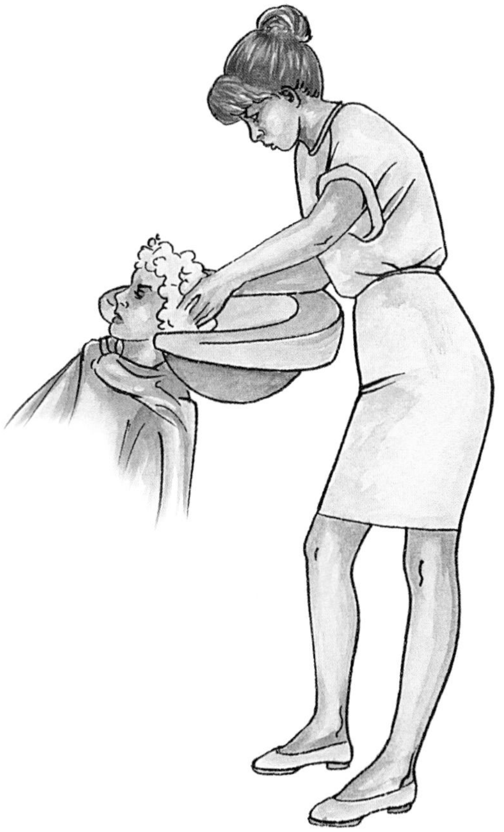

Figure 8.6 Poor posture

- Place your left heel close to the heel or instep of your right foot and point the toes slightly outward.
- Bend your left knee slightly inward (see Figure 8.7).

Basic stance for men

- Place your feet apart, but not wider than your shoulder width.
- Distribute your weight evenly over both feet.
- Your knees should be neither rigid nor bent.
- Your toes should point straight ahead or one or both feet should point slightly outward.
- For a more relaxed stance, bend one knee slightly while shifting some of your weight to the opposite foot (see Figure 8.8).

WHAT THE EXPERT SAYS By its nature hairdressing involves offering a service to others, our clients, so interaction with others is an essential aspect of this profession.

There are four categories of people with whom we interact, these being: our clients; those from whom we purchase goods and services which enable us to carry out the hairdressing process; those with whom we work and finally those who employ or manage us in our role. In order to be effective in our work we must work effectively with all these categories.

Your clients

As the hairdresser, you will control the relationship which develops between yourself and your client. You will be in the position of the 'expert' whom the client has visited to receive a service. You will set the scene. You will be the expert in your field, and will be responsible for providing your client with a service delivered in a style that will satisfy their expectations. You will be judged not only on your level of hairdressing skill but also on the efficiency and ambience of delivery of that skill, and what you do will determine the level of customer satisfaction.

Providers of goods and services

These people provide a support service. Effective communication with this group is essential to ensure that the correct level of support is provided. This support will include the provision of both products and equipment at the appropriate level at the appropriate time, and the provision of guidance and training in the correct and effective use of products. They may also keep you informed of emerging product developments.

Co-workers/colleagues

Most of us work with others at a variety of levels within a team. The team has a common goal, which must be the success of the team. Everyone within the team has a role to play and you can be more effective as a team than by working independently. In working as a team, members must respect each other. There are skills which must be developed by all members of the team. These include skills of working together and acknowledging each other's worth. People all have different characters and all work within a team in different ways, so the successful team will evolve by using each member's attributes most effectively. This can happen purely by chance, but it usually requires an expert in group dynamics to maximise the team's potential.

Employers/management

Employees interact with management and employers. To be successful the hairdresser must develop skills of negotiation and interaction with his or her managers. The hairdresser will negotiate terms and conditions of employment, scales and rates of pay, holiday periods and potential improvements in services offered within the salon. Due to the varied sizes of hairdressing businesses, the relationships that develop between management and workers will differ considerably between salons. However, the communication role between the hairdresser and the manager is two-way, and the hairdresser must be aware of the approaches available in the business.

A successful management will ensure that all of its staff are fully aware of this and that easy access to management is made available.

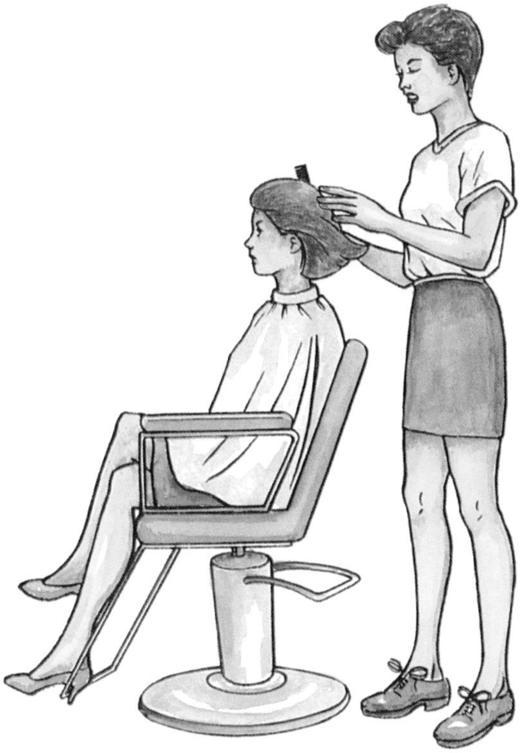

Figure 8.7 Basic stance for the female hairdresser

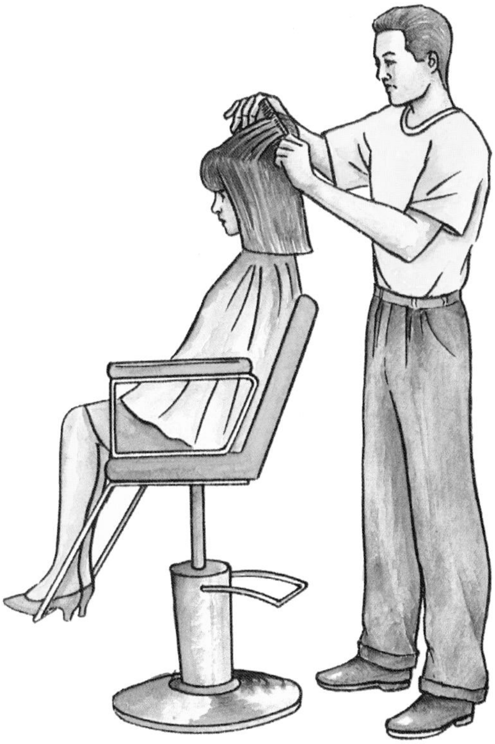

Figure 8.8 Basic stance for the male hairdresser

Desirable qualities for effective client relations

Emotional control

Learn to control your emotions. Do not reveal negative emotions such as anger, envy, and dislike. An even-tempered person is always treated with respect. 1

Take time to think through your response before responding, particularly when working in stressful situations. Control your body language: you may use it to defuse situations. A placid approach can calm a stressful situation. Remember, your clients come to you expecting a relaxed, enjoyable experience, not to hear about your problems or for you to vent your feelings upon them.

Positive approach

Be pleasant and gracious. You should have a smile of greeting and a word of welcome ready for each client and co-worker. A good sense of humour is also an important part of maintaining a positive attitude. A sense of humour enriches your life and cushions the disappointments. When you are able to laugh at yourself, you will have gained the ability to accept and deal positively with difficult situations.

The smooth running of the hairdressing salon is the result of teamwork. You must be able to work as a member of a team, being able to respect other people's points of view in matters of disagreement and finding workable solutions. These situations should be dealt with in the staff meeting or with the line manager, never in front of your clients. Within the view of the clients the team should always be supportive of each other, giving each other encouragement.

Good manners

Good manners reflect your thoughtfulness for others. Saying 'thank you' and 'please', treating other people with respect, exercising care of other people's property, being tolerant and understanding of other people's shortcomings and efforts, and being considerate of those with whom you work all express good manners. Courtesy is one of the keys to a successful career.

Good manners should not be viewed as a sign of weakness. As members of a team respect for each other is best gained by your actions towards each other. A well-mannered approach to a colleague is more likely to generate a similar response, whereas an ill-mannered approach is more likely to be met with a mirrored response that may then escalate or at least create resentment.

Mannerisms

Client care procedures, page 1

Gum chewing and nervous habits such as tapping your foot or playing with your hair and personal items detract from your personal effectiveness. Yawning, coughing, and sneezing should be concealed when in the presence of others. Control body language that reveals negative communication, for example, sarcastic or disapproving facial grimaces. Pleasant facial expressions and attractive gestures and actions should be your goal.

HUMAN RELATIONSHIPS AND YOUR PROFESSIONAL ATTITUDE

1 Human relationships involve the psychology of getting along well with others. Your professional attitude is expressed by your own self-esteem, your confidence in your abilities, and by the respect you show others.

Good habits and practices acquired during your training lay the foundation for a successful career in hairdressing.

Working with clients

The following are guidelines for good human relations that will help you to gain confidence and deal successfully with your clients.

- Always greet a client by name, with a pleasant tone of voice. Address a client by his or her last name (Mrs Smith, Mr Jones, Miss Allen) unless the client prefers first names and if it is customary to use first names in your salon (if you are in doubt check with your line manager). When greeting a new client introduce yourself to your client and establish their name as rapidly as possible either by consulting the appointment book or by asking your client direct.
- Plan your client's appointments to allow yourself adequate time to carry out the tasks with, if possible, time to react to any additional requests your client has. You should make an overall view of your appointments to try, if possible, to spread your workload evenly over your normal working times. This can help to reduce peaks of extreme pressure or quiet periods, provides a better pace of work and allows you to react to changing circumstances, such as the additional workload created by absence from work of colleagues.

Customer reception, pages 175–186

- Phasing client appointments to enable work to be carried out on more than one client at any one time, when relevant, will improve your efficiency. This can occur during the shampooing period, if this is carried out by an assistant, following consultation, while the processing of chemical treatments is taking place or while other specialists within the salon are working on your client.

- Be alert to your client's mood. Some clients prefer quiet and relaxation, others like to talk. Be a good listener and confine your conversation to the client's needs. Never gossip or tell stories.
- Topics of conversation should be carefully chosen. Friendly relations are achieved through pleasant conversations. Let your client be the guide in the topic of conversation. In a business setting it is best to avoid discussing controversial topics such as religion and politics, topics that relate to your personal life such as personal problems, or subjects relating to other people, such as another client's behaviour, poor workmanship of fellow workers or competitors, or information given to you in confidence.

> ***TIP*** Remember, while discussing issues with your client others with differing views may be listening.

- Confidential details about your clients, addresses, telephone numbers, holiday arrangements, should not be disclosed to others, unless authorised by the client or a responsible person in the business.
- Make a good impression by looking the part of the successful hairstylist, and by speaking and acting in a professional manner at all times.
- Cultivate self-confidence, and project a pleasing personality.
- Show interest in the client's personal preferences. Give your undivided attention. Maintain eye contact and concentrate totally on your client.
- Use tact and diplomacy when dealing with problems you may encounter.
- Be capable and efficient in your work.
- Be punctual. Arrive at work on time (give yourself sufficient time to prepare yourself for work) and keep appointments on schedule. Plan each day's schedule so that you manage your time effectively.
- Develop your business and sales abilities. Use tact when suggesting additional services or products to clients. Be aware of the features and benefits of products retailed within your salon. You should know salon prices so that you may easily inform your clients of their commitment.
- Avoid saying anything that may sound as if you are criticising, condemning, or putting down a client's opinions.
- Keep informed of new products and services so you can answer clients' questions intelligently.
- Continue to add to your knowledge and skills.
- Be ethical in all your dealings with clients and others with whom you come in contact.
- Always let the client see that you practise the highest standards of hygiene.
- Avoid criticising your competitors.

Be aware of your level of responsibility when dealing with clients. As a member of a team that provides services to members of the public, you may be able to make decisions on some issues but not on others. If you are in doubt check this with your line manager.

Do not allow concerns or problems raised by clients to be ignored: they should be dealt with immediately. If these must be referred to another member of staff, this should be done promptly and discreetly. Do not discuss clients or their concerns with colleagues or in front of clients.

Working as part of a team

1 The following are guidelines for good human relations that will help you to gain confidence and perform successfully with your colleagues.

- As a member of a team, you should make yourself aware of the structure of the team, who your line manager is, who is the overall team leader/manager and what are the responsibilities of the individual team members. There will be those who are responsible for particular tasks or functions within the salon.
- Find out precisely what is expected of you as a member of the team. What are your duties? Who are you responsible to? Who do you approach for advice and guidance? Be prepared to respond to requests for guidance, if this responsibility is within your capability and responsibility.
- 1 As a team member, you will interact with others. As a junior member of a team your role will be more responsive rather than initiative, but you will have a role with defined parameters of personal responsibility. As a more established member of a team your role will evolve often into a more responsible function and gradually may take on supervisory functions, at various levels.
- In the supervisory function, the needs of others should be anticipated and if possible advice and guidance given, or, if necessary, arrangements made for others to do this.
- 1 Requests for assistance by colleagues should be viewed positively. Take care to ensure that your own duties are not neglected in your attempts to assist others. If you are in doubt consult with your line manager about which tasks should be given priority. In an emergency, all possible help should be given, particularly when people may be at risk. Do not undertake tasks for which you are not trained, or use equipment with which you are unfamiliar.
- When you are not actively busy, as a member of a team you should be prepared to offer help and assistance in tasks that you can do to other members of the team.
- Deal with all disputes and differences in private. Take care of all problems promptly. If problems cannot be resolved your line manager should be informed.

> ***TIP*** If you are to carry out your role within the salon, you must ensure that you are aware of what is expected of you in your job.

Remember that the team is only as strong as its weakest member. Every member of a team is important to ensure success. Responsibilities, no matter how unimportant they may appear, should be taken seriously. As a team member ensure that you are fully aware of what is expected of you by the rest of the team. Should you be unable to undertake certain tasks, you should discuss this with your functional manager, to gain suitable training/instruction.

Team meetings are ideal occasions to raise issues that are relevant to the team. Be prepared to listen to others as well as putting your own thoughts forward. As a team member you must be prepared to accept justified constructive feedback, as well as being able to give this. When giving comment it can help to consider how you might best prefer to receive such comment and use this as guidance in how to undertake this.

> ***TIP*** Your line manager is that person to whom you are responsible in decision making, your functional manager is that person to whom you are responsible when carrying out specific tasks.

Personal career development

The following are guidelines for good human relations that will help you to gain confidence and perform successfully within your career in hairdressing. 1

For successful career progression you should have a planned route (Professional Development Plan). Consider what you wish to achieve within your career, and when determining this consider your strengths and weaknesses. Chart how you might achieve these goals. Consider what experiences and training you need to achieve these expectations, being realistic in considering a time scale. As you progress within your career, review your development plan. Be prepared to amend the plan in the light of your experience. It may turn out that you achieve milestones within your plan sooner than expected. This will necessitate a change in part of the plan. The reverse may also apply. In the experience of work you may decide that your original goals no longer apply and you wish to amend these. The Professional Development Plan is a dynamic document, always prepared to respond to change. In the light of changed expectations the route to achieve this will need to be mapped out. The entire process may be done either formally as part of a work review and appraisal process or very informally as a personal thought process. Without a Professional Development Plan, achievement will occur more by accident than by design, and time and experience may be wasted.

As part of your career development consider the following:

- Objectively review your performance.
- Identify your strengths and weaknesses; awareness of these can help you to capitalise on the former and address the latter.
- Make the most of opportunities to learn and develop skills;
- Always be prepared to watch specialists work (subject to available time).
- Participate in any available training activities.
- Be prepared to seek advice on issues relating to your job or your learning.
- Be prepared to participate fully in salon activities which will give experience through which learning will take place.

> ***TIP*** When setting your targets for personal achievements make them SMARTS.
> Specific
> Measurable
> Achievable
> Relevant
> Timebound
> Stretching
>
> Then you will recognise when you achieve and your achievement will support your development.

As part of your employment you may be involved in the process of appraisal and review. This is a quality opportunity, with your line manager or personnel officer or training manager, to review your performance since the previous appraisal, and plan future work. This process may focus on evaluating your performance to date and/or your career action plan and/or planning/responding to your training and development requirements. This becomes your opportunity to review your performance and to highlight those achievements that you consider noteworthy; advice may be given on areas of possible improvement (this should centre around your job description), and to negotiate and agree further training.

The hairdressing industry involves constant evolution of fashion, techniques and equipment. The experienced hairdresser must learn continuously if they are to maintain the currency of their skills.

FURTHER STUDY

- Awareness of body language can be an important tool in developing/controlling the client/hairdresser relationship. This area should be developed by the hairdresser.
- Maintain an awareness of emerging fashion trends and their associated techniques.
- Create your own Professional Development Plan and review this regularly.
- Draw up a list of what you consider to be your strengths (things you do well or are good at) and your weaknesses (things you do less well or are not so good at). Use this list to help to identify areas that you should develop.
- Find out what equipment is required for each process carried out in your salon that you are involved in.

1

REVIEW QUESTIONS

1. What is a Professional Development Plan?
2. How should exposed cuts be treated, while working with clients?
3. What style of heels are best suited to be worn by the hairdresser, while at work?
4. To reduce fatigue, how should the hairdresser's spine be positioned while working on the client?
5. What advantage is there in phasing customer appointments?
6. Suggest two topics of conversation that should be avoided, with your client.
7. Of what detail about retail products should the hairdresser be aware?
8. At what stage, during the hairdressing process, should clients' concerns be dealt with?
9. What is the ideal occasion to raise issues that are relevant to a working team?
10. Suggest one focus that an appraisal interview may follow.

CHAPTER 9

Effective use of resources

The information in this chapter affects all other areas in the book. It provides the essential knowledge to help you understand the concepts and practices of resource control in the hairdressing business.

Level 1	
Unit 104	
Element 104.3	Develop yourself within the job role
Unit 105	
Element 105.2	Support health and safety at work
Level 2	
Unit 209	
Element 209.2	Support health, safety and security at work

Contents

INTRODUCTION

1 Resources are the commodities that the hairdressing salon have to sell to produce an income. The most obvious resource, in addition to our skills, is the products that we use on our clients and the products that we retail to the public. To make the most effective use of this resource, which represents an asset of the business, it must be kept to the minimum level necessary to satisfy the demand, yet sufficient to ensure smooth operation. This resource must be stored and handled correctly to avoid wastage and damage.

A major resource of the salon, often overlooked as a resource, is the effective working time of staff. This places demands upon effective phasing and allocation of work and the provision of adequate facilities to encourage this.

PREPARATION OF THE SALON

Health, safety and security in the salon, pages 207–214

1 Before each working day and at stages throughout the day some preparation is required. This includes not only keeping the salon clean, but also the preparation of the materials and equipment required to undertake the work in the salon. Effective use of time is made if the correct quantity of product is in the right place at the right time, time and customer confidence can be lost if the stylist has to repeatedly leave the client to fetch items for use.

In preparing the salon for the day, ensure that there are adequate supplies of the products to be used. Shampoo and conditioning products should be topped up, and bottles and applicators cleaned. Racks and displays of products both for use in the salon and for retail should be topped up and free from dust. Always top up shelves by pulling forward the stock already in place and placing newer stock at the back. This process is known as *stock rotation*. Using the older stock before the new ensures that the resource does not deteriorate. This is particularly important when handling products that have short shelf lives, as they lose their effectiveness if left on the shelf too long. Exposure to sunlight for prolonged periods may cause products to fade, thus making them less effective and less attractive for sale.

> ***TIP*** When handling products and topping up containers, ensure that you observe all guidance given to you in correct handling techniques.

Supplies of clean laundry should be made ready, and should be checked throughout the day. Supplies of sterilising liquids should be maintained.

Take care if handling and topping up substances that may be corrosive including cleaning materials, hydrogen peroxide and sterilising liquids. They may burn the skin if spilled, or discolour clothing. Wear protective gloves and protective clothing. If you are in doubt consult with the person responsible for risk analysis within the salon. They will be identified in the salon's health and safety policy and procedures statement. If in doubt speak to your manager. Spillages should be wiped up immediately and any cloths used for this thoroughly rinsed clean or disposed of.

Having checked the day's appointments, it is possible to forecast the needs for certain items of equipment, for example perm rods. The perming trolleys should be prepared so as to save time at a later stage, possibly while the client is waiting. It is not advisable to mix products until they are required or before the consultation has taken place. These trolleys may be on display throughout the day and should therefore be maintained in a clean and ordered fashion. A tidy work station will also facilitate smooth working and can speed up processes.

STOCK CONTROL

The level of stock on display should be checked. There will be minimum levels of stock set, which 1
may be determined by the size of the retailing unit or by the quantity normally sold during the working day. Stock should be drawn from the main stock to top up these displays.

Your salon will have a system for the person responsible to record what stock is drawn for use. This list will be checked against the retail sales record and reconciled, to ensure that there is a balance between what is being drawn from stock and what is being sold. This will highlight theft, should it occur. Many salons now have computerised stock control systems, and some of these allow you to deduct retail stock from the stock record automatically when a sale is recorded. They can also prompt the purchase of fresh supplies (see Figure 9.1).

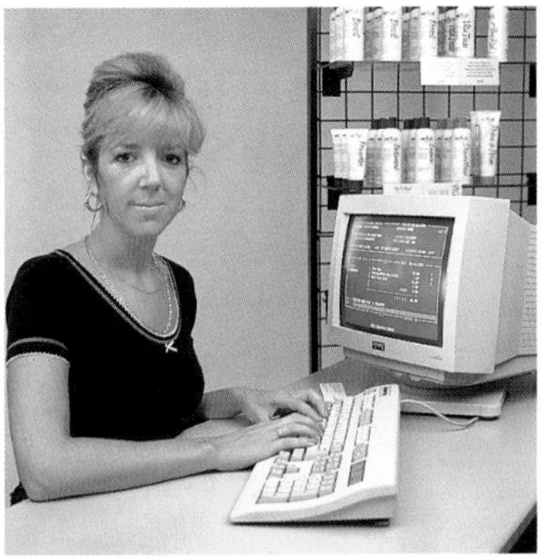

Figure 9.1 Computer terminal showing stock record

The retail display must be maintained in a manner which encourages clients to buy and therefore should always appear in best condition (see Figure 9.2). It is an advantage to selling if the client can handle the product, but this does increase the need to maintain the cleanliness of the products. Testers, which allow clients to sample products, must be kept clean at all times as they project the image of the product and will be subject to contamination. Product prices should be quite clearly displayed.

Levels of stock for professional use in the salon should also be maintained. Similar guidelines for maintenance of stock levels and the appearance of the stock apply. Records of rates of stock use will be used to monitor the effective use of stock. They will also help to predict the quantities of stock required. Your salon may have a policy on stock levels for these areas and how replenishment stock is obtained.

TIP All staff should be vigilant in monitoring retail stock and should theft or loss be observed this should be reported to the manager, who may then deal with it. Remember that product not paid for reduces the income of the salon.

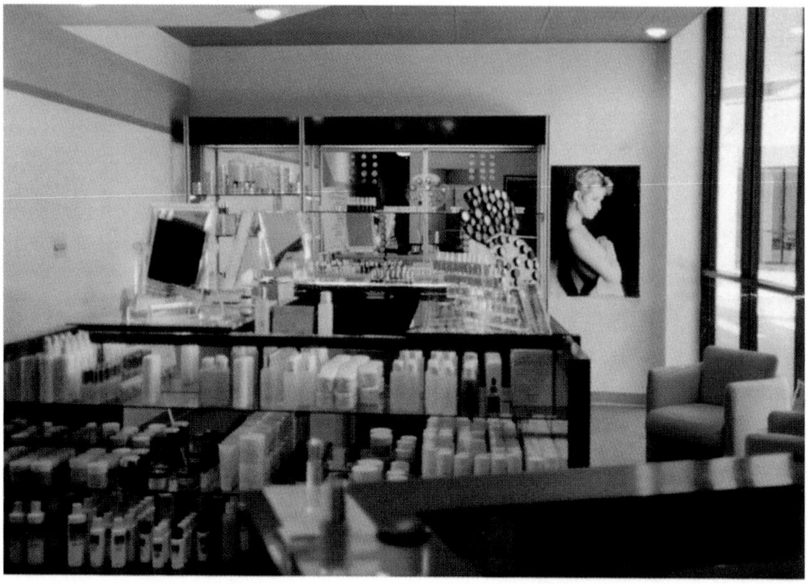

Figure 9.2 A retail display

Storage and handling of stock

1 Deliveries of stock should be checked against accompanying delivery notes and any product that arrives in a damaged condition or in variance from that listed should be reported, as soon as is possible, to the person who is responsible within the salon. They will then inform the supplier of this and make a claim for replacement or compensation. Pass all delivery notes and accompanying documentation to this responsible person.

> ***HEALTH AND SAFETY*** Products that release gases (such as hydrogen peroxide) are best stored in opaque plastic containers. If glass containers are used, a space for expansion must be left inside the container. The gases released cause increases in pressure which can cause the bottle to explode when handled. Light and heat can accelerate the release of gas.

As new stock arrives, the old stock should be drawn forward and the newer replenishments put behind this. Partially used containers, tubes of tint etc. should be used before new products are opened, provided that the product already opened is still in good condition. It may be necessary to obtain permission from the manager to dispose of part-used containers if they are no longer usable.

Quantities of stock should be stored in a secure area. This area should be dark, dry and cool with a minimum of temperature variance. This will avoid excessive deterioration of stock. Shelves containing stock should be secure. It is not advisable to store substances that are corrosive above eye level, in case they spill onto the user. Glass bottles may best not be stored above head height, to reduce the risk from breakage if dropped.

Inflammable substances may need to be secured in a flame-resistant cabinet.

Products that may react with each other should not be stored together. The salon owner/stock controller will have made assessments of any risks involved in the storage, movement and use of products. If you are in any doubt about how to handle stock seek advice from your manager or trainer.

Take care when moving stock and equipment. Lift heavy products with your back straight (see Figure 9.3) bending at the knees. Do not attempt to lift more than you can reasonably cope with; if in doubt seek assistance. If stock must be obtained from shelves above eye level, stand only on appropriate steps, do not overextend yourself, risking strain or a fall (see Figure 9.4)

➤ Health, safety and security in the salon, pages 207–214

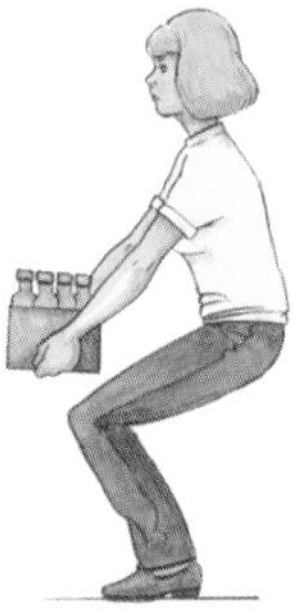

Figure 9.3 Always lift heavy items in the correct manner

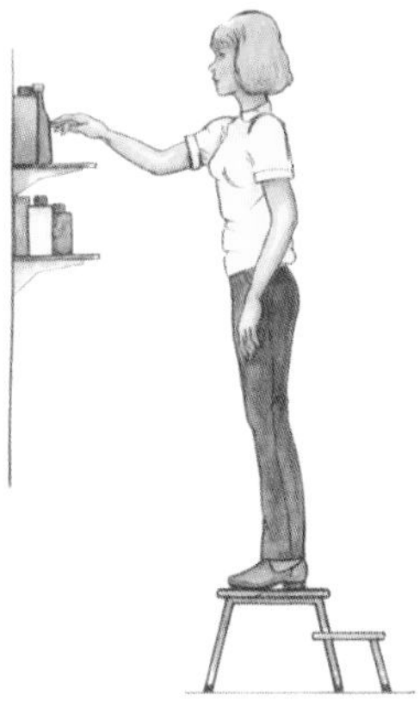

Figure 9.4 Do not over-extend yourself when handling stock above head height

EFFICIENT USE OF RESOURCES

> ***TIP*** Manufacturers provide guidance on the rate of use of bulk-supplied products and the number of applications that may be obtained. If you are unsure of the correct amount of a product to use, seek advice from your manager or trainer.

Wasteful use of any resource will have a detrimental effect upon the business. If you are in doubt about salon procedures and requirements regarding use of resources, consult your line manager or trainer. Here are some basic guidelines that should be adopted by all: 1

- Turn off electric lights when they are not required, provided that they do not produce a hazardous environment.
- When shampooing turn off the water supply while massaging.
- Apply only sufficient shampoo to cleanse: applying too much shampoo will result in additional time and water being wasted in removing the excess lather.
- Do not leave electrical appliances operating when no longer required.
- Rotate stock and use up previously started stock, provided it is still in good condition and not contaminated.
- Plan your appointments to make the most effective use of your time.
- The telephone is a link for the salon to its clientele; do not use it for personal calls, or extend telephone conversations which may prevent a potential client making contact.
- Following manufacturer's guidelines in correct methods of using equipment will reduce unintentional damage. 1
- To avoid wastage and maintain consistency use measured quantities of products.

There may be risks involved when intentionally using products and equipment for purposes other than for those for which they were intended. This may neutralise any responsibility that a manufacturer has for the products that it produces. It may also impact upon any compensation available, via insurance, should damage result from this. If you have been instructed in the correct usage and then misuse the product and equipment you may put yourself and/or your colleagues at risk and may also reduce any compensation that you may obtain should an industrial accident result.

Should you identify potential alternative or additional use of resources or identify improvements these should be communicated to your manager or trainer and their agreement and support gained before you implement them. These suggestions may form part of a development exercise for the salon's staff team at a later date.

FURTHER STUDY

1 ■ Review your own use of resources and try to act on any areas of potential improvement identified.
- Ensure that you are fully aware of your responsibility, within the hairdressing salon, with regard to the correct storage and display of products.

REVIEW QUESTIONS

1. Suggest two resource items that will require monitoring before each working day.
2. What is stock rotation?
3. How should you protect yourself when topping up potentially hazardous materials?
4. How should spillages of liquids be dealt with?
5. What are the ideal conditions for the storage of stock?
6. How should heavy products be lifted?

CHAPTER 10

Health, safety and security in the salon

The information in this chapter affects all other areas in the book. This chapter provides the essential knowledge to help you understand the current industrial and legal requirements regarding health, safety and security in the salon.

Level 1

Unit 105

Element 105.1	Follow emergency procedures
Element 105.2	Support health and safety at work

Level 2

Unit 209

Element 209.1	Follow emergency procedures
Element 209.2	Support health, safety and security at work

Contents

INTRODUCTION

The maintenance of health and safety at work is the responsibility of everyone. Each person working in the hairdressing salon has a legal requirement to take reasonable care of themselves and not intentionally to put themselves or others at risk by their actions or omissions. Employers have considerable responsibilities within this area, but all employees have a duty to comply with reasonable requests that employers may make of them in their efforts to make the workplace safe.

GENERAL SALON HYGIENE

1 A hairdressing salon, due to the warm, moist atmosphere and the numbers of people who pass through the doors each day, is an ideal place for the spread of infection and contagious disorders. Section 77 of the Public Health Act, 1961, empowers local authorities to make bye-laws for the registration of premises and health hygiene within them. These bye-laws may differ slightly between authorities, but they are all legally enforceable.

Hygiene within the salon is not only a legal requirement, it must also be highly desirable from everybody's point of view. Your clients visiting the salon will wish to feel safe from the risk of infection. As someone employed in the salon, and therefore spending much of your time in this environment, you too will wish to feel safe, and the salon owner will view this as an essential aspect for successful business.

It is not always satisfactory just to be hygienic: your clients must see that this is the case. This will be reflected by the hygienic behaviour of all staff in the salon, and the high profile given to hygiene. There are three aspects to hygiene in the salon:

- cleanliness and hygiene of the premises and its provisions for hygiene
- cleanliness and hygiene of the tools and equipment
- cleanliness and hygiene of those employed within the salon.

> ***TIP*** If your job is to clean surfaces and empty bins, look on this as part of the team's work to maintain the correct environment for your clients. Remember, your clients will not be impressed by floors that are littered with hairs or bins which are full to overflowing.

Cleanliness and hygiene of the premises and their provisions for hygiene

All surfaces should be easily cleaned. This includes work surfaces, basins, walls and floors. Hair clippings can be difficult to remove from some surfaces. Floors should be swept daily and cleaned at least once a week. There should be covered bins for hair clippings and other waste materials, and these should be emptied, once full, and at least once a day.

Remember, when cleaning work surfaces using cleaning products, always follow the manufacturer's directions, including the use of protective clothing if required. Products used for cleaning and sterilising surfaces are sometimes flammable.

Cleanliness and hygiene of tools and equipment

Gowns and towels used on your clients, should be freshly washed before use. Tools should be washed and sterilised between use on your clients. In the salon you will find various methods used to sterilise tools. These include; autoclaves, ultra-violet light cabinets and sterilising fluids. 1

The autoclave

This is a steamer that produces steam at high pressure, allowing high temperatures to be achieved. Due to the high temperatures used, the autoclave is only suitable for use on tools which are not damaged by heat. It is therefore not suitable for use on vulcanite or plastic combs, scissors with plastic inserts or for hair brushes.

Take care when using an autoclave. Always follow the manufacturer's directions for safe use. The outer casing will usually become hot, and you should always allow adequate time for the pressure within to drop and the temperature to drop before opening to remove tools.

> ***TIP*** Follow manufacturer's directions in the correct and safe use of sterilising equipment and products.

Ultra-violet cabinet

This cabinet uses ultra-violet light to sterilise those surfaces that the light rays touch. As a result it is only effective for tools that can be totally exposed to the light on all surfaces, so it may be necessary to turn tools to ensure coverage. To sterilise effectively, tools must be clean and dry when placed in these cabinets. You should not expose yourself to this light. 1

Sterilising fluids

These are possibly the most widely used means for sterilising tools in the hairdressing salon. Tools should be cleaned before being immersed in the fluids. Fluids should be changed regularly as they: 1

- rapidly lose their strength. Some have colour detectors to indicate their strength.
- lose their efficiency when the fluid becomes dirty.

Some fluids attack the surface of metallic tools and may make cutting tools blunt. Aerosol sterilising fluids are available which are particularly useful for use on cutting tools.

Before sterilising tools, always wash and dry them, as the presence of dirt, dust and moisture may impede the effects of the sterilising fluid.

> ***HEALTH AND SAFETY*** Some fluids may be poisonous; alcohol based fluids may be flammable or produce flammable vapour.

Cleanliness and hygiene of those employed in the salon

It is anticipated that hairdressers will be dressed appropriately, wearing protective overalls or uniforms that are worn exclusively at work. Overalls or protective clothing should be washable and kept hygienic for use at work. 1

Working with others, pages 187–200

The Personal Protective Equipment at Work Regulations 1992 (PPE) requires that suitable protective equipment is provided for employees who may be exposed to risk while at work within the hairdressing salon. This usually means the provision of protective gloves for your use when handling perm lotion, hydrogen peroxide, tints and any other product where the manufacturer's directions indicate this. Protective goggles may also be required in certain circumstances. **As an employee, you should report to your employer any loss or damage to personal protective equipment.**

> ***TIP*** Spillages should be cleaned away immediately. Take care to dispose of contaminated cleaning items correctly. If in doubt, seek advice.

SAFETY IN THE SALON

1 Safety legislation requires that all employers should provide a safe working environment and as an employee you have a responsibility to work within the guidelines of safety for the salon. If your salon staff team has five or more people in it, there will be a written health and safety policy. This will give you guidance about:

- who is responsible within the salon for aspects of health and safety
- reporting accidents
- first aid procedures
- emergency procedures.

You may receive training about health and safety and in the particular provisions and procedures for your salon. Some features of safe working may be common sense but may not be apparent to all. In the sketch (see Figure 10.1) there are a number of unsafe practices: can you find them?

1 The following is a list of some features for safe working practice within your salon.

- Always mop up spillages of liquids immediately.
- Hair can make floor surfaces slippery, so sweep up hair clippings and place in a covered bin.
- Do not tamper with fire extinguishers or other safety items.
- Do not block doorways, emergency exits or stairways.
- Do not decant products into unmarked or incorrectly marked containers.
- If you are unaware of how to use products and equipment correctly seek advice or read the manufacturer's directions.
- Before using electrical equipment check for any obvious damage to the casing, flex or plug connections. Any identified damage to equipment should be reported to the responsible person and that item taken out of use until checked and repaired.
- Do not trail electrical cables across walkways in the salon.
- Find out where the salon's first aid box is and if there is a trained first aider for the business.
- Find out what the procedures are for the safe evacuation of the salon in an emergency.

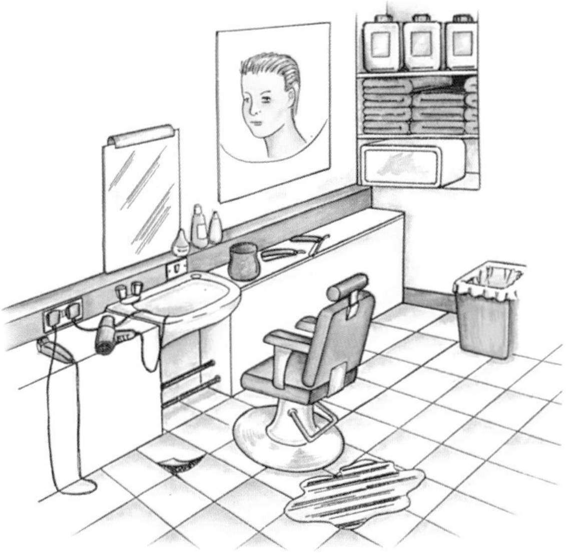

Figure 10.1 Unsafe practices

SAFETY LEGISLATION

The Health and Safety at Work Act 1974 (HASAWA) 1

The employer has a duty of care to employees and others within the salon, or those affected by the work of the salon. Employees have a duty not to intentionally endanger the health, safety and welfare of themselves or others. Employees must not interfere with or misuse any items provided in the pursuance of health and safety.

The Workplace (Health, Safety and Welfare) Regulations 1992

Originally applied to all new workplaces which had opened since 1992, and now applies to all workplaces, effective from January 1996. It focuses mainly upon a minimum standard of facilities and the provision of safe premises to work in.

The Manual Handling Operations Regulations 1992

Requires that employers make an assessment of individuals' capability to carry or move stock and for guidance to be provided in safe working practices.

The Personal Protective Equipment at Work Act 1992

Requires employers to provide, free of charge, suitable personal protective equipment to employees who may be exposed to risk at work. Employees must report to the employer any loss or damage of these provisions.

The Provision and Use of Work Equipment Regulations 1992

Requires that an employer should provide equipment that is suitable for its use, that it is properly maintained and that staff are trained to use it safely.

The Control of Substances Hazardous to Health Regulations 1988 (COSHH)

Requires employers to consider potential hazards to people exposed to substances within the salon. This includes assessing substances for potential hazards, having identified any potential hazard to consider possible alternative less hazardous substances which may be used and to set up safe working procedures.

A Guide to the Health and Safety of Salon Hair Products (fourth edition) is produced by the Hairdressing and Beauty Suppliers Association. It provides good advice on the contents, potential hazards and good practice in the use of a range of substances used in the hairdressing profession.

The Electricity at Work Regulations 1989

These cover the fitting, maintenance of electrical systems and equipment.

The salon is required to ensure that all electrical equipment is regularly tested, it is recommended that this should be done at least once a year. The salon should ensure that all electrical equipment is individually numbered and that a list of all this electrical equipment and their numbers is kept. All equipment tested should have a label attached indicating the last test date.

A member of the salon staff should, in addition, carry out a visual check of all electrical equipment. Any tools brought in by members of staff, for use in the salon, must also be tested and this recorded in the same manner.

EMERGENCIES

These may be described as 'a sudden state of danger'. While emergencies cannot be forecast, you should be aware of basic procedures and the salon's policy on how to act in these circumstances. Emergencies should be reported to your functional manager as quickly as possible. Emergencies may include:

- fire
- bomb alerts
- suspicious persons and packages
- flood
- gas leaks
- security risks

The extent of your actions will depend upon your own personal level of responsibility. Advice should be sought from your manager, and your level of responsibility may be defined in the salon's health and safety policy statement.

> ***TIP*** Always follow the salon's guidelines in dealing with emergencies while at the same time safeguarding your own safety.

Fire

Your salon may have a fire alarm system. This should be sounded, (check on your salon's guidelines for dealing with a fire emergency). A minor fire may be dealt with using the appropriate form of fire extinguisher (see Figure 10.2); all fires should be reported to the responsible person in the business.

Note: If in any doubt, premises should be evacuated and the emergency fire service called.

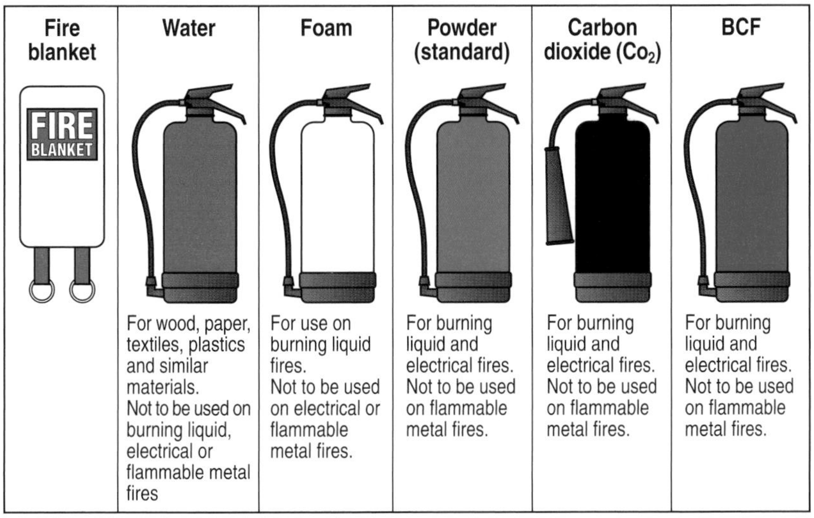
Fire blanket
FIRE
BLANKET
Water
For wood, paper, textiles, plastics and similar materials. Not to be used on burning liquid, electrical or flammable metal fires
Foam
For use on burning liquid fires. Not to be used on electrical or flammable metal fires.
Powder (standard)
For burning liquid and electrical fires. Not to be used on flammable metal fires.
Carbon dioxide (Co2)
For burning liquid and electrical fires. Not to be used on flammable metal fires.
BCF
For burning liquid and electrical fires. Not to be used on flammable metal fires.

Figure 10.2 Appropriate fire extinguishers

Fire extinguishers

There are a range of fire extinguishers available today. For some the body of the extinguisher is colour coded to indicate the type of fire on which they may be used.

Other fire extinguishers may be labelled with a code letter (A, B, C, D) which denotes the type of fire on which they may be used.

Fire extinguisher ratings:

Class A Extinguishers will put out fires of ordinary burnable items including wood, paper and textiles.

Class B Extinguishers should be used on fires of flammable liquids including grease, petrol, oil, etc.

Class C Extinguishers are suitable for electrical fires or fires on electrical equipment.

The fire brigade may be contacted by dialling 999 on the telephone. The emergency service will wish to take some details about the nature and location of the emergency and may ask you to stay by the telephone.

Flood

Report to a designated person, who will turn off the water supply at the mains, and using dry hands turn off any electrical appliances that may be wet. Check on the salon's guidelines for dealing with a flood emergency. If water has flooded through the ceiling, electrical circuits may have been affected, so turn off the electricity supply at the mains. Contact a plumber. 1

Bomb alerts

Check on the salon's guidelines for dealing with a bomb emergency. This will possibly result in the evacuation of the premises and the authorities being informed. 1

Gas leaks

Report to a designated person, who will turn off the gas supply, both at the appliance and at the mains (by the meter). Check on the salon's guidelines for dealing with a gas emergency. Open windows, vacate the premises and report the leak to the local gas suppliers using their emergency number. Take care not to use a telephone (including mobile phone) in the affected area. Do not look for the gas leak using a naked light, nor turn on electric switches or use electrical machines as this may cause a spark which may ignite the gas.

Suspicious persons and packages

Any person acting suspiciously should be reported to the salon manager or your supervisor, check on the salon's guidelines for dealing with a security emergency. It may not always be wise to approach a person acting in a suspicious manner; depending on the circumstance it may be necessary to call the police or a security guard for assistance. This will normally be a management decision.

Suspicious packages should always be reported to your manager.

Failure to follow emergency procedures could result in injury or damage to people or property. Procedures will have been developed to reduce the risk to all in the event of an emergency. Businesses are required to show that emergency evacuation procedures are in place and are practised by the staff team (fire drills etc.). Failure to comply with them may also invalidate any insurance policy.

FURTHER STUDY

- Find out about the contents of the products that you use in the salon, and what should be done with them in the case of accident.
- Find out what types of fire extinguishers are available in your salon and how they should be effectively used.
- Ensure that you are aware of your salon's procedures in dealing with an emergency.
- First aid procedures can save lives. Consider taking a course of training in this area.

REVIEW QUESTIONS

1. Who is responsible for undertaking COSHH risk assessments for a business?
2. Which method of sterilising in the salon uses moist heat at high pressure?
3. How should the hairdresser cover any exposed cuts when working on a client?
4. How often should floor surfaces be swept?
5. How should tools be prepared before being placed in an ultra-violet sterilising cabinet?
6. What protective clothing should be used when handling perm lotion?
7. What responsibilities do employees have with regard to the Personal Protective Equipment at Work Regulation 1992?
8. What are the possible consequences of not following accident, emergency and evacuation procedures?
9. How should damaged equipment be treated in the salon?
10. What risk is there in failing to sweep up hair clippings from the floor?

CHAPTER 11

Setting and dressing hair

This chapter will provide the essential knowledge necessary for understanding a variety of techniques for setting and dressing hair, including long hair.

Level 2	
Unit 201	
Element 201.1	Consult with and maintain effective relationships with clients
Unit 203	
Element 203.1	Maintain effective and safe methods of working when drying and setting hair
Element 203.3	Set and dress hair to style
Element 203.4	Dress long hair to style
Unit 209	
Element 209.2	Support health, safety and security at work

Contents

INTRODUCTION

Setting hair is the traditional method of wet styling ladies' hair. While it may not be fashionable with younger clients today, its use is quite widespread and offers a range of styling not so easily achieved by blow-drying techniques for a wide range of clients. The techniques are often adapted for fashion use.

Setting allows a wide range of temporary shapes to be introduced into the hair. These shapes are usually curved or wavy. In some cases they create volume for the hair at the root area and/or in the middle lengths and ends of the hair strand. As it is the shape that the hair is in while it is dried that produces the final style, the possibilities are endless. The hair is wetted, usually with water, stretched into a new shape, and dried into this shape. The hair retains the new shape until it becomes moist again.

Drying hair into shape, pages 37–52

There are a number of techniques for introducing shape into hair by setting. These include:

- roller placement, wrapping hair around a cylinder form to produce a curl or wave
- pin curling, shaping the hair into round forms, either flat to the head or with lift at the roots and securing these in place using clips
- finger waving, shaping wet hair into a wave form, against the scalp to produce flat waves.

These techniques may be used on their own or may be combined together to produce the required finished look (see Figure 11.1).

SETTING TOOLS

The actual type of tool selected for use when setting will depend mainly upon personal preference. Do remember, however, that poorly-made tools may have sharp surfaces that damage the hair or scalp, or may be made of materials that are adversely affected by heat from the hair-dryer. Select tools that are easily kept clean and may be sterilised.

Hair rollers

Hair rollers are cylindrical in shape and vary in diameter. Within a range of diameters there may be several lengths of roller (see Figure 11.2).

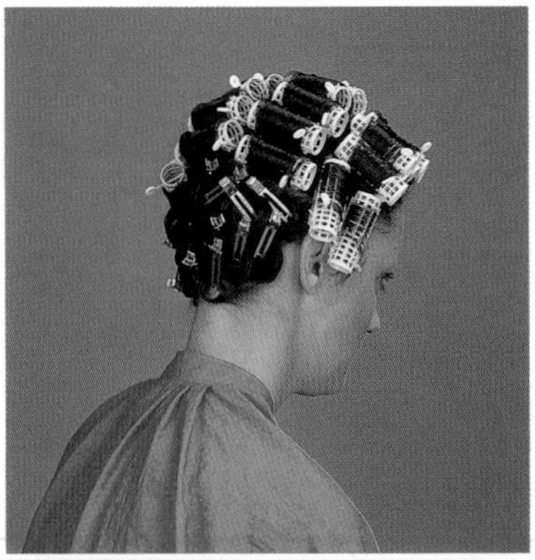

Figure 11.1 Hairset in progress

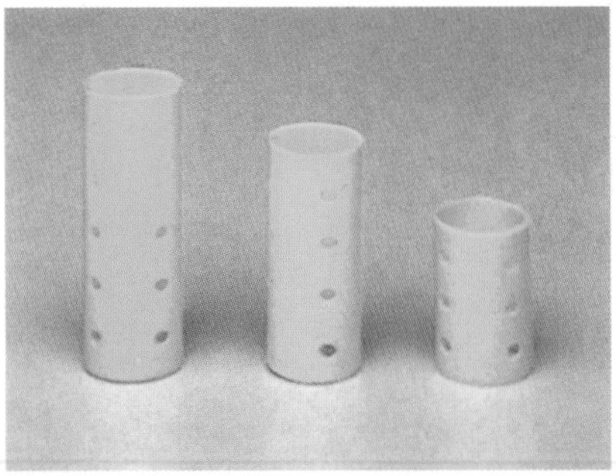

Figure 11.2 Rollers of similar width and various lengths

Roller selection

The diameter of the curler will dictate the degree of curl or wave achieved in the hair, as well as affecting the amount of root lift produced. Rollers that have small diameters will produce tight curl and little height in the hair. Large diameter rollers will produce a soft wave movement in hair but with root lift.

Rollers may be made of a variety of materials, with a range of surface finishes:

- Smooth plastic: ideal for use on porous hair, which may mark easily. The ideal roller for competition use as it leaves a smooth finish on the hair. It may be difficult to retain in place on the head.
- Spiked plastic: will grip the hair more easily. Avoid very long or too numerous spikes as these may mark the hair, cause distortion in the hair or may become entangled in long hair.
- Sponge rollers will produce a soft set, but due to the porous nature of some they can extend the drying time of hair.
- Metal mesh rollers, will grip the hair, they may mark very porous hair. Take care that these rollers do not rest directly on the skin as they may become very hot and burn the client's scalp.
- Flexi/bendy rollers, usually made with a plastic-coated, stiff copper wire centre, covered either by foam or cloth. These are easily placed in the hair, do not mark and by bending when positioned do not require any additional fixings to hold them in place.

Some rollers are tapered, which enables them to fit curved, pivotal setting patterns on the head (see Figure 11.3).

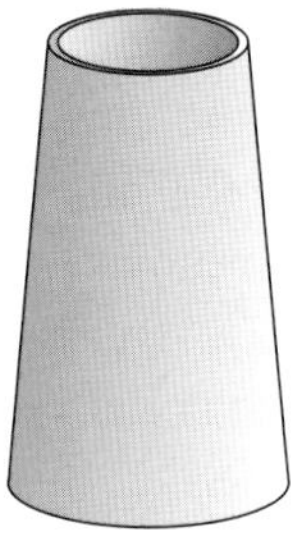

Figure 11.3 Tapered roller

Roller pins

These are available in metal, plastic or plastic-coated metal. The metallic pins have a coating which prevents them from rusting while on the hair. Take care when using metal pins as they can become very hot under the hairdryer and may burn your client's scalp. Pins are available in a range of lengths, which may be selected to suit the diameter of roller being used. When placing roller pins to hold the roller in place, take care not to distort or break the hair.

Pin curl clips

These clips are usually made of aluminium with a ferrous metal spring. There are a number available which are made of plastic with a metal spring. Clips are available either with single or double prongs. In selecting, choose the smallest-sized clip necessary to hold the curl in place, as clips can mark the hair. Contoured double-pronged clips are available for use on very thick hair, and have the advantage of being able to close around the hair without flattening the hair or sliding off the curl.

> **NOTE** Pressure marks from clips and pins will show as indentations in the finished style. Very porous and bleached hair is particularly susceptible to this.

Combs

The actual comb used when setting may be determined by personal preference or by salon policy. The comb should enable you to control and mould the hair. When roller setting a tail comb is often used, as this provides fine-set teeth to comb the hair into place and the pin-tail end to help when sectioning hair and when wrapping the hair smoothly around the roller.

Styling tools, page 43

For pin curling the tail comb or a setting comb may be used. The setting comb has fine-set teeth at one end and coarse-set teeth at the other. This style of comb may also be used when finger waving. Combs should be made of materials that are not affected by the chemicals used in hairdressing. They should not damage the hair or cause static electricity. The most suitable material is Vulcanite and the teeth of the combs should be saw cut.

PREPARATION

Client consultation, page 3

Whatever techniques of setting are used, for ease of dressing and to prolong its life the set should follow the direction of the intended style. The required style should be determined before commencing, by consultation with your client.

Hair sets most effectively when it is thoroughly wet and may be stretched easily into a new shape and then dried into that shape. Shampooing allows the hair to be wetted most effectively, allowing stretching to take place. Stretching and then thoroughly drying the hair allows a new shape to be introduced to the hair. Other techniques are less effective: the less wet the hair is made, the less the hair may be stretched and therefore the softer the set achieved. Hair may be set from dry, applying heat from a hairdryer to induce the set, or heated rollers may be used. Once wrapped around the heated rollers, the natural moisture in the hair is heated, inducing a temporary curl in the hair. The heated rollers may be used in conjunction with fast-drying sprays which moisten the hair, allowing it to be stretched and moulded into shape, and which then dry very quickly.

Hair that is in its unstretched state consists of 'alpha' keratin; when stretched it becomes 'beta' keratin, remaining in this state until it absorbs moisture and returns to its natural shape and its 'alpha' keratin form.

Preparing your client

Following consultation gown your client to protect their clothes, and shampoo if appropriate.

Setting aids

The set will last longer if the hair is protected from the effects of atmospheric moisture, which will cause the hair to spring back to its original shape. Setting aids usually coat the hair with a soluble, water resistant coating, which will slow down the effects of atmospheric moisture on the hair. They also often contain ingredients that will help the hair to dry, and which help to reduce static electricity and make the hair controllable.

TIP As the hair retains the shape in which it is set, any misshapen or distorted ends will also be retained in the finished hairstyle.

Setting lotions

These liquids often contain a thermoplastic, polyvinyl pyrollidone, which coats the hair with a film. This gradually breaks down with brushing and is washed away with shampooing. Setting lotions are available with a range of holding powers which offer from a strong hold through to a gentler, mild hold.

Shampooing and conditioning the hair and scalp, pages 18–36

When selecting appropriate setting lotions you will often find that when setting fine, delicate hair you need a setting lotion which is not too heavy, but that when controlling strong hair you may need a stronger lotion. Setting lotions are usually applied to towel-dried hair, by sprinkling onto the hair direct from the bottle. When applying, gently massage the hair and scalp; this will help to spread it and prevent it from running down the client's face and neck. Spread the application throughout the head, combing to ensure even distribution.

Drying hair into shape, pages 37–52

Points to remember

- Hair sets best when the hair has been shampooed.
- The hair set will last longer and be easier to dress if it follows the direction of hair growth.
- The set will last longer if protected from atmospheric moisture. Setting lotions can do this.

SETTING TECHNIQUES

The three setting techniques are:

- roller setting (winding)
- pin curling
- finger waving

These three techniques may be used independently or in conjunction with each other to achieve different effects in the hair.

Roller setting (winding)

The placement of rollers usually follows the direction in which the root area of the hairstyle moves. The hair should be long enough to be wrapped around the roller at least $2\frac{1}{2}$ times. This will ensure that it will holds firmly in place.

To ensure maximum root movement and control over the hair the roller section should be the same size as the roller to be used. Remember that the size of roller used will determine the strength of curl and degree of root lift achieved.

Using a comb, take a mesh of hair and comb away from the scalp so that the front of the

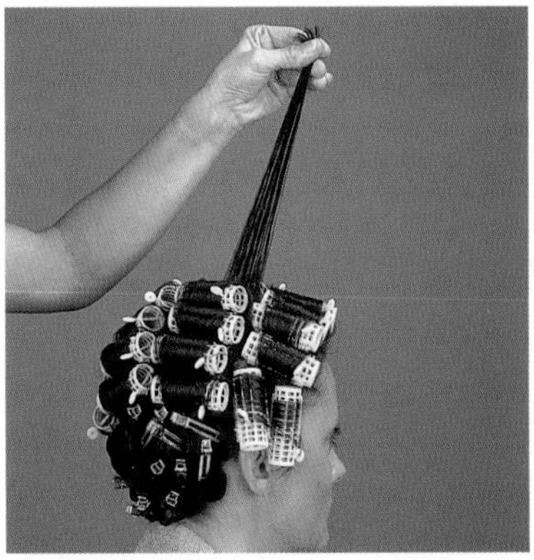

Figure 11.4 Placing rollers

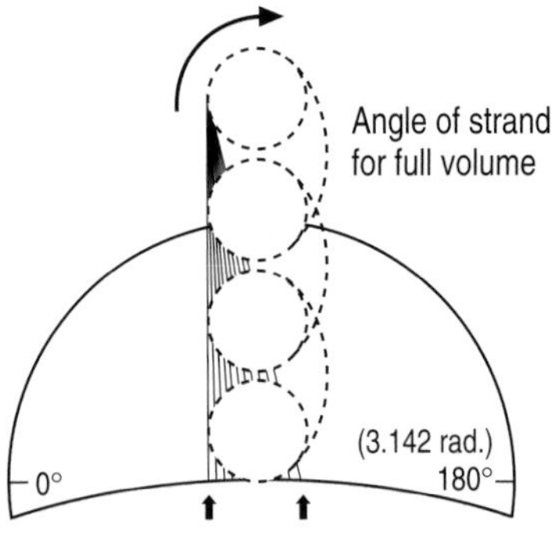

Figure 11.5 Roller set for full volume

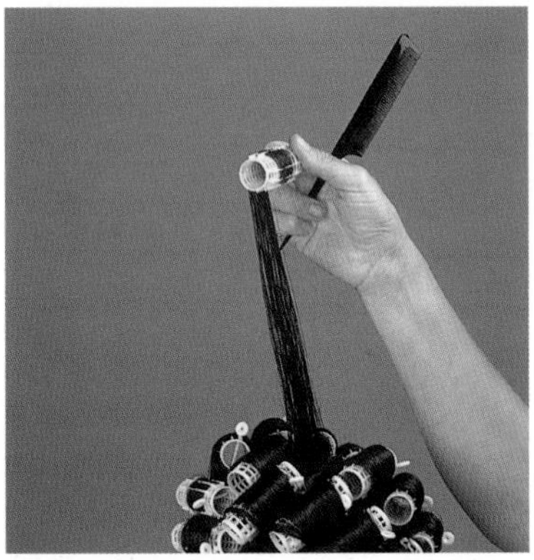

Figure 11.6 Placing roller against mesh

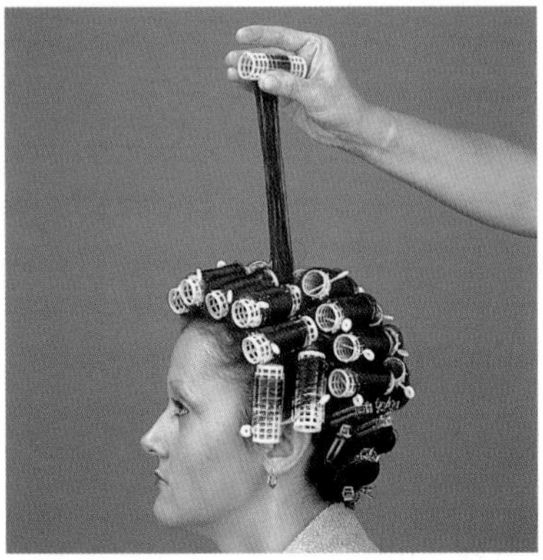

Figure 11.7 Smoothing hair point ends against roller

mesh is at slightly more than 90 degrees to the scalp (see Figures 11.4 and 11.5). Hold the hair firmly and place the roller against the mesh (see Figure 11.6) near the point ends. The mesh of hair should be held centrally but without the points bunched together. Smooth the hair point ends around the roller (see Figure 11.7).

When using rollers with spikes, rotating the roller against the hair can help to ensure a smooth wrap for the hair ends. With the hair point ends wrapped smoothly around the roller, wind the roller down towards the scalp with the hair around it, without bunching. Allow the hair to spread across the width of the roller and ensure that there are no distortions in the hair as it is wrapped (see Figure 11.8).

> ***TIP*** Buckled hair point ends or distorted hair lengths will not dress smoothly into the finished hairstyle.

The angle at which the hair is held when the roller is placed at the ends can vary the degree of lift achieved in the finished style. Over-directing the mesh away from the direction of the style (see Figure 11.9), allows the hair to be controlled further towards the root, and is ideal when working on very curly hair.

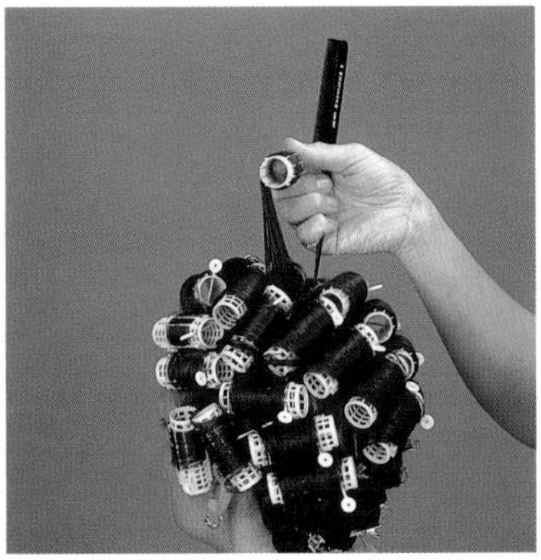

Figure 11.8 Winding roller towards scalp with hair on it

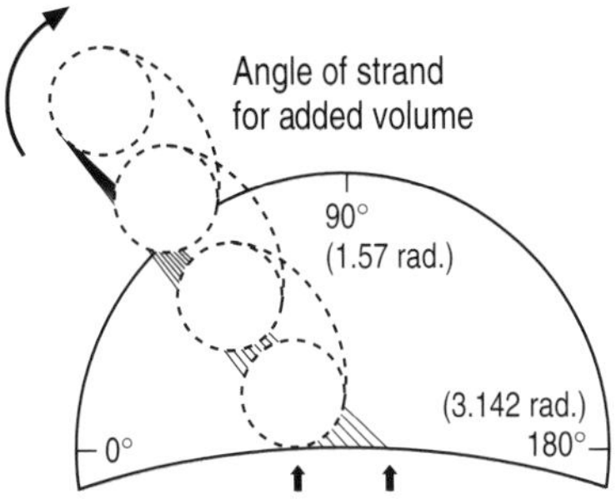

Figure 11.9 Overdirecting for added volume

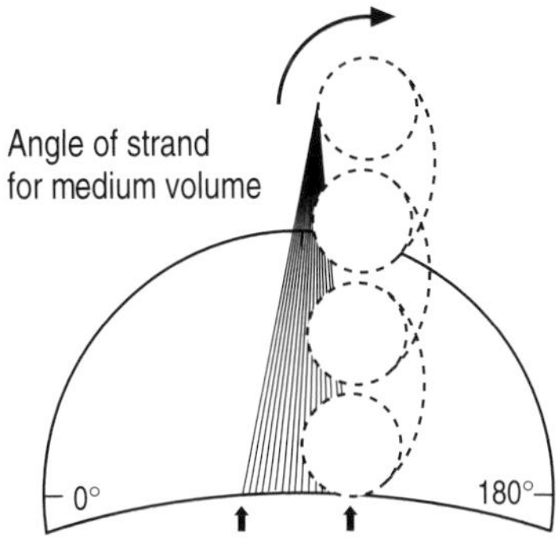

Figure 11.10 Medium volume

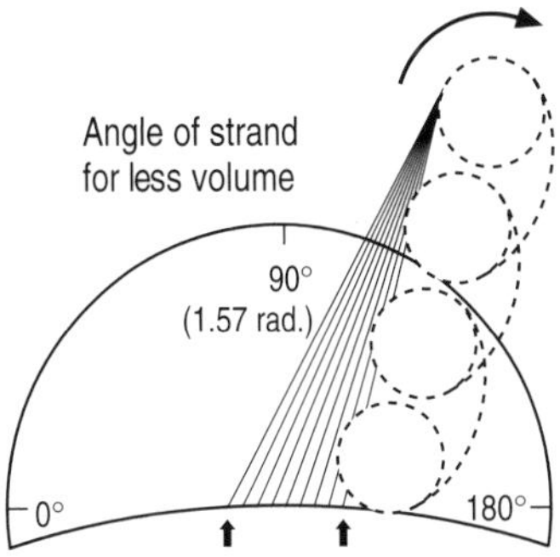

Figure 11.11 Less volume-root drag

Holding the mesh of hair at less that 90 degrees will flatten the root area (see Figures 11.10 and 11.11). This technique may be used when setting overly thick hair to reduce volume without thinning. In cases when no root lift is required at all, the hair may be combed flat to the head, and the roller may be placed on top of the mesh and wound back towards the root area (see Figure 11.12). This technique may be alternated with that in Figure 11.5 to produce deep wave movement at the scalp on long hair.

Features of good practice

- Never take sections with too much hair as this will extend the drying time and relax the curl strength towards the roots.
- For control roller sections should be no wider than the roller being used.
- Ensure that all the hair is wrapped with even tension, across the width of the curler.
- Spread the hair across the width of the roller as it winds.
- Avoid damaging or distorting the hair when placing the fixing pin (see Figure 11.13).

Pin curl setting

Pin curling enables you to place curled hair in the exact position, with the exact degree of curl and with the exact direction of root movement required for the finished dressing. There are three types of pin curls:

- barrel pin curls – a constant degree of curl throughout the length of hair (see Figure 11.14)

- stand up barrel curls – the same effect as that of a hair roller (see Figure 11.15)
- clock spring pin curl – a curl which gets tighter towards the hair points (see Figure 11.16).

Other than the 'stand up' curl, all others produce little or no root lift. There are three parts to the pin curl: the stem, the body and the base (see Figure 11.17).

The stem direction will determine the direction in which the hair moves, and will normally be determined by the required hairstyle. The size and direction of the body of the curl will determine the degree of movement and how the hair moves from the stem. The size and shape of the base will be determined by the required hairstyle, the thickness of the hair and the direction of the stem.

Barrel curls

Take a section of hair and comb to remove any tangles. Mould the stem of the curl in the required direction and, holding the hair mesh at the point where the stem joins the curl body, form a rounded curl shape of the required size (see Figure 11.18).

Ensure that all of the hair is smoothly moulded into place and then secure the curl, locating a curl clip over the curl body. Place the clip over only as much of the curl body as is necessary to hold the curl. This will avoid unnecessary pressure marks on the hair (see Figure 11.19). When locating the clip avoid distortion of the stem and root area.

The stems may be directed to support the style, either with a long shaped stem (see Figure 11.20) to produce a flat, directed effect, or over-directed to deepen a movement (see Figure 11.21).

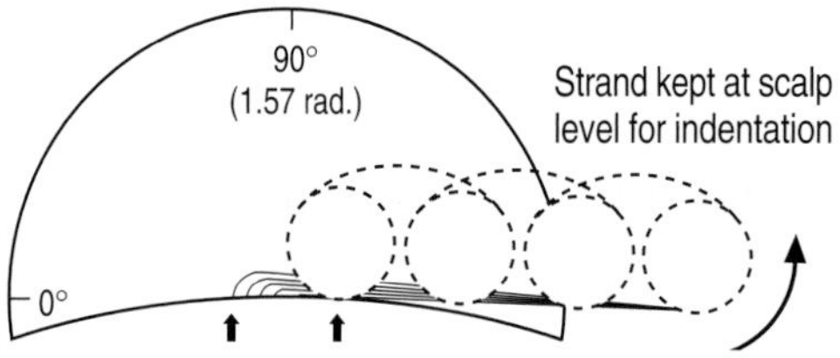

Figure 11.12 Strand curled at scalp level

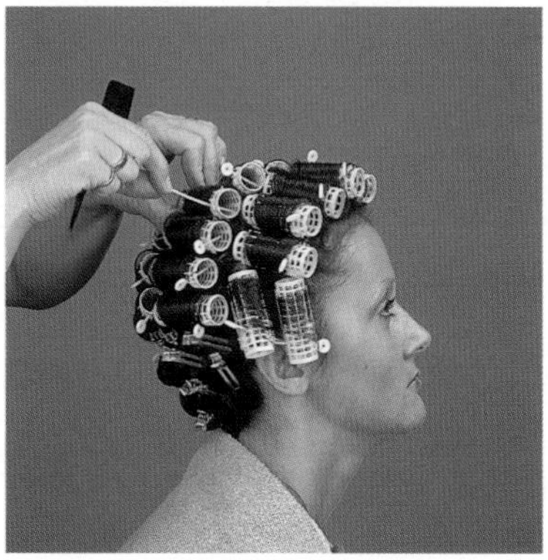

Figure 11.13 Placing fixing pin

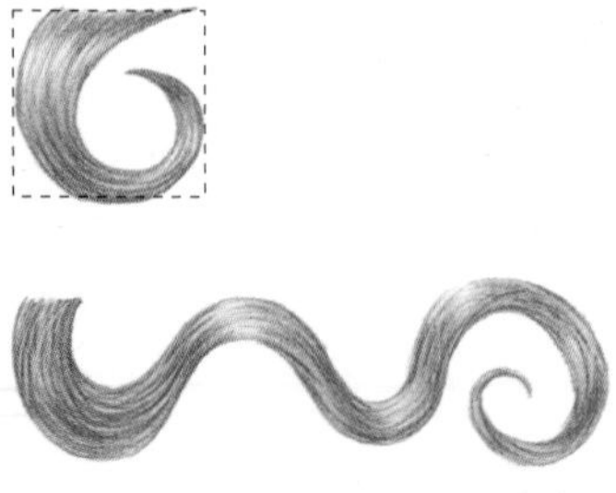

Figure 11.14 Barrel pin curls

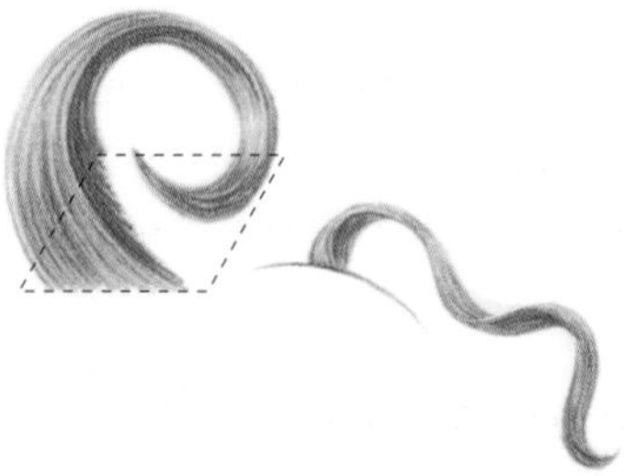

Figure 11.15 Stand up barrel curls

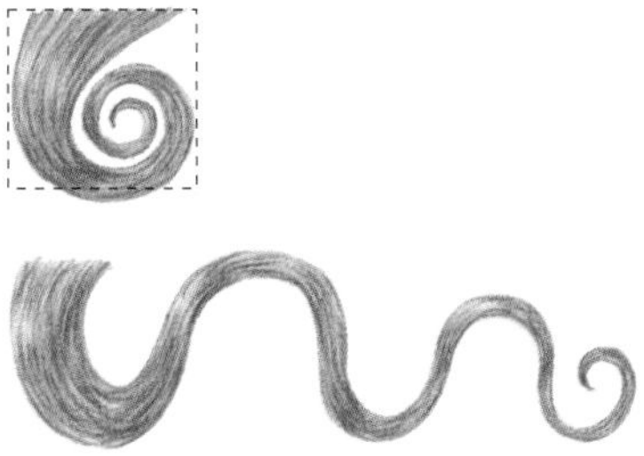

Figure 11.16 Clock spring pin curl

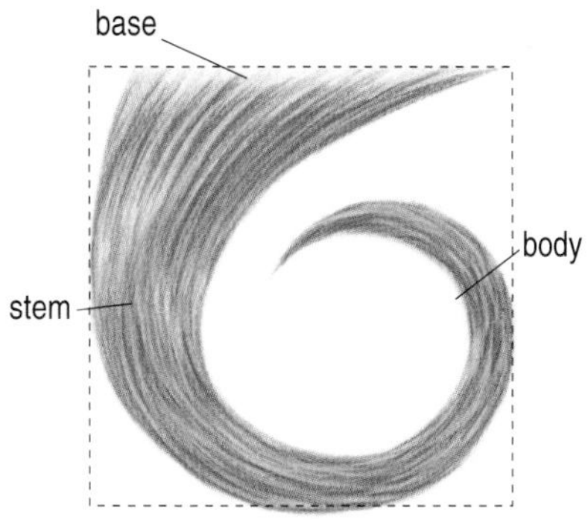

Figure 11.17 Parts of a curl

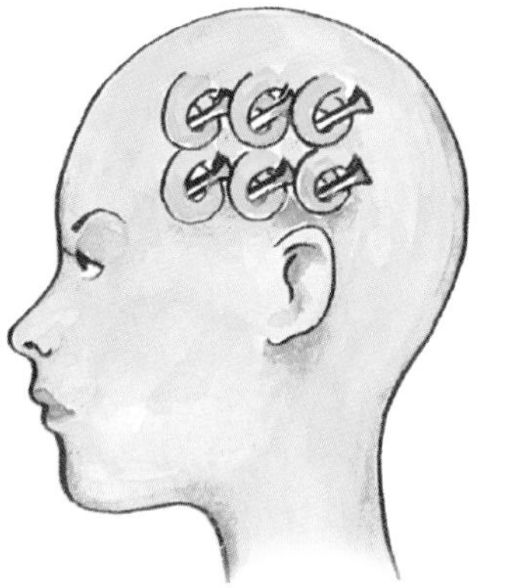

Figure 11.18 Forming barrel curls

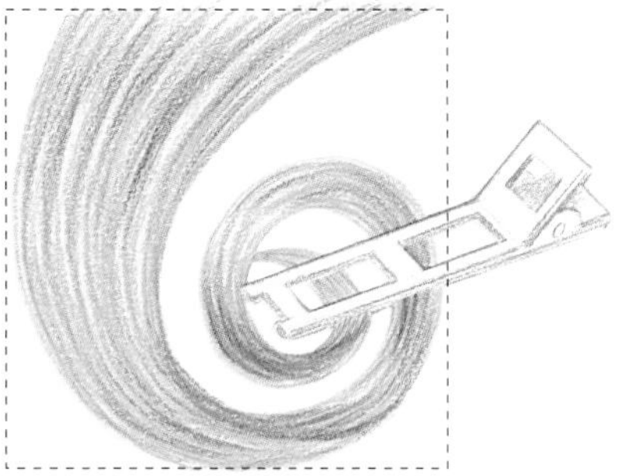

Figure 11.19 How to clip curls

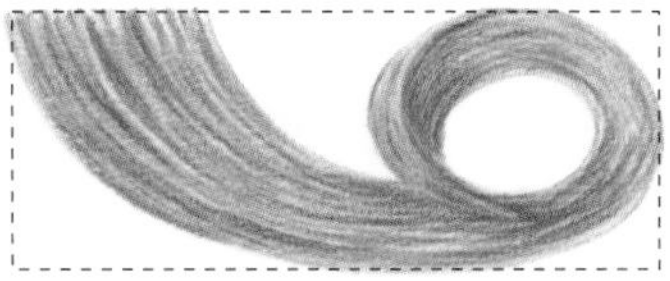

Figure 11.20 Curling to produce a flat, directed effect

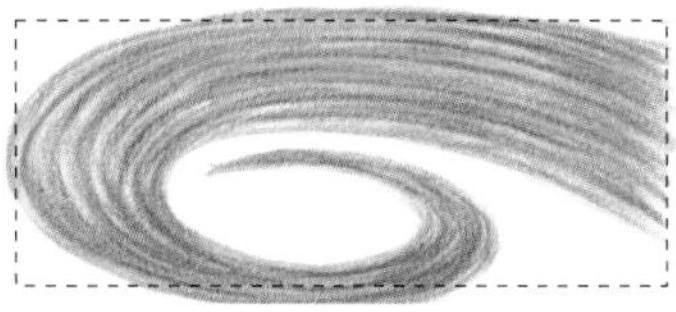

Figure 11.21 Overdirection for a deeper movement

Barrel curls may be used to produce a flat waved effect in hair, known as reverse pin curling. Rows of curls, placed with the body of the curl following the direction of the wave, may be dressed into a corresponding wave movement. The hair may first be moulded into a wave shape, and then the ends of the hair picked up and curled into the wave shape and secured (see Figure 11.22). Alternatively, section the hair into rows at the scalp and then subdivide the rows into pin curl sections. Pin curl the bodies of the curls for each row in alternate directions (see Figure 11.23).

Stand up barrel curls

Take sections of hair of a similar depth as that you would take for a hair roller, to produce a similar degree of curl. The width of the section should be no wider than the prongs of the securing

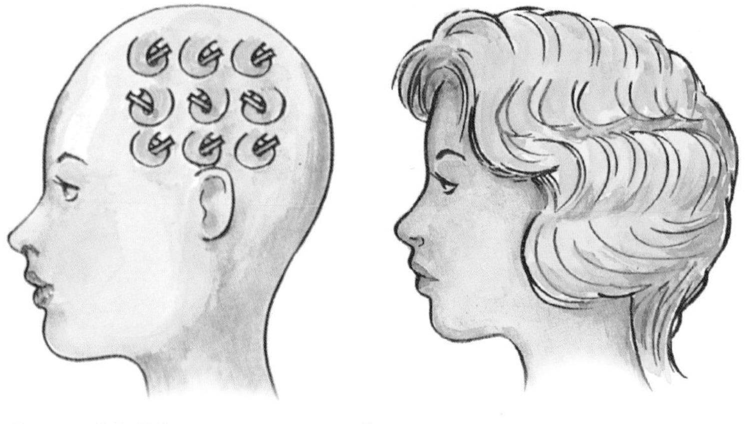

Figure 11.22 Reverse pin curling

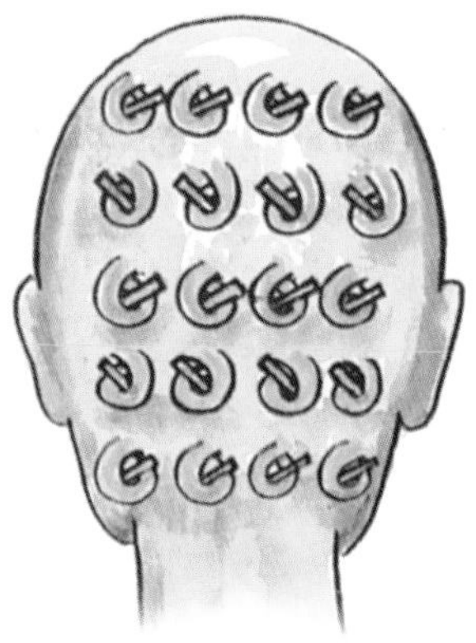

Figure 11.23 Reverse pin curling

clip. Hold the hair up from the scalp and comb to remove tangles and mould the hair together. As for hair rollers, the hair may be over-directed to gain maximum control of hold at less than 90 degrees to produce less root lift (see Figure 11.11).

Holding the points of the hair, create a rounded shape of the required size and rotate the hair until it rests at the scalp. Locate the securing clip through the curl onto the base of the section. Take care not to mark or indent the curl stem (see Figures 11.24 and 11.25).

Barrel curls may be produced which combine aspects of both the flat and the stand-up effects. This give subtle degrees of lift where a full effect may not be required (see Figure 11.26).

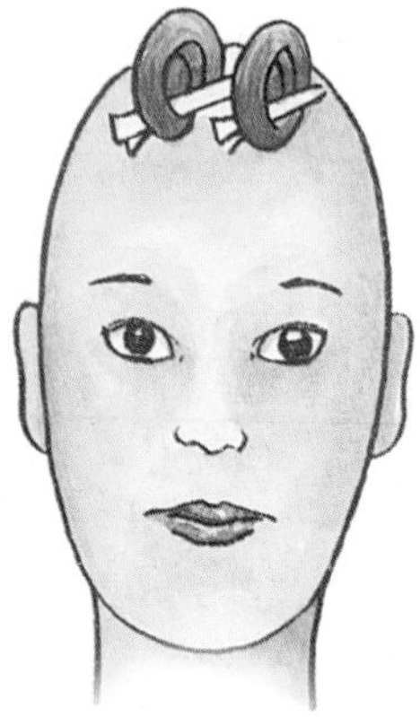

Figure 11.24 Forming stand up barrel curls

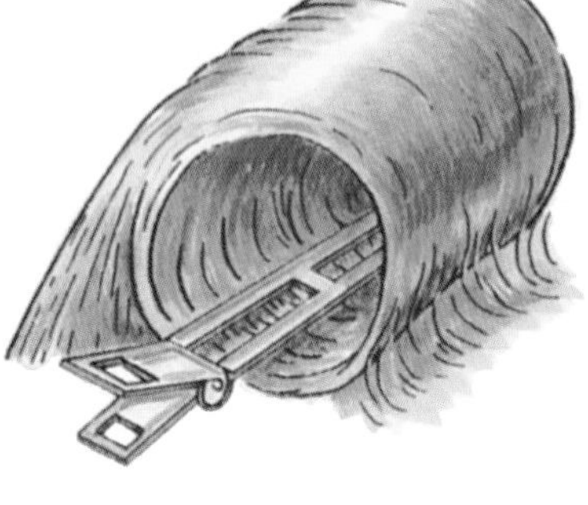

Figure 11.25 Clip on stand up barrel curls

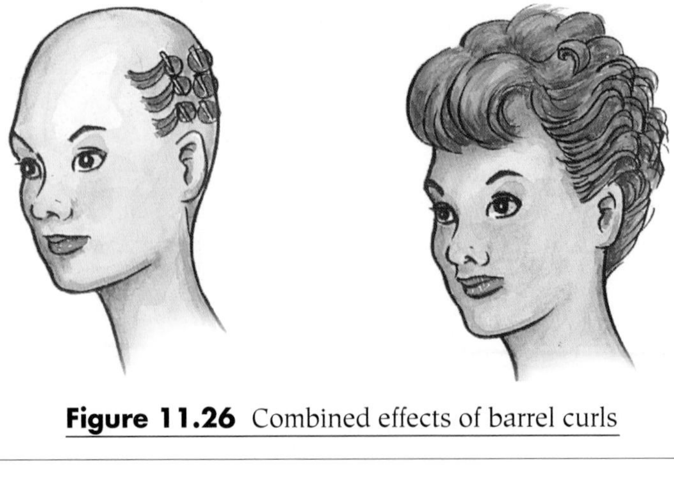

Figure 11.26 Combined effects of barrel curls

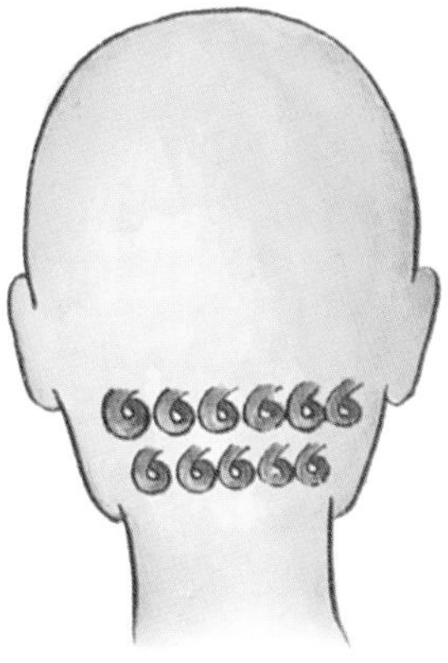

Figure 11.27 Clock spring curls

Clock spring curls

Clock spring curls are produced in a similar way to barrel curls, but the body of the curl is generally tighter, with the curl getting tighter towards the ends (see Figure 11.27). This type of curl is little used in modern hairstyling.

Finger waving

Finger waving is the technique of moulding and shaping the hair into wave movements using just fingers, comb, waving lotion and hairpins, clips or tape.

Apply waving lotion to towel-dried hair. Use an applicator bottle to apply the waving lotion and comb through to distribute. This allows the lotion to be distributed smoothly and evenly. Do not use an excessive amount of waving lotion as this may run onto the client's face and neck, causing them discomfort.

To determine the natural hair growth, comb the hair off the face, and push hair forward gently with the palm of your hand; the hair will fall into its natural growth pattern.

> ***TIP*** Apply lotion to one side of the head at a time; this prevents it from drying before completion and requiring additional applications.

Shaping the top area

Using the first finger of your left hand as a guide, shape the top hair with a comb, using a circular movement. Starting at the front hairline, work towards the crown in 3.7 to 5 cm sections at a time until the crown has been reached (see Figure 11.28).

Place the first finger of the left hand directly above the position for the first crest. With the teeth of the comb pointing slightly upward, insert the comb directly under the first finger. Draw the comb forward about 2.5 cm along the fingertip (see Figure 11.29). With the teeth still inserted in the crest, flatten the comb against the head in order to hold the ridge in place (see Figure 11.30). Remove the left hand from the head, place the middle finger above the crest and the first finger on the teeth of the comb. Raise the crest by closing the two fingers and applying pressure to the head (see Figure 11.31).

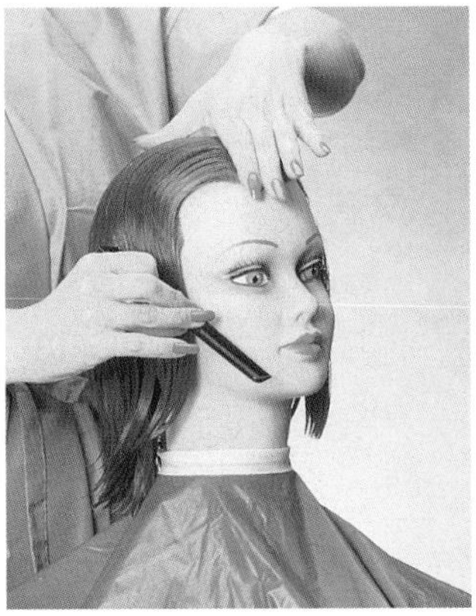

Figure 11.28 Shaping the top area

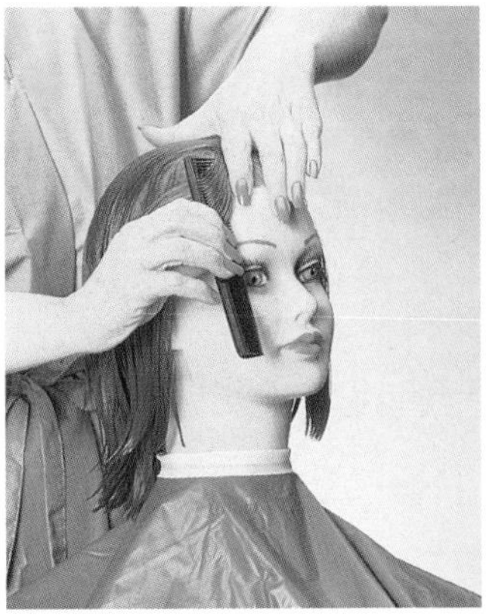

Figure 11.29 Draw hair towards finger

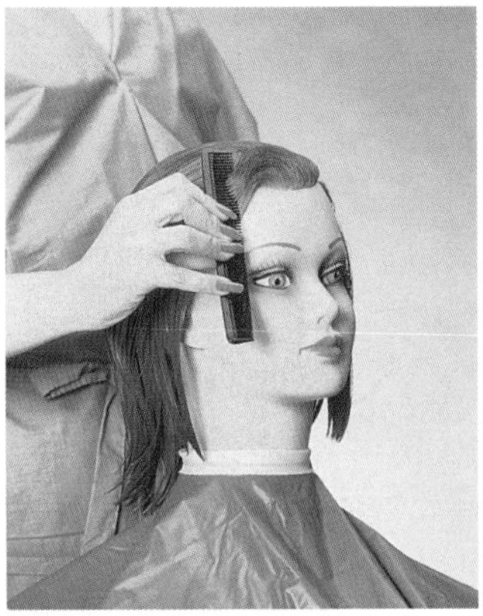

Figure 11.30 Flatten comb against head

Without removing the comb, turn the teeth downward, and comb the hair in a right semi-circular direction to form a dip or trough in the hollow part of the wave (see Figure 11.32). Follow this procedure, section by section, until the crown you reach, where the crest phases out (see Figure 11.33).

The crest and wave of each section should match evenly, without showing separations in the crest and trough part of the wave.

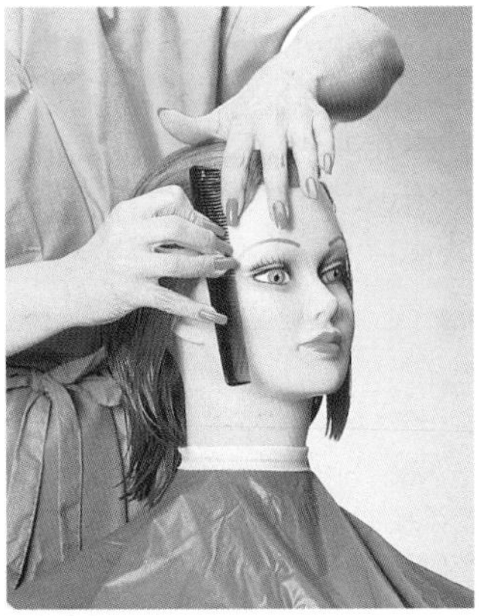

Figure 11.31 Emphasize ridge

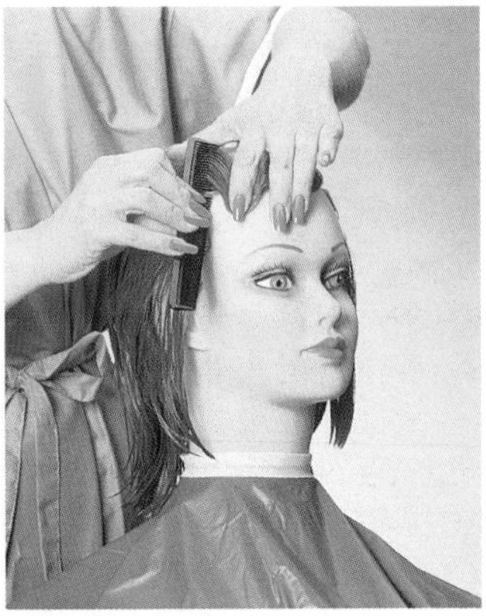

Figure 11.32 Comb hair in semi-circular direction

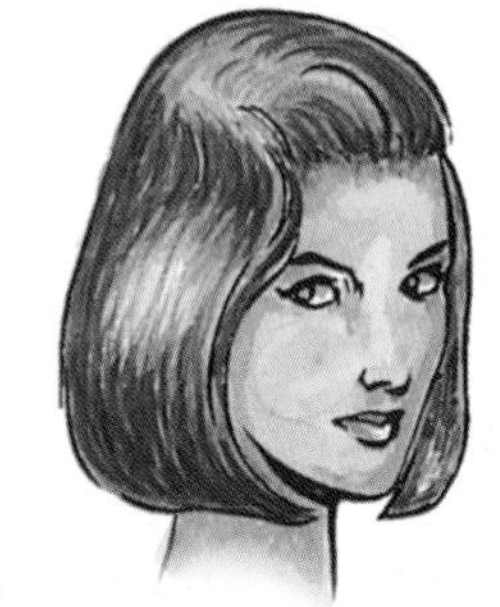

Figure 11.33 Complete first ridge at the crown

Forming the second crest

Start at the crown area (see Figure 11.34). The movements are the reverse of those followed in forming the first crest. The comb is drawn from the tip of the first finger towards its base, thus directing formation of the second ridge. All movements are followed in a reverse pattern until the hairline is reached, therefore completing the second crest, (see Figure 11.35).

Forming the third crest

Movements for the third crest closely follow those used in creating the first crest. However, the third ridge is started at the hairline and extended back toward the back of the head, (see Figure 11.36). Continue alternating directions until the side of the head has been completed, (see Figure 11.37).

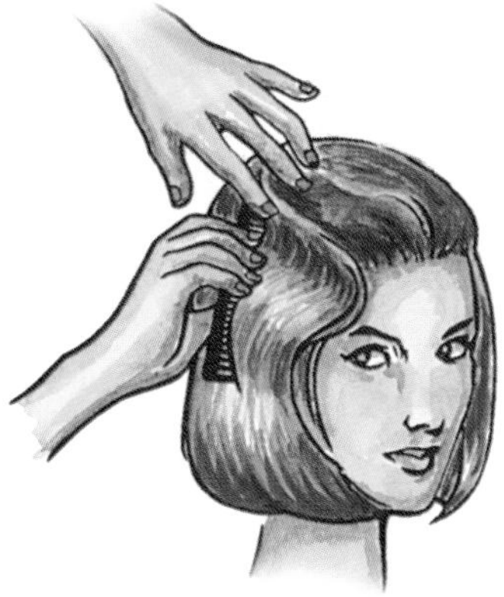

Figure 11.34 Starting the second ridge

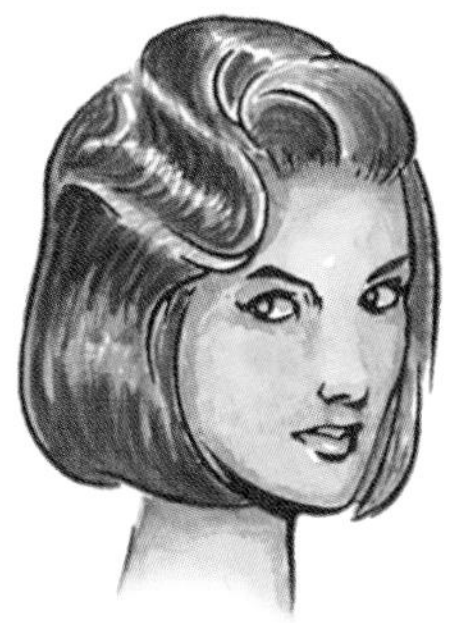

Figure 11.35 Complete second ridge

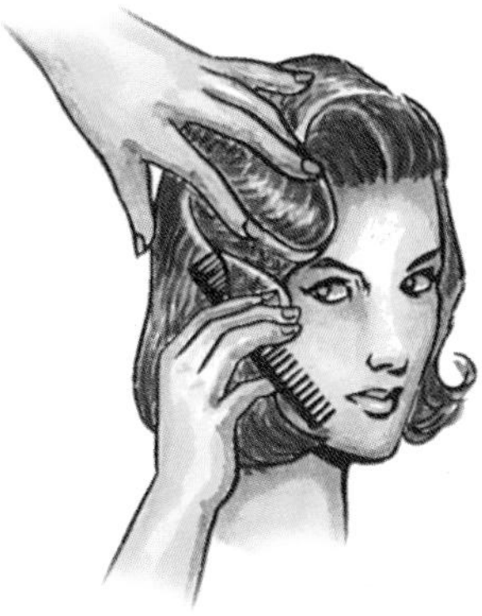

Figure 11.36 Start the third ridge

Completion

Continue to create these wave movements around the head. The ends of the hair may require pin curling if the hair is too long for you to mould into the nape or onto the side of the face. The waves may be held in place while you are drying them by placing setting tape along the wave troughs or using clips or fine hair pins. Place a net over the hair, taking care not to allow the net to press onto the hair, particularly on the front or on the nape, as this will result in marks on the finished hairstyle. Dry the hair thoroughly, using a hood hairdryer. Once dry remove your client from the dryer, remove the net and any pins or clips and allow the hair to cool. Using a bristle brush, brush the hair in the direction of the style. Dressing creams or wax may be applied to the hair (to give control) and then using a dressing comb reform the waves as they were set. Use the dressing mirror to check the balance of your hairstyle.

DRYING THE HAIR

Always pre-heat the hairdryer. This will speed up the drying process as well as making it more comfortable for your client. If required, place a setting net over the hair set. Secure this ensuring that the net does not press onto any area of the set, as this may mark the set and affect the finished dressing (see Figure 11.38).

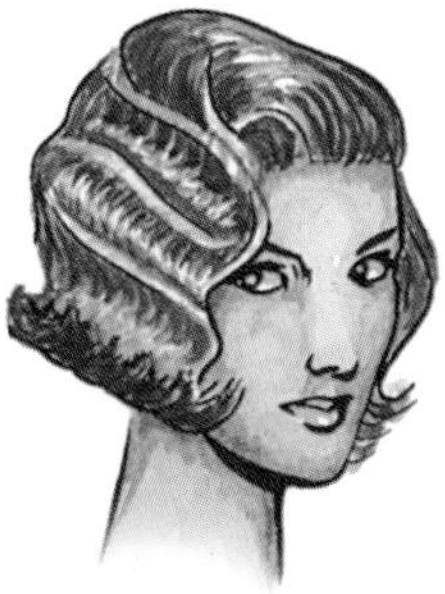

Figure 11.37 Complete right side

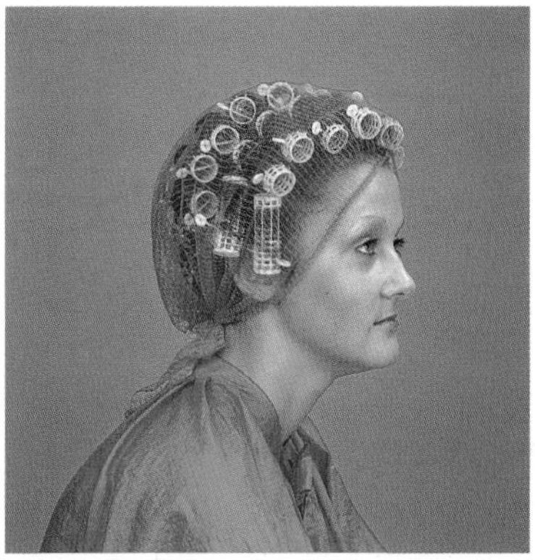

Figure 11.38 Setting net in place

Check that no pins or metal items are pressing onto your client's scalp or hairline. If so, remove them or place a protective pad between the tool and the scalp. Locate the hood of the dryer over the scalp area, ensuring that all of the scalp area is enclosed without it resting on your client's neck or on their face. Inform your client of how to regulate the heat setting and set the timer for the desired time.

Avoid over-drying the hair as this can unnecessarily damage it. However, the hair must be thoroughly dry if it is to be dressed satisfactorily. Allow the hair set to cool slightly, before removing the rollers and pins. While the hair is hot the shape may be relaxed.

Having removed the setting tools, brush the hair thoroughly in the direction of the intended style, using a bristle brush.

> ***TIP*** For some fashion styling techniques, once the setting tools are removed the hair is combed using only the stylist's fingers. This retains the separate effect on the curl.

DRESSING HAIR

Hair must be thoroughly dry when dressing into style. You may be dressing hair following a wet set or you may be dressing hair which has been set using heated rollers or you may be dressing hair which has little remaining set. It is a distinct advantage to have some set in the hair as this will give you control over the hair.

Thoroughly brush the hair, using a bristle brush, following the direction of the intended hairstyle. Care may be necessary when initially brushing the hair, not to cause discomfort when breaking down the crisp effect created by the use of a setting lotion (on freshly set hair) or the effects of hair-fixing spray and tangle (from previously set and dressed hair).

Hair may be moulded into shape using a bristle brush or a wide-toothed comb. Follow these guidelines:

- To achieve control, brush the hair holding the brush flat to the head.
- To achieve volume, slowly lift the brush or comb from the head allowing the hair to fall from the bristles (see Figure 11.39).
- To achieve curve under, place the brush under the section of hair and draw the hair in rolling under (see Figure 11.40).
- To achieve wave, use a comb or brush incorporating a finger wave technique (see Figure 11.41).

> ***TIP*** For control, use a dressing cream, oil or wax to control the hair and add shine.

Back combing

Control and volume may be achieved in hair by back combing. Hair that has been tapered or has a natural taper can be back combed more easily. When building a hairstyle, just as when building a house, build from the bottom up. Use a comb with both widely- and closely-set teeth; there are specialised combs made with alternate longer and shorter teeth to aid back combing.

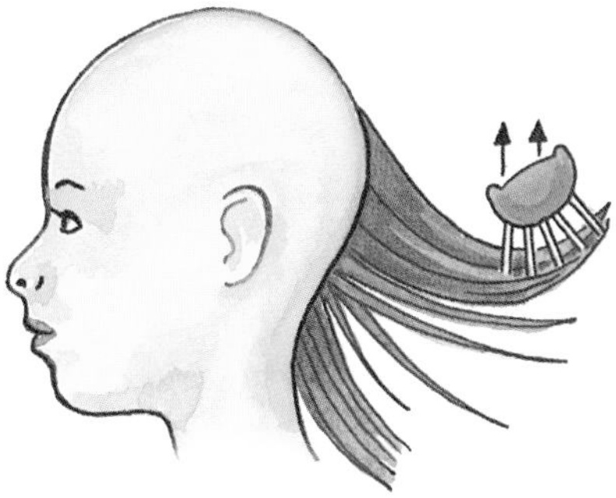

Figure 11.39 Using brush or comb to achieve volume

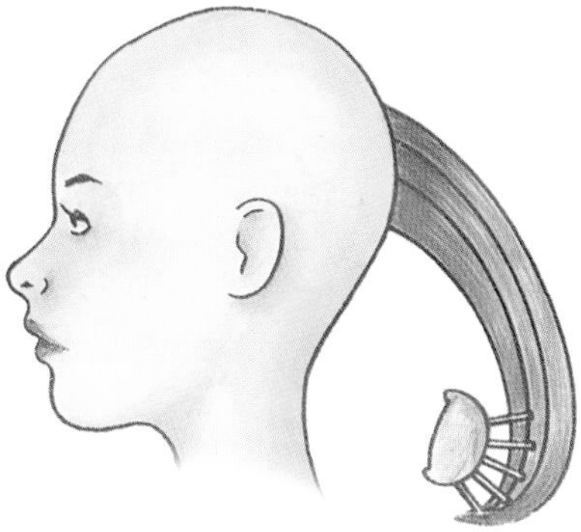

Figure 11.40 Using brush or comb to achieve curve under

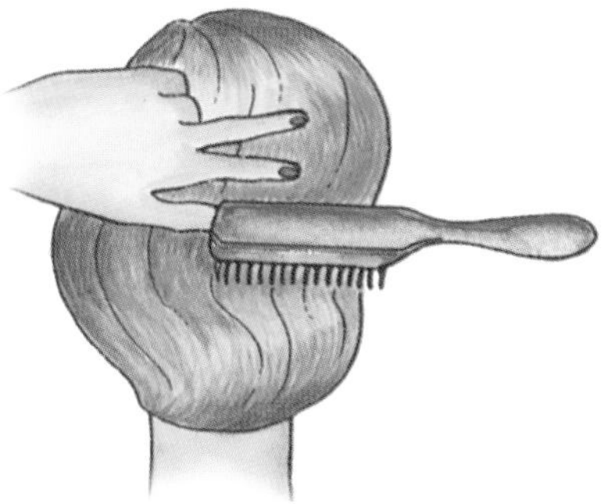

Figure 11.41 Using brush or comb to achieve wave

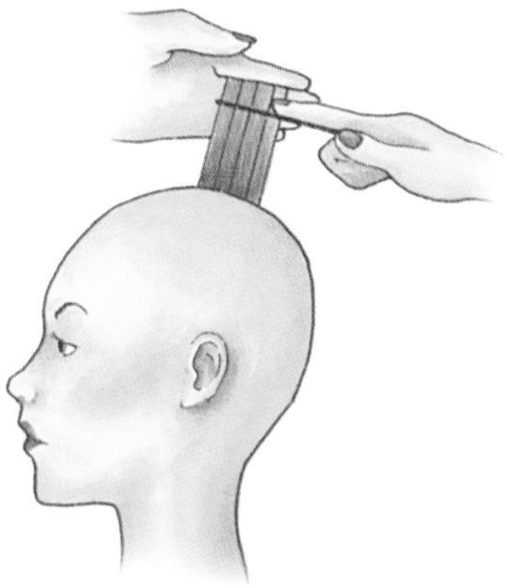

Figure 11.42 Taking mesh for back combing

Take a mesh of hair, sufficiently small to be able to hold firmly, and grip towards the points using the first and second finger (see Figure 11.42). The thumb pressing onto the side of the first finger provides added grip. Comb and hold the hair at the angle you wish it to lie; so if you want height, hold the hair in an upright position, and if you want control and flatness hold the hair closer to the head.

Insert the comb, approximately one-third of the length out from the root, into the mesh and push down towards the root (see Figure 11.43). Some of the hair will matt. Continue to do this until the required degree of back combing is achieved, gradually extending the start position further from the hair root area.

When one section has been back combed take an adjacent section and continue. Stagger the section like the bricks in a wall. This will help to prevent gaps and partings in the finished dressing.

Some stylists back comb all or at least an area of the head before then using the wide teeth of the comb or a hair brush to dress the surface of the hair (see Figure 11.44). Others dress each mesh of hair in turn.

The surface of the hair is smoothed while the back combing is retained beneath.

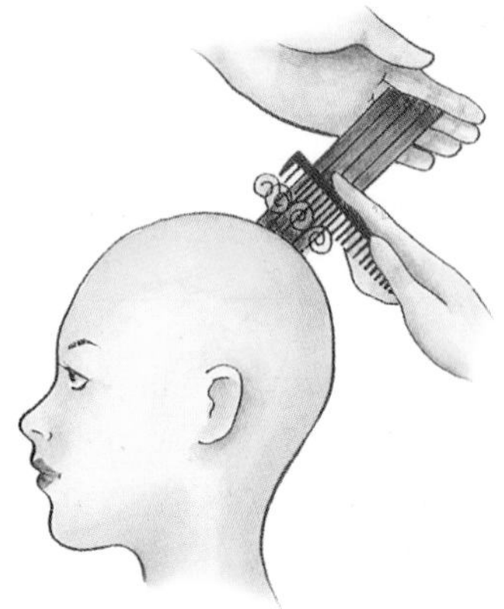

Figure 11.43 Inserting comb for back combing

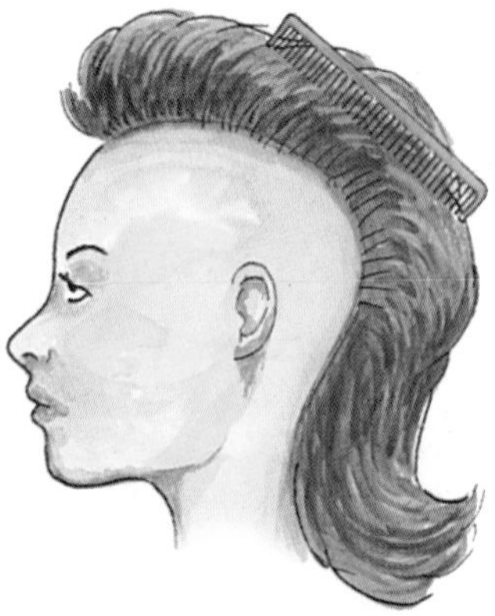

Figure 11.44 Dressing the surface of the hair

TIP When dressing hair, check the balance of the style using the dressing mirror.

Back brushing

A stiff-bristled brush may be used in a similar technique to back combing. Alternatively a bristle brush may be used on the surface area of the hair to create volume and control.

Starting at the top of the hairstyle, take a controllable mesh of hair, gripping as for back combing. Hold the hair in the direction and position that you wish to dress it. Lay the bristles of the brush on the top of the section and push towards the root area, rotating the brush slightly, in a flicking action (see Figure 11.45). The higher the section is held from the head the greater the volume potentially created. Before all of the hair within the mesh is used, pick up additional hair from the mesh below. This will produce a continuous back brushed effect. To control rather than create height, the 'flicking' action is reduced. Once completed the hair may be dressed into place by smoothing the surface and dressing into place using a brush or comb (see Figure 11.46).

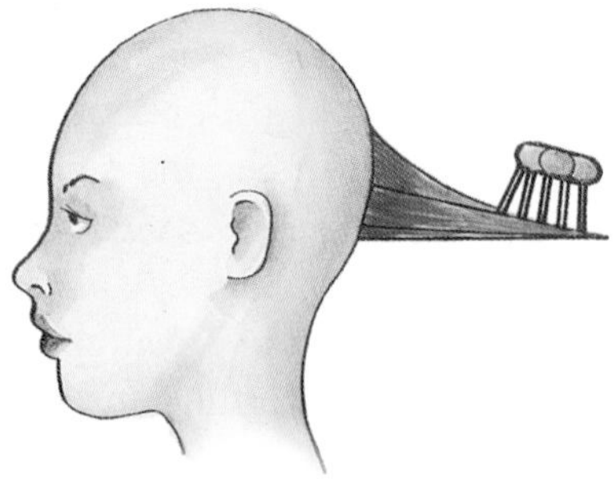

Figure 11.45 Back brushing

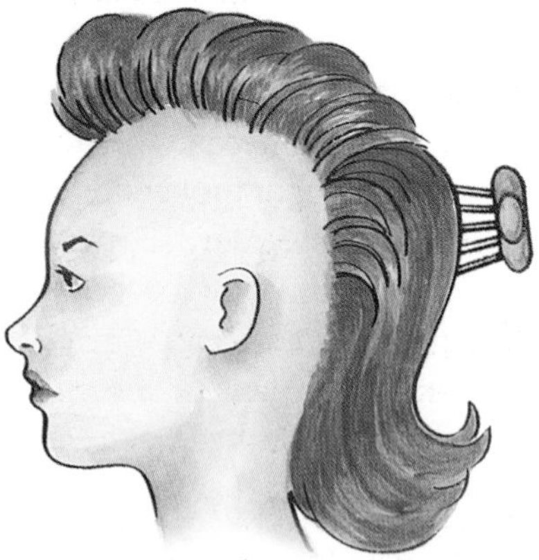

Figure 11.46 Dressing back brushed hair

DRESSING AIDS

There are a number of control and gloss products available. Some may require care in application to avoid over-use. Oil-based products may make the hair appear greasy if too much is used.

A variety of mousse or gel-based products may be used to control and add texture to the hair. These are usually applied either to individual strands of hair (using the fingers) or by spray on the dressed hair. An individually stranded effect may be achieved in the hair by carefully drawing the strands of hair between fingers coated with liquid finishing products, the fingers providing the shaping and the product producing the finish and the hold.

Hair-fixing spray may be used to hold the hairstyle in place. There are a number of types of hair-fixing sprays available. Always follow the manufacturer's directions for safe use. Shield the client's face and neck from the effects of the sprays (see Figure 11.47).

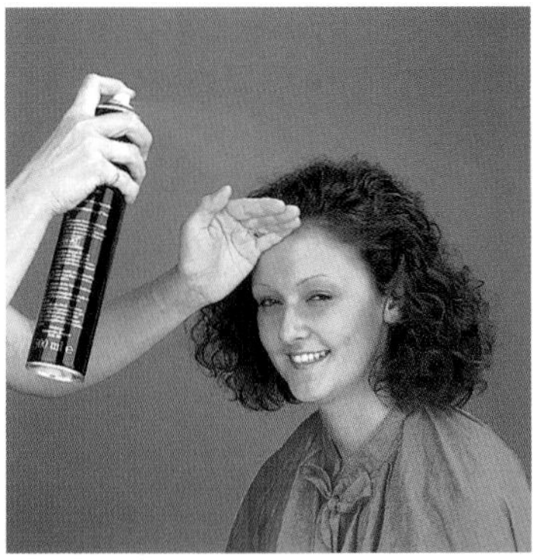

Figure 11.47 Spraying dressed hair

When applying spray to the finished, dressed hair, take care not to disturb the hair. On very smooth styles direct the spray with the direction of the hair and follow this by carefully drawing the palms of the hands along the hair in the direction of the hair fall. This can smooth down any stray hairs which may otherwise detract from the effect.

DRESSING LONG HAIR

Long hair may be dressed without the need to pre-set, but some preparation will enable you to work more easily and improve the achieved result. If the hair is not to be set beforehand (either wet set or set using heated rollers or tongs) it should be clean, though ideally not freshly washed, as this can make the hair very slippery and more difficult to secure firmly.

The styles that may be achieved will depend not only on your client's wishes but also on the length, texture and density of their hair.

> ***TIP*** Take care when using aerosol sprays with clients or colleagues who may suffer breathing problems. Never use them near a naked flame.

The plait

You can plait hair so that it either hangs from the head or becomes part of the hairstyle against the head. For this effect the hair does not normally require any pre-setting, but very fine hair can be crimped to add volume. You can achieve different effects by carrying this out on wet instead of dry hair, using gel to produce a crisp-look finish as well as providing control.

Simple plait

Draw the hair together, by brushing, towards the back of the head, and divide the hair into three sections of even volume.

Gripping the three strands of hair between the fingers, pass the outside left strand over the centre strand (now to form the centre strand). Now pass the outside right strand over the middle strand (now to form the middle strand). Continue to do this down the length of the hair. Maintain an even tension at all times, holding the plait in the position in which it will lie. The ends of the hair may be secured with a cotton-covered band, a ribbon or a specialised clip.

For variation the outer strands may be passed beneath the middle strand. The hair may be secured in a 'pony tail', before being plaited. The basic three-stranded plait may be extended to include any uneven number of strands. The greater the number of strands required, generally the longer the hair should be.

French plait or braid

There are a number of techniques that may be used to achieve the french plait, giving a range of results. The basic principle is the same as for a simple plait: the plait is started at the top of the hairstyle and fresh supplies of hair are added to the plait.

1. Take a small section of hair at the start of the braid and divide this into three even-thickness strands. The hair beneath should be tangle free. Cross these strands over as for the plait (see Figure 11.48)
2. Cross the outer strand 1 over strand 2, which now becomes the central strand; then cross strand 1 with strand 3, (see Figure 11.49)
3. Add additional hair from beneath 2 to strand 2 and then cross over strand 3 to form the central strand (see Figure 11.50).
4. Pick up additional hair to add to strand 3 (see Figure 11.51), and continue in this way.

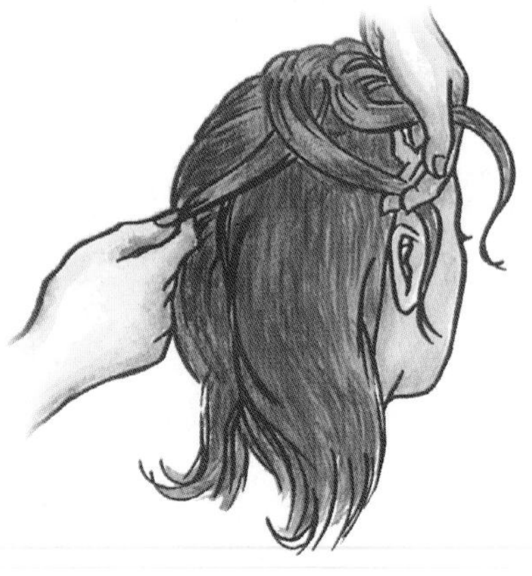

Figure 11.48 Divide into three strands

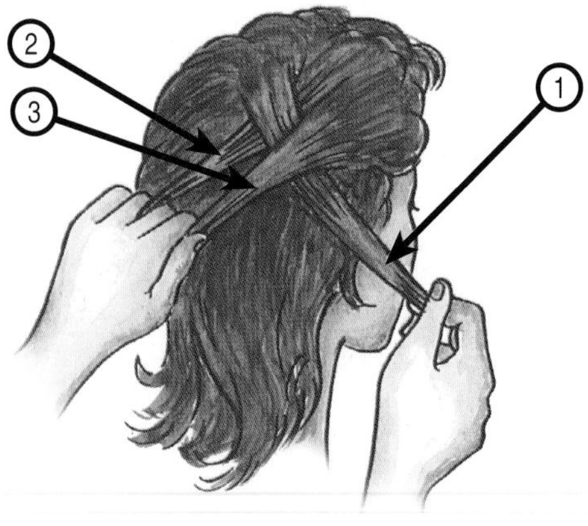

Figure 11.49 Starting the braiding

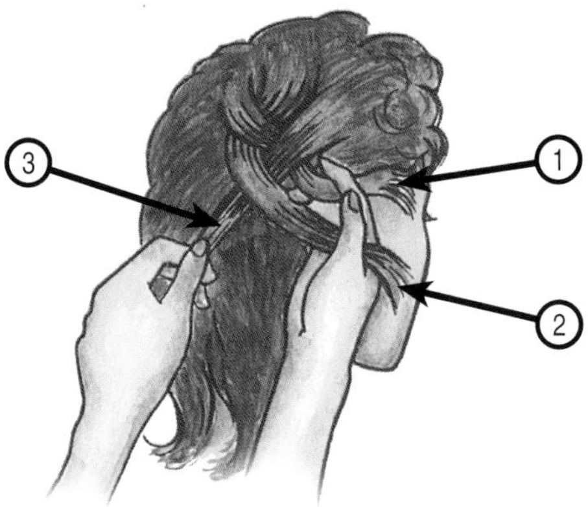

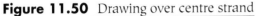

Figure 11.50 Drawing over centre strand

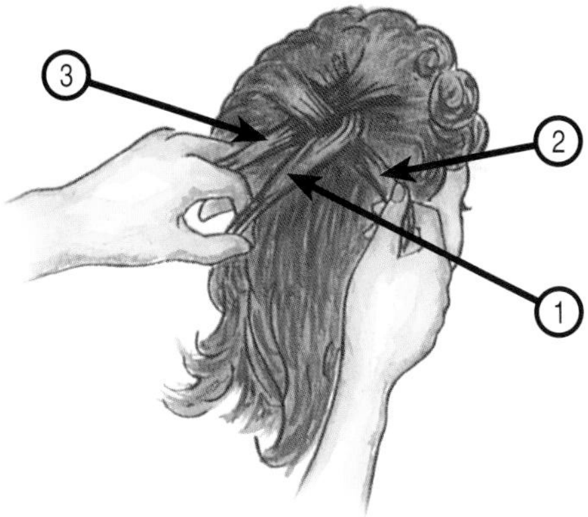

Figure 11.51 Pick up strand

For a tight, close effect this is best carried out on moist hair, with the hands holding the hair close to the scalp. The hairstyle may be completed by securing the ends of the braid and rolling and securing them under the braid.

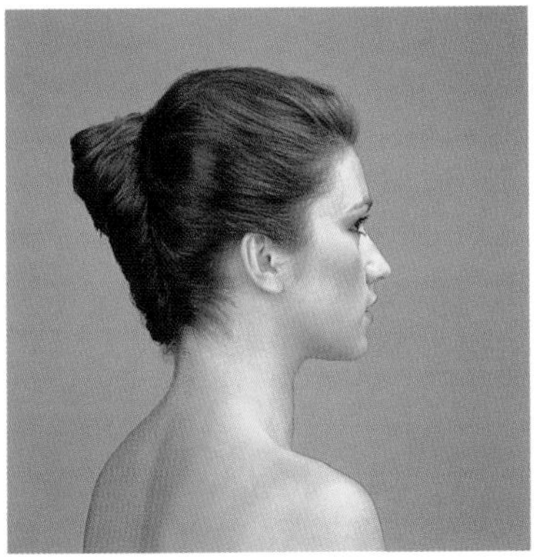

The pleat

The pleated effect is obtained by twisting long hair up the back of the head to form a line. This may be carried out on long hair without pre-setting or following a set (see Figure 11.52).

Figure 11.52 Completed French plait

Flat pleat

For a pleated effect on hair that is to lay smooth to the head, brush the hair, using a bristle brush, to form a 'pony tail' at the back of the head. Twist this 'pony tail' at the same time pulling the hair in a upward direction (see Figure 11.53).

Use larger roller pins to hold the hair in place while the hair is dressed and then replace them with fine way pins once the pleat is positioned (see Figure 11.54)

The ends of the hair may then be dressed to style.

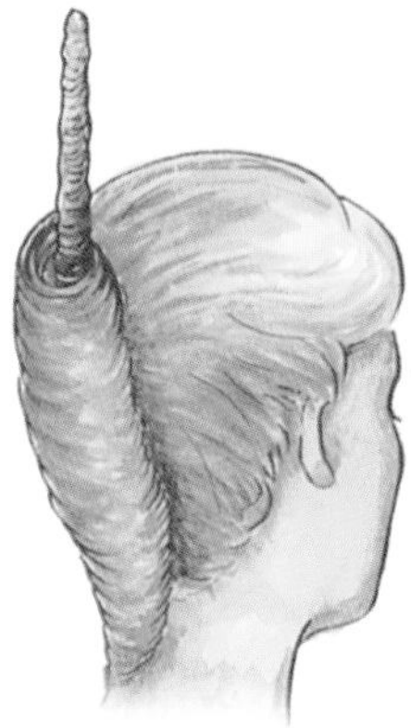

Figure 11.53 Flat pleat

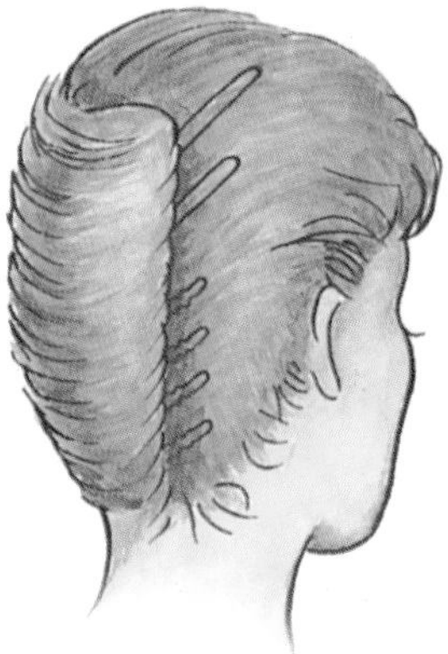

Figure 11.54 Hair in pleat

Full pleat

For this technique the hair is often back combed or back brushed prior to dressing.

1. Brush the hair across, horizontally at the back, and locate a row of overlapping hair grips in a line, slightly off-centre, going vertically (see Figure 11.55).
2. Brush the hair back across the back of the head, then in the opposite direction, and twist the hair to form a vertical line up the back of the head. Smooth the hair using a brush or comb, retaining any volume required for the profile shape.
3. Use fine pins to secure the pleat, placing the pins in the edge of the top section of hair pointing towards the pleat line, so that the pins penetrate to the lower section. Push the pin into the hair, turning it now away from the pleat line. This will place tension on the pin. Take care not to place the pin under too great a tension as this may cause your client discomfort.

The roll

A roll may follow either a horizontal or vertical line. The technique is similar to that of a pleat. Close-fitting effects may be achieved on wet hair and softer, fuller effects on dry hair, which may have been set. For full effects a pad may be used to provide volume and control.

Vertical roll

This is usually produced on the top of the head at the side. For maximum effect it is often located on the 'corner' of the head.

1. Brush the hair over the top of the head from one side to the other and secure a line of hair grips, slightly below the roll line.
2. If required locate and secure a pad of shape over which to build the hair.
3. Dress the hair over the roll's shape, twist the hair ends or tuck them under and secure using fine hair pins (see Figure 11.56).

Horizontal roll

The roll is usually located across the back of the head or in the nape.

1. Brush the hair back and down and secure a row of hair grips horizon-tally across the head at a position slightly below the edge of the role.
2. Secure a pad or shape if required.
3. Shape the hair over the pad or dress the hair, twisting it to produce the roll's effect across the back (see Figure 11.57).
4. Secure with fine pins as for a pleat, tucking in the hair ends to add to the volume of the roll.

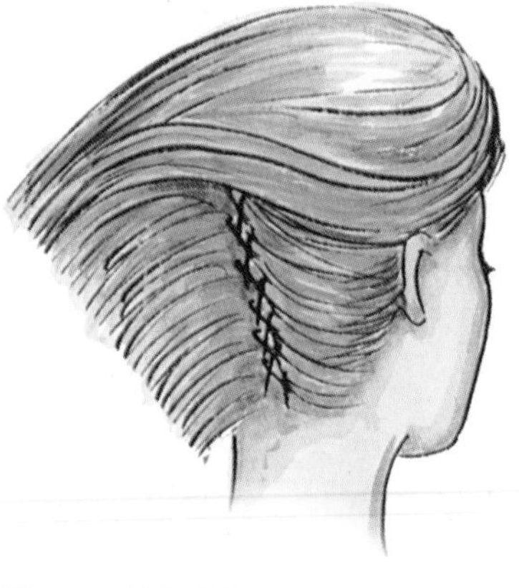

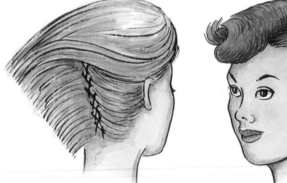

Figure 11.55 Full pleat

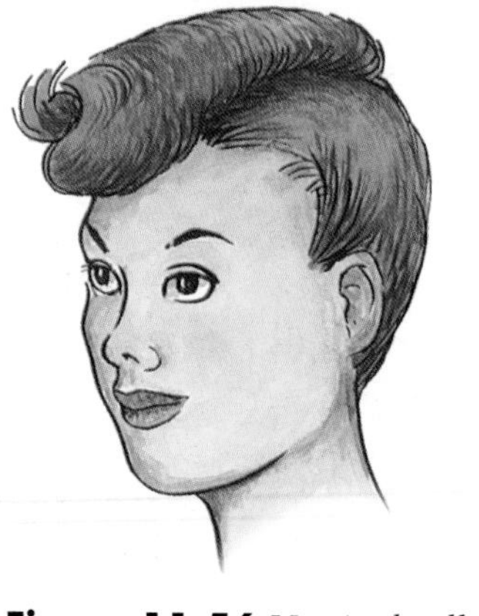

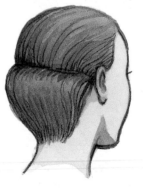

Figure 11.56 Vertical roll

Figure 11.57 Horizontal roll

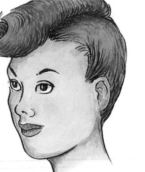

Helpful hints with long hair

1. When placing hair pins, ensure that they point downwards, as this will prevent them from loosening.
2. To prevent hair grips from loosening, overlap or cross them.
3. Avoid using large quantities of hair spray until the style is complete.

Ornamentation

Ornamentation may be used to change the style from a style suitable for day wear to a style suitable for a special occasion. The use of ornamentation should enhance the hairstyle and not be allowed to cover or substitute. Ornamentation may take the form of:

1. specialised pre-formed hair ornaments, attached to the hair by combs or clips
2. flowers which may be added to the hair
3. various items of haberdashery, ribbons, buttons etc. which may all be secured into the hairstyle (see Figure 11.58).

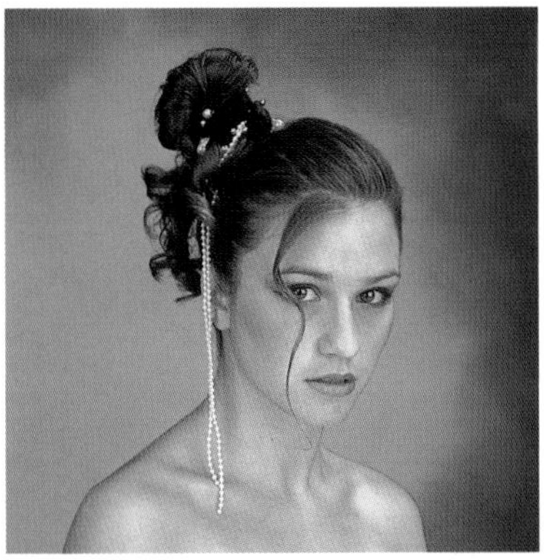

Figure 11.58 Ornamented hair

FURTHER STUDY

- There are a large range of styles of professional hairdressing combs. Visit your wholesaler or trade exhibition to see them and try them out.
- Hairdressing competitions are a good way to test your skills. Watch competition workers competing and learn the skills of hair control from them.
- Modern hair setting techniques use a variety of tools around which to form the hair. Find out more about the currently emerging fashion setting techniques.

REVIEW QUESTIONS

1. For how long is a set retained in the hair?
2. Which type of hair roller is most likely to mark bleached or very porous hair?
3. When roller setting, what determines the strength of curl achieved?
4. What size is the section taken for a hair roller?
5. Hair in its unstretched state consists of what sort of keratin?
6. What is meant by the term 'over-directing' when setting hair?
7. In what direction should the hair be brushed prior to dressing?
8. What direction should back combing follow?
9. How should your client be protected during the application of hair-fixing spray?
10. How should fine pins be located in a finished hairstyle so that they do not fall out?

CHAPTER 12

Barbering

This chapter provides the essential knowledge you need to develop barbering skills, and provides you with guidance in the procedures and techniques used in this important area.

Level 2	
Unit 201	
Element 201.1	Consult with and maintain effective relationships with clients
Element 201.2	Advise clients on salon products and services
Unit 203	
Element 203.1	Maintain effective and safe methods of working when drying and setting hair
Element 203.2	Dry and finish hair to style
Unit 204	
Element 204.3	Cut hair to achieve a variety of layered looks
Unit 208	
Element 208.2	Develop and improve personal effectiveness within the job role
Unit 209	
Element 209.2	Support health, safety and security at work
Unit 210	
Unit 210.1	Maintain effective and safe methods of working when using barbering techniques
Element 210.2	Cut hair to achieve a variety of looks with different neckline shapes
Unit 211	
Element 211.1	Maintain effective and safe methods of working when shaving and massaging the face
Element 211.2	Remove hair by shaving

Unit 212	
Element 212.1	Maintain effective and safe methods of working when cutting facial hair
Element 212.2	Cut beards and moustaches to shape
Unit 213	
Element 213.1	Maintain effective and safe methods of working when drying hair
Element 213.2	Dry and finish hair

Contents

INTRODUCTION

Those traditional skills closely associated with men's hairdressing include developing graduation and sculptured looks, and shaping and removing facial hair. Traditionally the shapes produced in men's hair are squarer and much sharper than those usually associated with other forms of hair-styling. They are produced using techniques that facilitate the easy manipulation of short hair on the scalp or face using the comb and either clippers or scissors.

Barbering invariably involves attention to facial hair, whether it is to level sideburns or, at the other extreme, to shape a full beard and moustache. Facial hair may be used to enhance the wearer's appearance just as with scalp hair. It can alter the apparent shape of the face, drawing attention to or minimising the effects of a range of facial features.

To ignore the total appearance of your client when barbering would be a great error. Having styled the hair on the scalp, neglect of any facial hair, subject to your client's agreement, would equate to failure to complete a hairstyle.

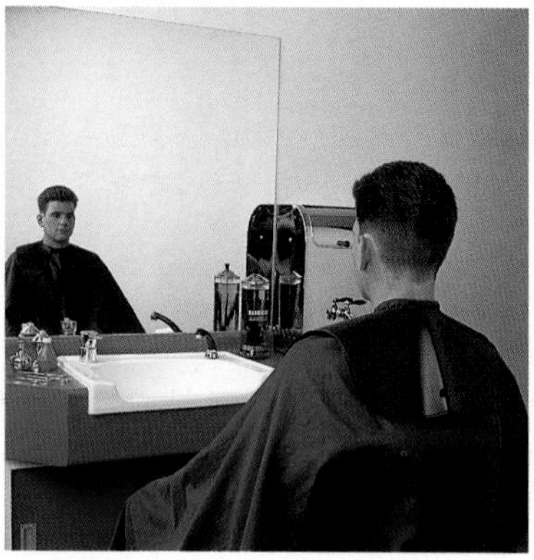

Figure 12.1 A barbering situation

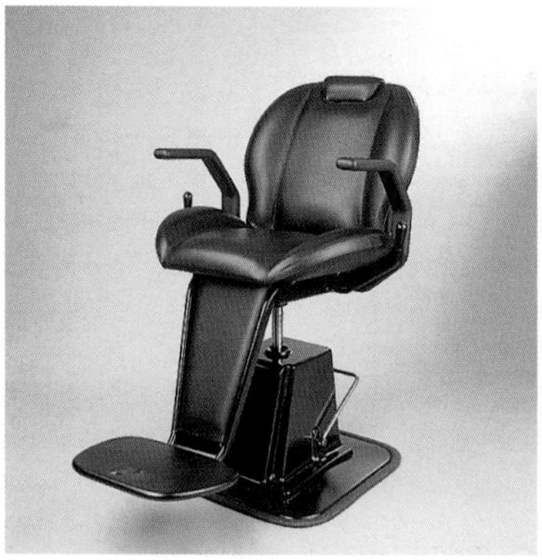

Figure 12.2 Hydraulically operated chair

PREPARATION

Seating your client

Barbering skills usually require the use of a hydraulically operated chair for the client (see Figure 12.2).

This allows you, the barber, to raise or lower your client and position him to a height and angle which allows you easy and comfortable access to all areas of his scalp and face, no matter how tall he is. To shape facial hair your client should be slightly reclined, as this makes the chin area of the face more accessible. A chair that allows you to do this is a great advantage for the barber and keeps your client comfortable.

HEALTH AND SAFETY If you are uncertain of the safe working of the chair ask for guidance from your line manager or trainer.

Always ensure that the hydraulic chair is clean and free from hair cuttings. Lower the chair to its lowest position. At this height the chair is at its most stable and least likely to tip or move. In the case of a manual hydraulic chair this may be done by depressing the foot pump and holding it down while the chair falls. Some pressure on the chair may be required to encourage it in its downward journey. Once it is at the desired height, pull the foot lever upwards by placing a foot beneath the chair and pulling upwards. This locks the chair in position and prevents it from revolving. Electronically operated chairs are available and the manufacturer's directions for use should be followed.

Ensure that the back of the chair is in an upright position and, if you are about to cut the scalp hair, remove the head rest, if attached (its location can often prevent you from working with ease in the nape area of your client's hairstyle).

When your client is seated, the chair may be adjusted to a height to suit your work. Pump the foot pedal to do this.

Client consultation

Client care procedures, pages 1–17

Discuss with your client the treatment to be given. Listen to you client.

Gowning your client

The cutting cloth or cape is usually a square or rectangular shape with a slit in the middle of one side. This slit is to fit your client's neck, being tucked into the client's collar. Ensure that the gown covers your client's clothing.

When cutting, tuck a strand of clean cotton between the gown and the neck. This forms a seal to prevent hair clippings from passing down the neck. A cutting collar may also be used to hold the gown in place while cutting.

When shampooing at a front wash basin it is advisable to protect your client by placing a towel around their chest, followed with a second around the back. At the completion of the shampoo use the towel at the back to towel-dry the hair, and move the one from the front to the back.

Shampooing and conditioning the hair and scalp, page 18

Personal hygiene

It is particularly important to be aware of your personal hygiene when shaping facial hair, as you will be very close to your client and often facing into his face. Body odour can offend your client, as can over-liberal use of strong-smelling perfume and cologne. Oral hygiene is also very important. Breath that smells of strong-tasting foods, cigarette smoke or the effects of halitosis or decaying teeth can be very unpleasant to your client.

> ***TIP*** Always keep your breath fresh, particularly when working closely with your client or colleagues.

BARBERING TOOLS

All the tools that you use should be of good quality and hygienically clean. At the work station there should be a method of easily sterilising tools between clients. Usually you will need a second set of tools, so that you can sterilise one set while continuing to work.

Scissors

These are described in chapter 4. It is advisable to use scissors of 5$\frac{1}{2}$ inches in length or over when graduating over a comb. The additional length enables the scissors to be held correctly while close to the head.

Combs

A range of combs are required. Some should have both fine and coarse-set teeth and vary in size. Fine, flexibly backed combs can flex and fit against the contour of the scalp and neck. This is particularly necessary when close graduating. Rigid-backed combs can cope with strong hair. Combs set with even teeth may be used when producing flat surfaces on the hair (see Figure 12.3). Fashion styling effects may be achieved using specialist styling combs.

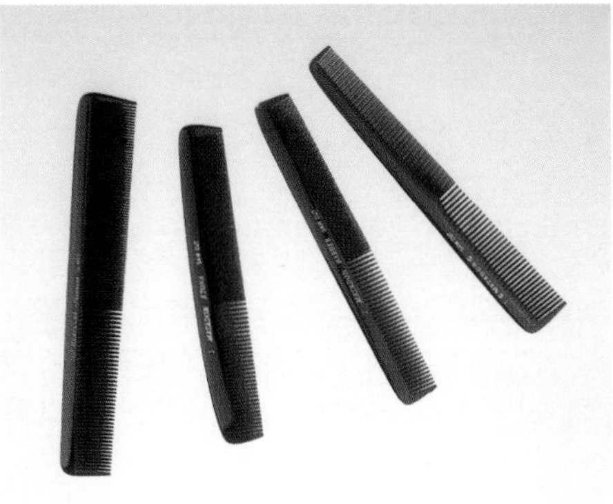

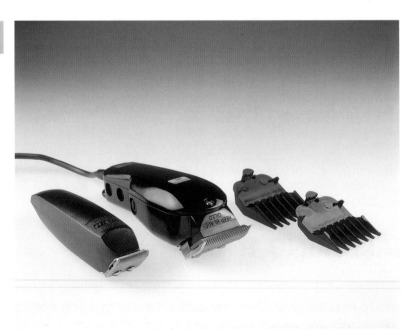

Figure 12.3 Barbering combs

Hair clippers

These act as shears, cutting the hair (see Figure 12.4).

Some ranges of electric hair clippers have grader attachments. The grader sets a gap between the scalp and the cutting blade, enabling a consistent length of hair to be cut. The

▶ Haircutting, page 53

Figure 12.4 Hair clippers

graders vary in size, the smallest (producing the closest cut) being 'number 1' progressing to the much larger 'number 8'. There are graders available which have a graduating effect on the hair if the clipper is inserted sideways into the hair mesh.

Brushes

A range of brushes are required. Closely set bristle brushes can pick up and hold short graduated hair. Coarser-set bristle may produce textured effects in completed dressings.

You will need a neck brush, to dust hair clippings from your client's skin, and you may need other items, such as:

- a talc puffer, to add talc to the skin, aiding the removal of clippings
- a pair of thinning scissors (see information in chapter 4)
- a razor (see information in chapter 4).

Tools used for haircutting, page 54

SHAPING FACIAL HAIR

To carry out a haircut and neglect the extremities of the hair on the face, for example the base of the sideburns, or to neglect the concept of the total look would be an error. To present the male client, the barber must consider the total appearance of the head and face together. When cutting and shaping facial hair, remember that you are producing a three-dimensional shape on the face, which itself is made of irregular shapes over which you must work.

Discuss the desired shape and effect of the facial hair fully with your client before commencing to shape.

Tools for use

Facial hair may be shaped using;

- haircutting scissors and/or electric clippers, over a comb, to shape
- freehand cutting using the scissors, to cut outlines or shape small areas
- inverted clippers, to outline the perimeter shape
- a razor, to remove unwanted facial hair around the perimeter of the shape.

Beard shaping

Client preparation

Following consultation, place a lightly coloured towel diagonally across your client's chest. Tuck in one side of the collar, and fold the towel to enclose the other side of the neck. The light towel will reflect light up under the chin area, as well as providing a contrasting surface against which to check the profile of the beard (see Figure 12.5). Ensure that there is no gap between the neck and the towel.

Recline, slightly, the back of the chair and then protect your client's eyes from hair clippings by either placing moist cotton wool pads on them or by draping a small hand towel across the eyes. A clean tissue should be placed across the head rest (if in position) to reduce the risk of infection from one client to the next.

Comb the beard to remove tangles. In some cases it may be necessary to lightly moisten the beard to soften dressings. Take care not to over-moisten, particularly if you intend to use electric clippers. While combing the beard, check for any strong or uneven growth patterns that may affect the finished shape. Strong patterns may have an impact upon the beard shape.

TIP If your client wears a full beard, it may not be necessary to define the outline. Consult with your client.

Outline shaping

1. Comb the hair thoroughly to lift it from the face. Check for any areas of thinness that may require special attention. Using the inverted clipper define the outline shape, by pressing the cutting edge into the beard at the required point (see Figure 12.9).
2. Using the clipper, remove the excess hair from this area.
3. Shave this area free of hair using those techniques described in chapter 13.

Shaping the bulk of the beard

Comb the hair to allow it to lay in its natural position. Insert the teeth of the comb at the position of the required cut and then using either scissors or clippers cut the hair to the level of the comb (see Figures 12.7 and 12.10).

Shaving and face massage, page 256

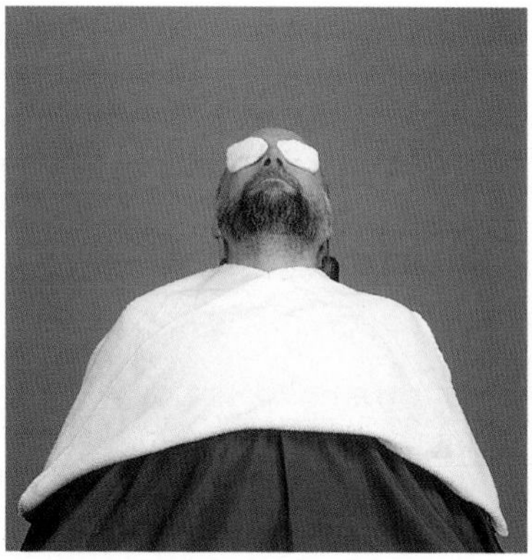

Figure 12.5 Client with cotton wool pads on eyes

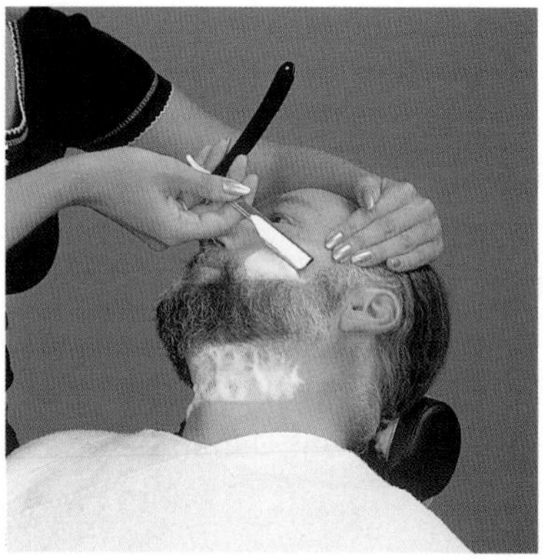

Figure 12.6 Beard shaping

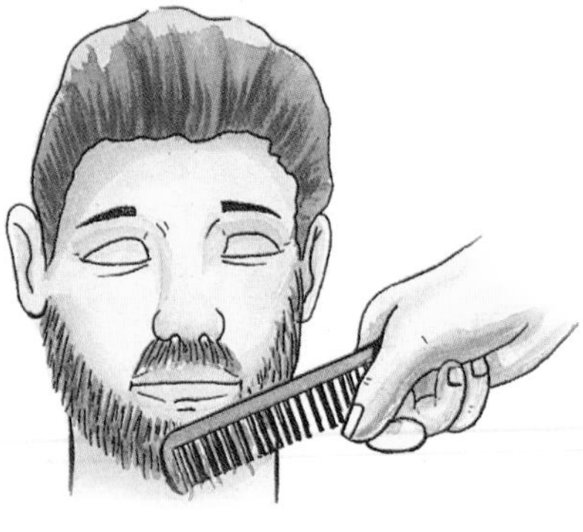

Figure 12.7 Combing beard

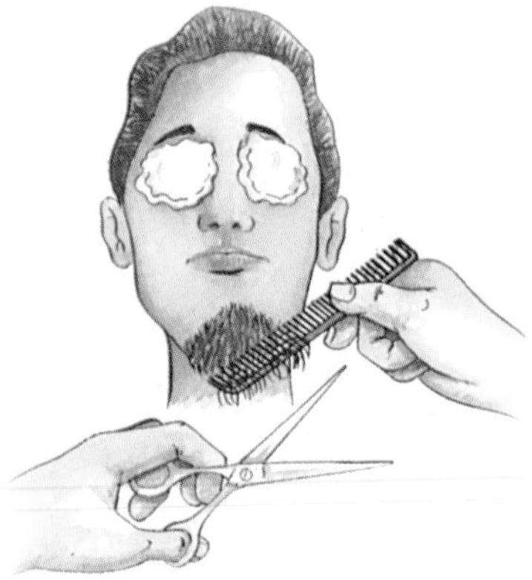

Figure 12.8 Trimming goatee beard

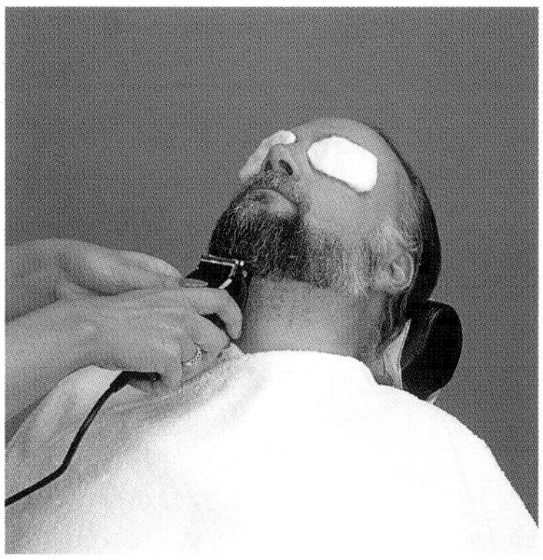

Figure 12.9 Outline shaping

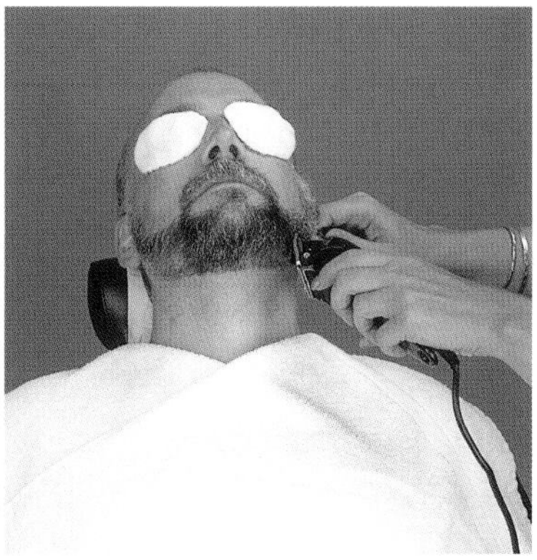

Figure 12.10 Shaping the bulk of the beard

Your choice of cutting tool will depend upon:

- personal preference
- the coarseness and thickness of the beard. A coarser beard is easier to cut using electric clippers
- the shape to be produced.

> ***TIP*** When cutting very curly facial hair, allow for the hair to spring back into place, producing a closer shape.

Move the comb slowly over the beard shape describing the shape required, and cut at this point. Take care to observe the profile and balance of the shape being produced, using the mirror and by checking against the light surface of the protective towel. Remember that the beard shape may appear different when the client's head is upright.

Shaping normally commences at the side of the beard, where it joins the hairstyle on the scalp. In most cases the two should flow together. The shape produced on the face may not be that of the face, so care must be taken in holding the comb in the correct position to follow the beard shape. Take care not to shape too short in areas where the beard is thin: the area where the moustache joins the beard is often thinner. Hair in the area beneath the chin will often appear shorter when the head is reclined and once the head is upright will still appear quite full. Take care not to take away corners or points if they are required in the finished shape.

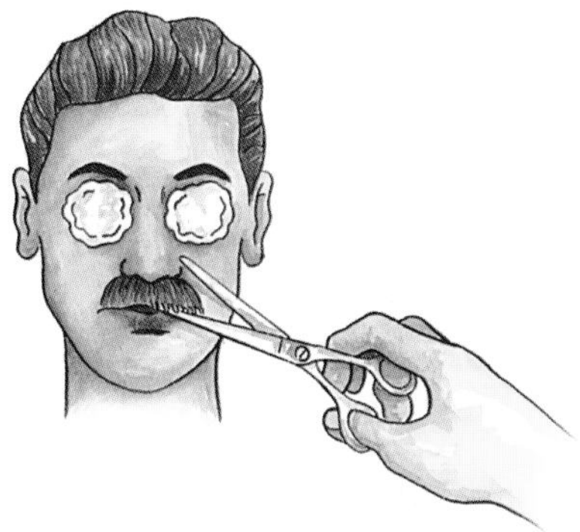

Figure 12.11 Outline moustache

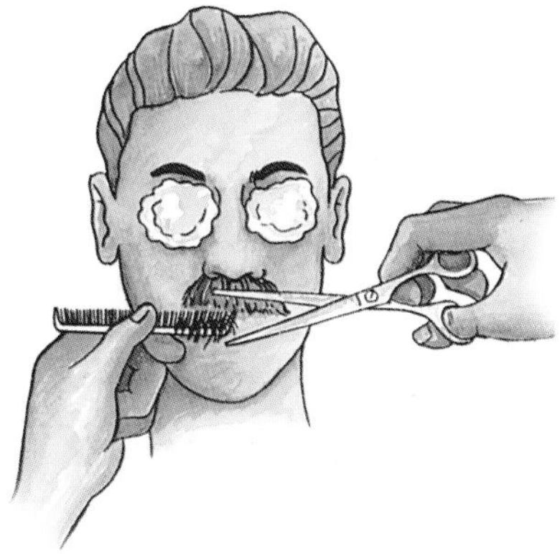

Figure 12.12 Trim moustache

Remove clippings from the neck continuously, avoiding a build-up of clippings that may become trapped between your client's skin and clothing.

The line along the top lip of the moustache is defined using either the inverted clipper or by freehand cutting using scissors.

Completion

Comb the facial hair fully to remove any loose hair clippings. Remove any protective pads from over your client's eyes and wipe any clippings from the face using a tissue. Dust the clippings from your client's neck area and remove the protective towel, taking care not to allow clippings to pass down the collar.

Gently raise the back of your client's chair, and then pass your client a hand mirror with which to view the beard.

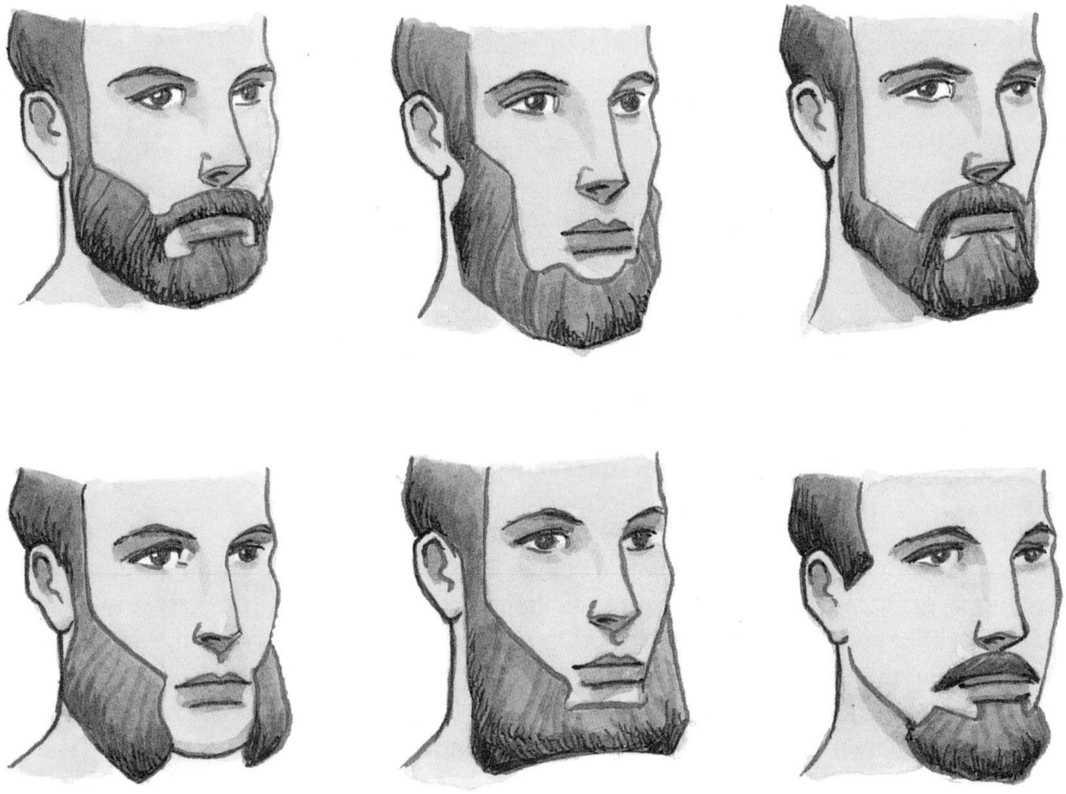

Figure 12.13 A range of beard shapes

Moustache shaping

When trimming the moustache, it may not be so necessary to gown your client with a lightly coloured towel as the moustache will be viewed against the face, not the towel.

Having reclined the back of the chair, outline the shape of the moustache area using clippers. The shaping may be carried out above the moustache or between the moustache and the lips. This area may then be shaved free of hair.

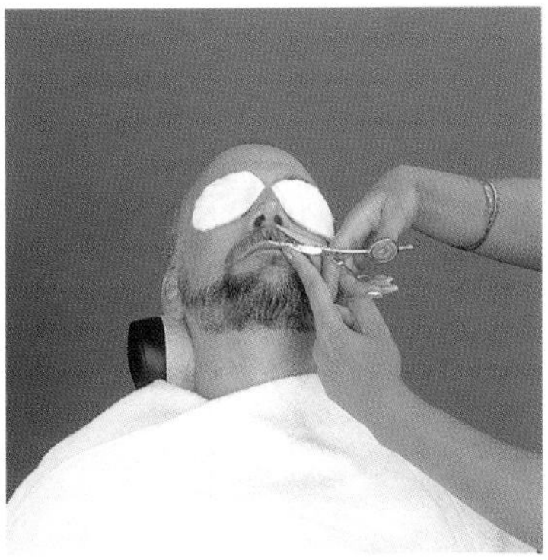

Figure 12.14 Trimming the moustache

Many moustaches have hair that is shaped to extend past the area of actual growth. Take care not to remove this. Comb the hair into place and cut the required length over the lip, if the hair projects onto the lip, scissors should be used, taking care to use the free hand to steady the blades.

Check for balance and evenness of length. Beards may require the application of dressing to produce the required result. Moustache wax may be applied to stiffen the hair to enable 'handle bar' effects to be achieved.

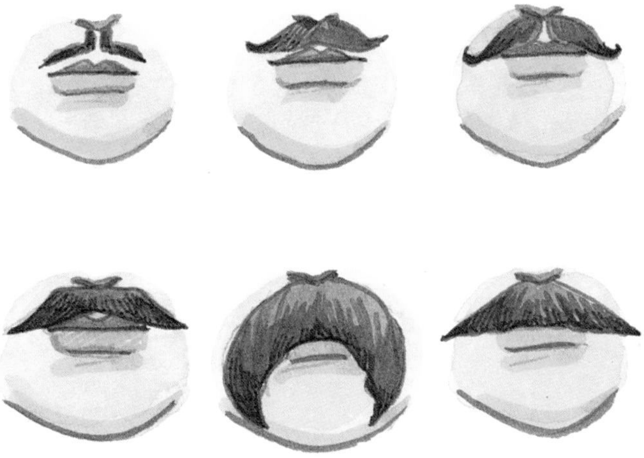

Figure 12.15 A range of moustache shapes

Sideburns

For all barbering the finished length of the sideburns must be checked, adjusted and made even. Sideburns that may have appeared quite flat before the haircut will require reduction to be in proportion when the scalp hair has been trimmed. The barber must be able to offer this service.

Following consultation with your client, and cutting using either scissors or clipper over the comb, reduce the bulk of the sideburns. Invert the clipper to cut the lower edge (see Figure 12.16), using the mirror to check balance. Having cut the lower line it may be necessary to soften the line with slight graduation.

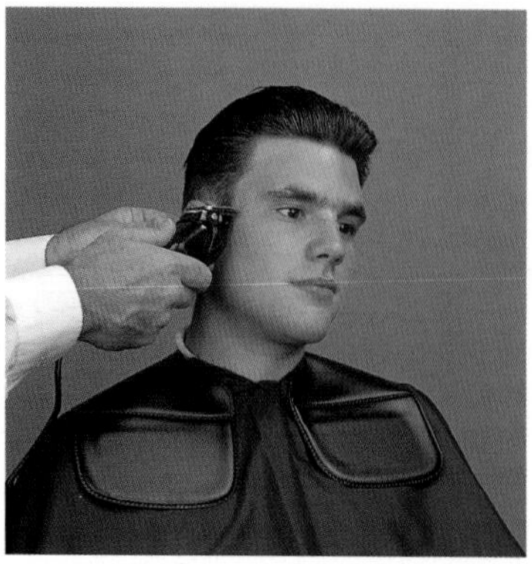

Figure 12.16 Using inverted clipper on sideburns

Sideburns may be used to add shape to the face. You should consider both their lower line and their profile shape. When removing the bulk, use the comb over which you are cutting to determine the profile shape being achieved. Use the mirror to monitor the progress in the shape. The outline shape of the sideburn may require shaving once complete.

WHAT THE EXPERT SAYS Cutting men's hair using barbering techniques requires specific skills. The shapes cut into men's barbered hair tend to differ from others, in that they are more angular, flattening the occipital area, taking the roundness off the crown.

In most cases the hair is cut using a scissor or clipper-over-comb technique, allowing effects to be achieved which are shorter than those which can be achieved by holding the hair between the fingers.

In recent years there has been a resurgence in barbering techniques, which has been brought about by shorter, more masculine hair designs.

Facial hair must be considered as all part of the total look of your client. Most men have hair growth on the face, some choosing to grow this and others preferring to be cleanly shaved. If a client has facial hair you must be able to work with this. Even the cleanly shaven face will require those areas of the hairstyle that join to the beard area to be cut and cleanly lined.

Facial hair

An increased use of facial hair has developed in recent years. With the longer hair looks of the 1970s, this was generally full-bearded looks that often did not receive too much shaping. As hairstyles have become shorter and more clearly defined, the facial hair has followed suit. Men once again sport a range of beard and moustache shapes. They may do this for a number of reasons.

When consulting with your client you should remember that there will be a number of reasons for the use of facial hair. Facial hair may be used purely as a fashion tool, enabling the wearer to produce a particular look for the moment.

Facial hair may also be used to cover blemishes or scarring. The apparent shape of the face can be altered considerably by the use of facial hair and in discussing and carrying out a beard or moustache trim it is essential that you identify the requirements of your client before proceeding.

Professional skills

Remember, shaping facial hair evenly and cleanly is something that your client may find difficult to undertake for themselves, as they can only observe the beard from one angle. You have the advantage in being able to offer the client something that they may not be able to undertake themselves to the same level of proficiency.

The complete service

As the professional barber, remember your client's total look. Be prepared to offer to remove hair from the ears, using the clippers or with extreme care using the points of the scissors. Be prepared to trim eyebrows and to produce clean even lines around your hairstyle. This includes the bases of sideburns, around the ears on very short hairstyles and the nape both behind the ears and on the neck. Remember that your client may not always wear a high-collared shirt: there may be times when he may wear a tee shirt, so you may need to remove neck hair to a lower level or to blend a clean neckline with a hirsute back.

THE BARBERED HAIRCUT

There are two styles of haircut described in this section: one which requires a closely graduated natural hairline effect and one which requires a more sculptured, artistic look, the latter being more closely associated with traditional men's hairdressing competition looks.

While both haircuts may be carried out on dry hair, and in the commercial salon often are, they may also be carried out from wet. Wet cutting gives more control over the hair and reduces the effect of hair clippings flying over yourself and your client.

Gown you client with a cutting cloth, cotton wool and a cutting shoulder cape (see Figure 12.17).

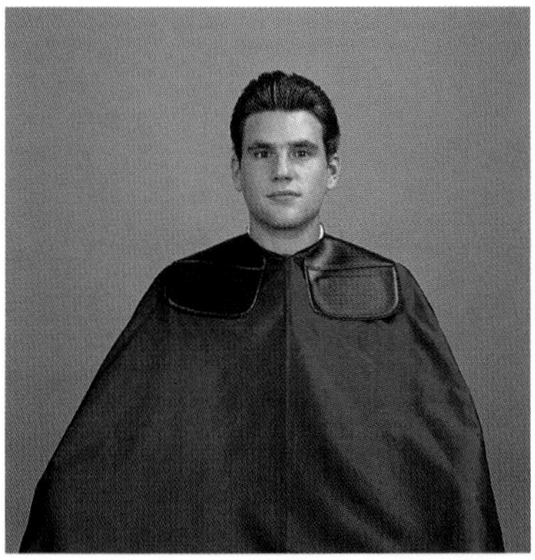

Figure 12.17 Client gowned for cut

Following a consultation check the hair for strong hair growth patterns, degree of curl, length and texture. The hair should be pre-shampooed if required: this is recommended. You should be aware that within a barbering context there will be a number of clients who do not wish to have their hair shampooed and it may be necessary to lightly spray the hair with water or styling lotion to achieve effective control. Avoid wetting the hair when cutting using electrical clippers.

HEALTH AND SAFETY Corded clippers should only be used on dry hair, owing to the risk of electric shock.

The graduated cut 'classic style'

This style is the classic closely graduated hairstyle, having a nape hairline that blends with the neck. The exact point at which the haircut ends and the neck line begins is almost indiscernible.

1. With the hair slightly moist or almost dry, and starting at the centre back of the head, slide the points of the scissors through the hair, close to the scalp at the outermost point of the occipital bone.
2. Lift the hair section and place it onto the comb.
3. Lift the mesh out from the head at 90 degrees and cut to the required length. Note the position of the back of the comb in the hair (see Figure 12.18).
4. Moving down the head, slide the scissors through the hair at the scalp, 0.5 cm beneath the previous section and place the hair onto the comb.
5. Lift the mesh of hair, together with the previously cut mesh out from the head, at less than 90 degrees and cut to the same length as the previously cut hair (see Figure 12.19). The lower the hair section is held the shorter the subsequent section of hair cut will be. Therefore you control the hairstyle.
6. At all times the section for the meshes should be taken at right angles to the hairline (see Figure 12.20).

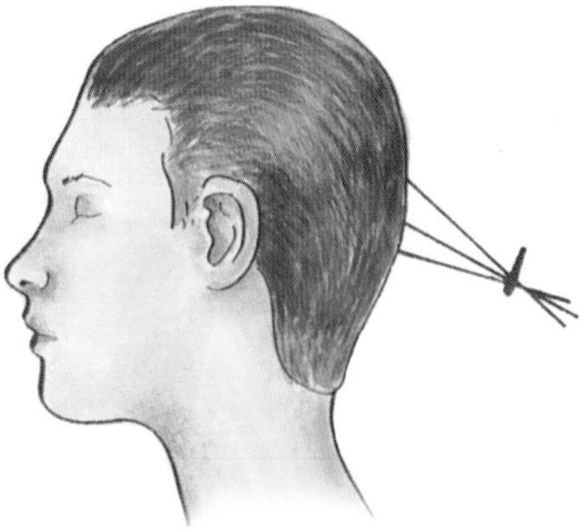

Figure 12.18 Lifting mesh for graduated cut

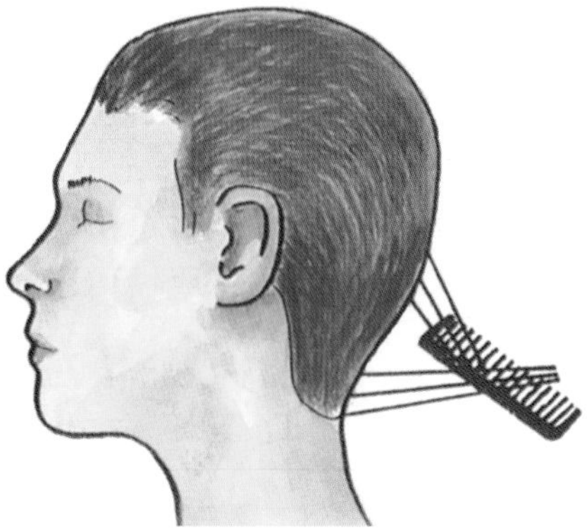

Figure 12.19 Next mesh in graduated cut

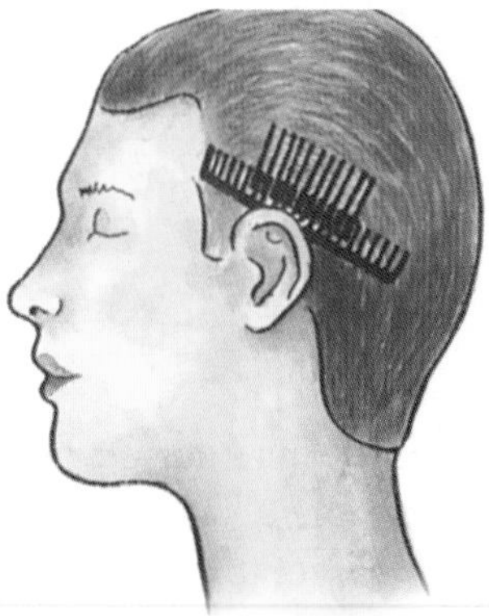

Figure 12.20 Taking section for meshes at right angles to hairline

7. Continue down the head in the same manner until the hairline is reached. Then, at the hairline, insert a fine-toothed, flexibly backed comb and, pressing it against the scalp with the comb teeth projecting slightly out, move the comb upwards and gradually out from the scalp, cutting continuously with the scissors as you go. A steady and continuous movement of the comb, coupled with a continuous cutting action, will ensure a smooth, even graduation without steps or cutting marks.
8. Move to a point adjacent to the first section cut and repeat the process. Always include a small section of the adjacent cut mesh of hair as a guide to the cut line.
9. Continue around to the side of the head in this manner, remember that the sections and your comb must follow the design or hairline. Ensure that your comb is parallel to the hairline at all times (see Figure 12.21).

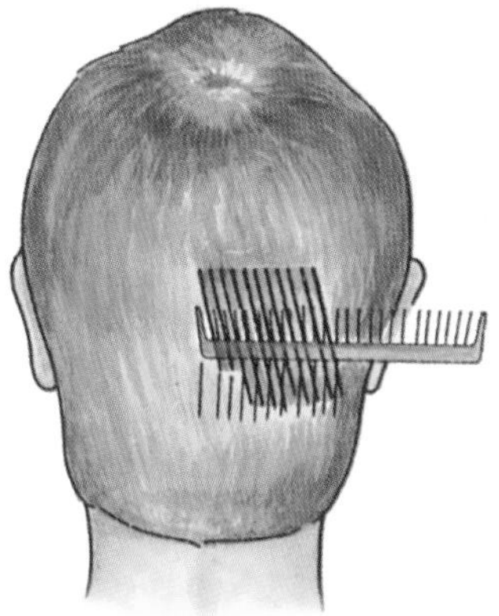

Figure 12.21 Following round head with graduated cut

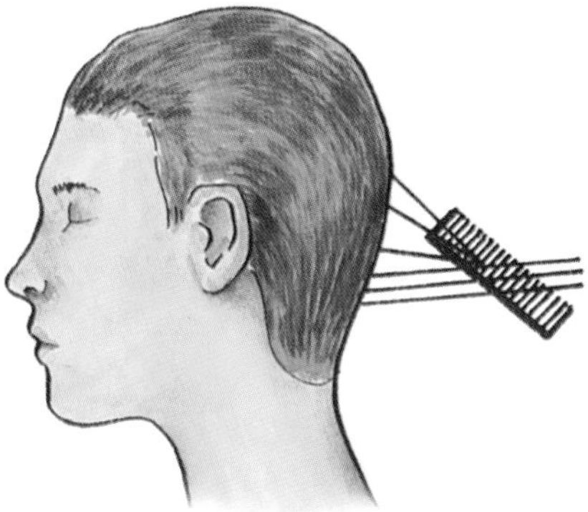

Figure 12.22 Cutting to occipital area

10. Once the front hairline is reached, return to the centre back and commence the movement to the other side of the head.
11. Once the lower areas of the hair are cut, the top should be addressed. Starting at the front hairline, take sections of hair 1 cm in depth, hold out at 90 degrees and cut to the same length as the very first cut at the occipital bone (see Figure 12.23).

TIP Remember that for your client's comfort, hair clippings should be dusted from the neck area regularly.

12. Taking small sections, continue from the front in columns, taking meshes of hair at 90 degrees and cutting to the same length as the previous sections until the occipital area is reached (see Figure 12.23). Always include a small mesh of hair that has already been cut within the mesh to act as a guide to the cutting line.
13. Having completed this with one row, start at the front hairline and work back with another row, and continue to do so until the top area of the hair is cut and blends with the graduated side areas. The top area will now have a uniform layer and the side and back a graduation.
14. It may be necessary to thin the hair where the uniform layer meets the graduation on the curve of the head, as within this area there will be a considerable volume of hair.
15. For a truly graduated hairline the nape area must be closely blended. This may be achieved by the use of the electric clippers. Using clippers with a variable cut setting, set for the longest cut and slide the clipper up the neck into the hairline, gradually

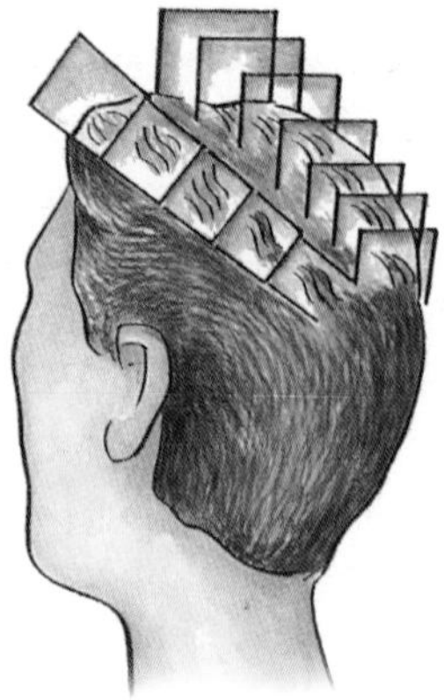

Figure 12.23 Top section blends with sides

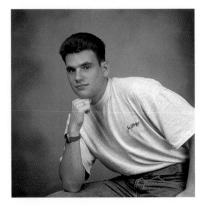

Figure 12.24 Finished graduated haircut

pivoting the cutting blade away from the hair. Repeat this several times, each time reducing the gauge of the cut and the distance up the hairline that this progresses.

This task may also be carried out using the very fine teeth of the comb, pushing the comb flat to the neck, gradually tilting the teeth and moving the comb away from the neck and scalp and cutting the hair that projects through the comb's teeth as you go.

A truly graduated haircut will have a blend with no obvious demarcation lines or 'steps' (see Figure 12.24).

The exact end of the hairstyle and the beginning of the neck area should be almost indistinguishable (see Figure 12.24). When a very short-haired result is required, particularly on dark hair, it may be necessary to shave away the hair from just above the ear, behind the ear (on the hairline) and the nape, without producing a definite hairline.

Shaving and face massage, pages 256–257

The sculptured haircut

This cut is generally less graduated than the previous, being more of a uniform layer. The hair is often cut wet, starting with the hair being thinned. This may be achieved by using thinning scissors or a razor.

> ***TIP*** Remember to consult your client throughout the cutting process to check for satisfaction and to consult on shape and length.

Thinning scissors

Systematically work over the head, cutting each mesh of hair using the thinning scissors. Avoid over-thinning the front hairline, parting area and the crown. To avoid a line of demarcation, use the thinning scissors lightly several times along the entire length of the hair rather that just the once.

Razor thinning

The razor should be used only on wet or moist hair. Having checked the scalp for any protrusions, section the hair off, starting at the nape, using sections 1 cm deep. Use a co-ordinated comb and razor action (see Figure 12.26).

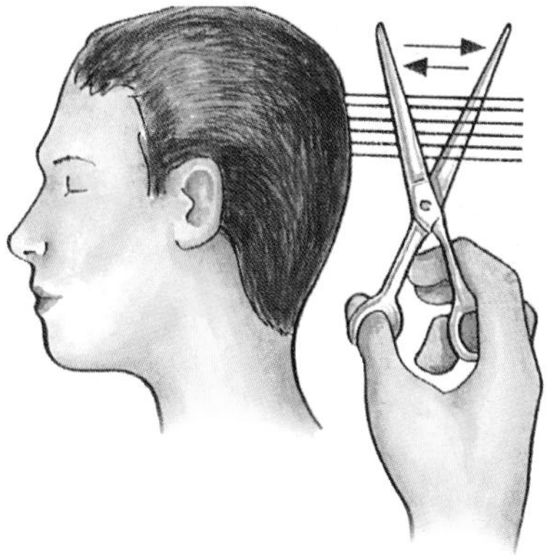

Figure 12.25 Thinning technique

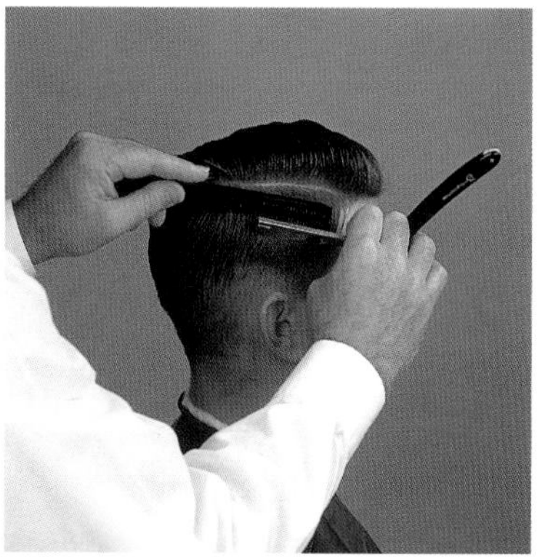

Figure 12.26 Razor cutting

Draw the razor over the last three-quarters of the hair's length in the direction in which the hair will lie. Complete this section by section throughout the haircut, taking care in areas where the head curves, as these areas may be over-thinned if a sharp razor is used. The hair of the top of the head is normally combed forward and thinned in this manner and the hair at the side is combed forward so as to avoid your client's ears.

The curl of over-curly hair may be reduced by thinning the ends of the meshes in this manner, and very straight hair may be styled more easily.

TIP Before razor thinning the hair, always check the scalp for any lumps or bumps.

The layering

The haircut may commence at any part of the head. This is often the nape or front hairline. Take a mesh of hair, comb it at 90 degrees out from the head and cut to the required length. Continue over the head in this manner, using a previously cut mesh of hair as a guide to the cutting line.

Remember that a square or angular shape is usually required for men, do not round off corners at the side curvature of the head or at the crown.

Once the layering is complete, the hair may require additional thinning to compensate for hair that has been removed by the cut.

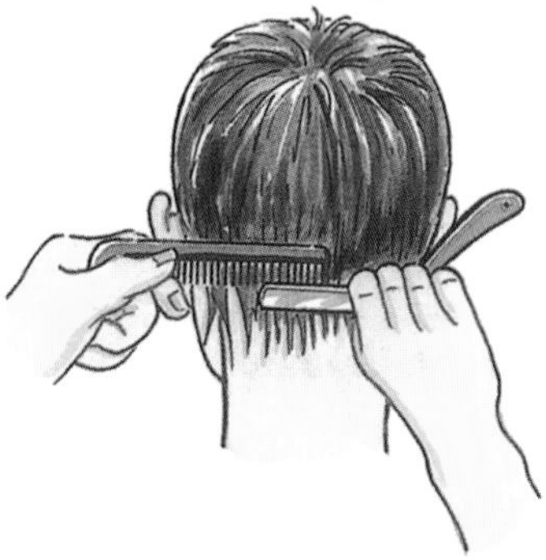

Figure 12.27 Razor cutting techniques (1)

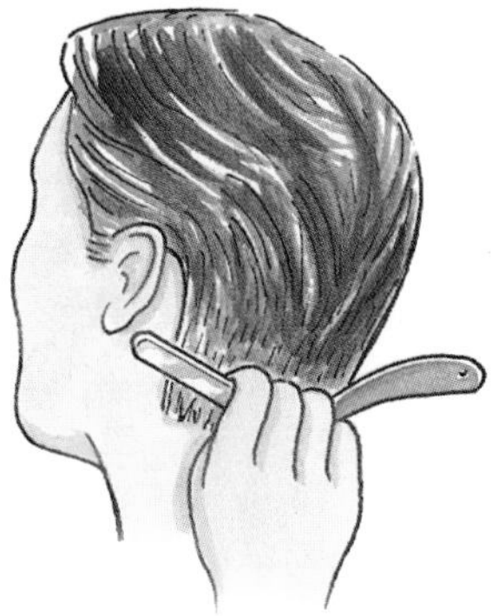

Figure 12.28 Razor cutting techniques (2)

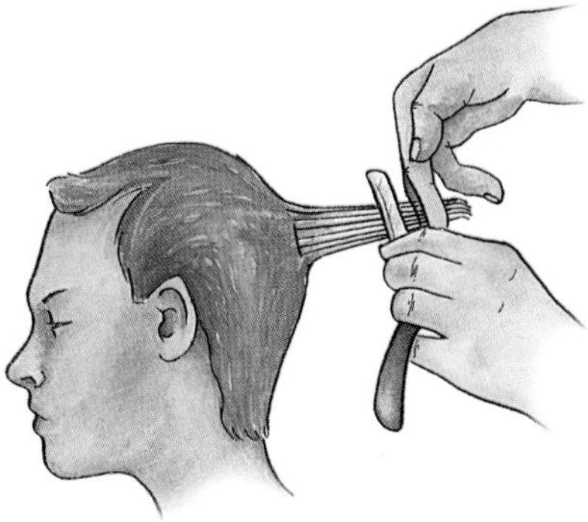

Figure 12.29 Razor cutting techniques (3)

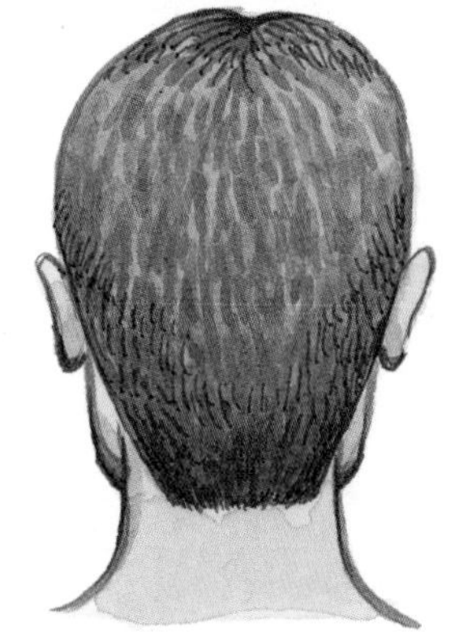

Figure 12.30 Graduated tapered nape hairline

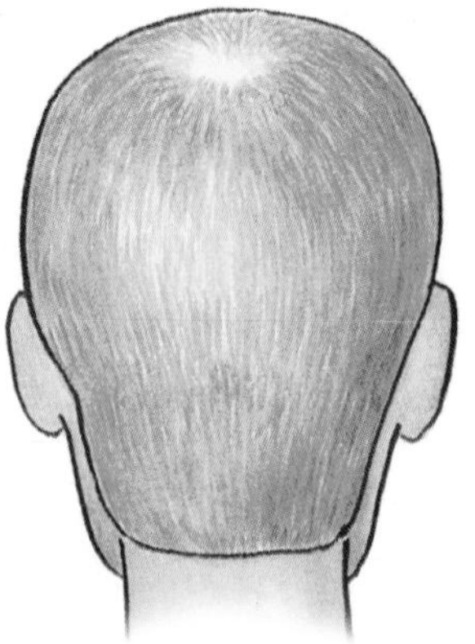

Figure 12.31 Boston neckline

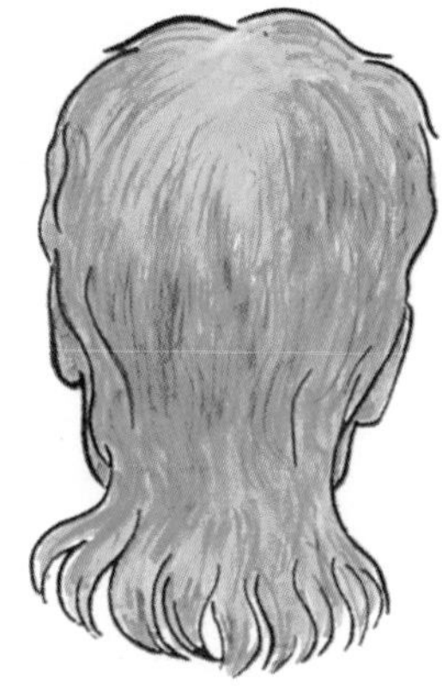

Figure 12.32 Lion's mane neckline

You must now outline the hair. Do this by moistening the hair and combing down, using the back of the comb to flatten the hair against the skin. The scissors or inverted clippers may then be used to cut the outline shape. Remember that most men's hairstyles have square-shaped necklines. These are either definite square shapes, the line behind the ear being cut in a downward line using the scissors, pointed from the ear down to the nape and then squared across the nape using scissors or inverted clippers, or downward lines either side of the nape with a graduated neckline.

A 'Boston' neckline is a heavy abrupt napeline across the back of the nape, curving slightly to accentuate the width.

FASHION STYLING 1 (see Figure 12.33a)

1. Commence the haircut lifting hair from the head in the comb at less than 90° (see Figure 12.33b).
2. Using the previously cut section take a section below this and hold the hair at less than 90°, cutting the hair using the previous section as a guide.
3. The result of using a less than 90° angle is that hair will be graduated shorter as you proceed down (see Figure 12.33c). By using the previous section as a guide prevent steps in hair length (see Figure 12.33d).
4. A close result is achieved at sides and nape by sliding the comb up into the hair line and tilting the comb's teeth outwards and cutting the hair as it protrudes between the teeth (see Figure 12.33e).
5. Comb back resting against the scalp, teeth pointing diagonally out enables hair to be cut closely to the scalp while blending with longer hair within the hair line.
6. The hair of the top is cut by taking sections from the crown working forwards using the previous cut section as a guide (see Figure 12.33f). Pulling the mesh slightly back at the front hairline will leave a little more length at this point.
7. Taking small square sections, twisting these and sliding the scissor blade along the outside of this twist develops a textured result in the style (see Figure 12.33g).
8. Using the points of the scissors the front hairline may be point thinned (freehand cutting) to provide a softer edge (see Figure 12.33h).

FASHION STYLING 2 (see Figure 12.33i)

1. At the occipital area take a section of hair holding out, in the comb, at less than 90°. Cut the hair as it protrudes through the teeth of the comb (see Figure 12.33j).
2. At the hairline the hair should be graduated into the hairline. As you progress towards

the hairline use the previously cut hair section as a guide to the cutting point. For each section hold the hair at less than 90° (see Figure 12.33k).

3. The nape and side hairline may be closely graduated by inserting a comb into the hairline with the back of the comb resting on the scalp, the comb's teeth tilted upwards and outwards and the hair protruding through the teeth may be cut (see Figure 12.33l).
4. The hair from the occipital to the crown area the hair is brought down in sections and cut like the position of the first cut. This may be followed around to the sides (see Figure 12.33m).
5. The top hair may be cut by combing sections of the hair up and connecting it into the hair at each side. This will produce a look with lift and movement (see Figure 12.33n).
6. Alternatively the hair may be combed flat to the head and cut to the base line. This will produce a heavy straight look (see Figure 12.33o).

The front hairline may be texturised by free hand cutting. Sliding the scissors either down the hair shaft while closing the blade or by point thinning, cutting into the hair from outside of the hair style (see Figure 12.33p).

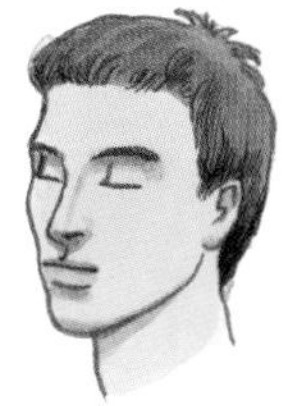
Figure 12.33a

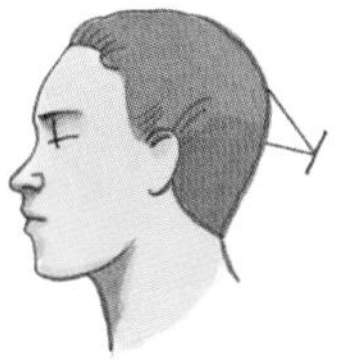
Figure 12.33b

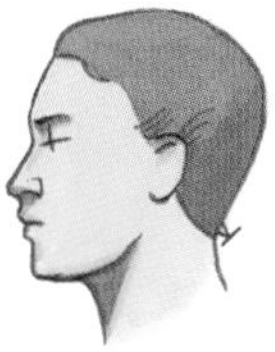
Figure 12.33c

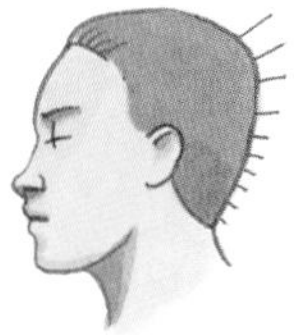
Figure 12.33d

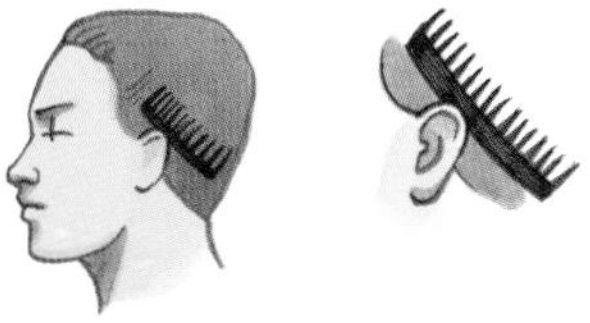
Figure 12.33e

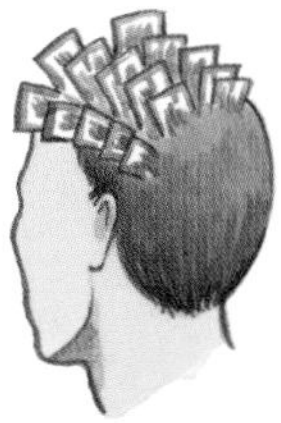
Figure 12.33f

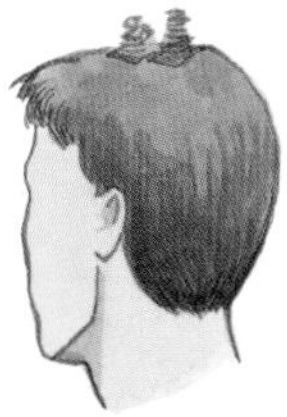
Figure 12.33g

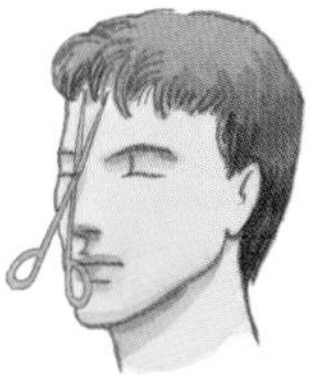
Figure 12.33h

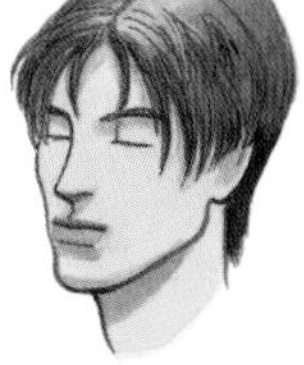
Figure 12.33i

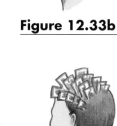

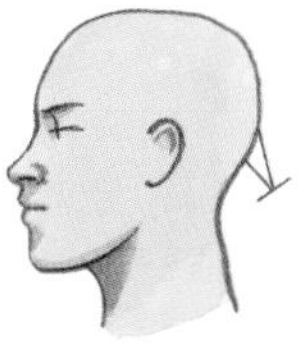
Figure 12.33j

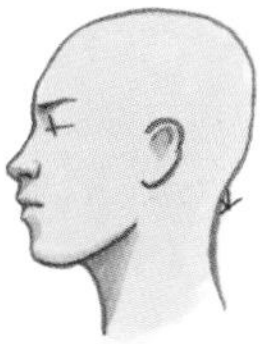
Figure 12.33k

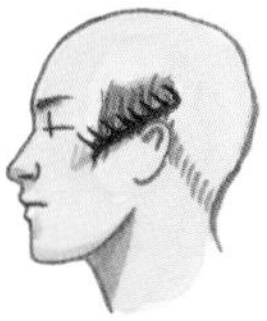
Figure 12.33l

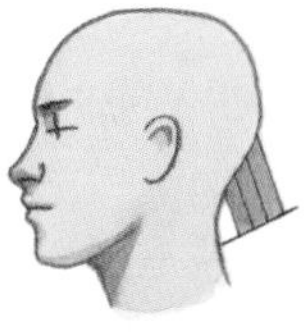
Figure 12.33m

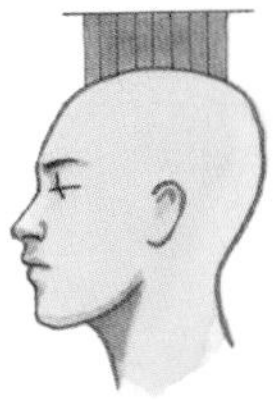
Figure 12.33n

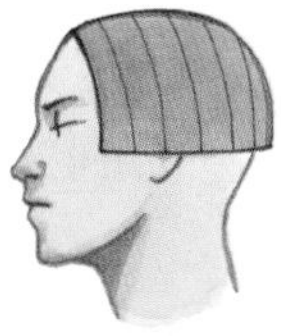
Figure 12.33o

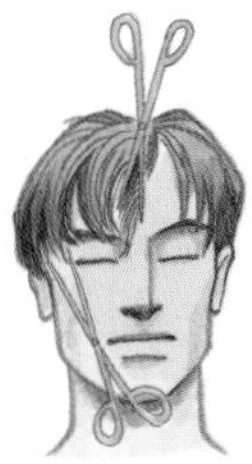
Figure 12.33p

DRYING THE STYLE

In order for the style to be created the hair must be dried in place. Remove the cutting cloth and remove all cut hair from your client. Take care when removing the cape not to drop cuttings onto your client, and use the neck brush on the nape area to remove clippings.

Styling aids, page 41

Replace the cutting cloth, and commence the dry. Apply any styling aids.

A closely set bristle brush or heat resistant comb may be used to guide the hair, together with a blow dryer with a fishtail nozzle to give control over the air flow. Commence the dry at the nape, taking care not to burn the scalp by allowing the air flow to rest in this area. Use the brush or comb to raise the roots where required to produce the shape and to tuck in the ends. For a smooth result direct the airflow in the direction of the style. Adjust the position of the fishtail nozzle so that it does not touch your client's scalp or face during the drying.

Once the dry is complete, apply any hair dressings required and then dress the hair into position. A number of combs and brushes are available that will give textured effects to hair, if required. First brush the hair at 90 degrees to the desired direction and then firmly brush in the finished direction.

Finish by showing your client the result, having removed the gown and any protective clothes and by using the back mirror (see Figure 12.34).

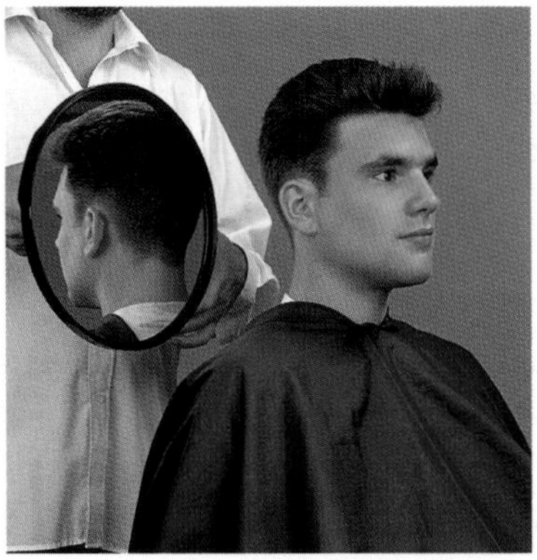

Figure 12.34 Using back mirror

STYLE VARIATIONS

Partings

When a parting is used in the hairstyle it is usual to cut to this, leaving one side, the heavy side, longer than the other. The heavy side may require more thinning than the other.

Fringes

Fringes will normally be outlined by cutting on the forehead. Additional length may be required if the fringe is to cover a receding hairline.

Off-face styles

Hair often dresses more easily back off the face if left a little longer than the rest of the hair.

Over-ear hairstyles

When cutting hair that will lay over the ear, allowance must be made for the hair to lay out over the ear and yet lay level with the rest of the hair. Often hair must be shaped around the ear or left substantially longer in order not to 'stick out' over the ear.

Added hairpieces

When cutting hair to fit with a hairpiece, additional thinning may be needed so that the hair blends with the lengths of the added hair. Take care not to cut the added hair at the same time as the client's natural hair. Once complete ensure that the two do blend together.

Areas of hair loss

Often additional length of hair must be left to allow an even line to be achieved over an area of hair loss. Discuss the requirements with your client before commencing the cut. Remember tact must be used at all times as hair loss can, for some, cause considerable mental anguish.

FURTHER STUDY

- There are a number of beard and moustache shapes, most of which have names that are used to identify them. Find out more about these and learn those more usual ones.
- Find out more about modern tools that can help you produce textured effects in barbered hairstyles

REVIEW QUESTIONS

1. How should the electric clipper be used to outline a beard?
2. In what position should the hydraulic chair be in when the client is invited to sit?
3. Why is a lightly coloured towel used when beard trimming?
4. What is the largest size clipper grader available?
5. Why is a tissue placed on the chair's head rest while trimming the beard?
6. When beard trimming, will the area beneath the chin appear longer or shorter when the head is upright?
7. Why is the scissor-over-comb method used in preference to holding the hair with the fingers?
8. For safety, should hair be wet or dry when using electric hair clippers?
9. What is the essential feature of a graduated neckline?
10. Should a razor be used on wet or dry hair?

CHAPTER 13

Shaving and face massage

This section provides the relevant essential knowledge about preparing for and carrying out a wet face shave and a facial massage. This includes the procedure for a complete facial shave and an outline shave, and will enable you to select appropriate tools and products and be aware of the correct procedure for carrying the process out safely.

Level 2	
Unit 201	
Element 201.1	Consult with and maintain effective relationships with clients
Unit 209	
Element 209.2	Support health, safety and security at work
Unit 211	
Element 211.1	Maintain effective and safe methods of working when shaving and massaging the face
Element 211.2	Remove hair by shaving
Element 211.3	Massage the face
Unit 212	
Element 212.1	Maintain effective and safe methods of working when cutting facial hair
Element 212.2	Cut beards and moustaches to shape

Contents

INTRODUCTION

The traditional art of the barber includes shaving and face massage. Evidence of shaving the beard may be found in the earliest civilisations. To many, these may appear to be skills that are no longer relevant, but they are undergoing a renaissance. Wet shaving is a skill that is still in demand in certain communities and geographic areas. Fashions in facial hair require the skill of outline shaving as part of the shaping process. The skills of shaving may also be applied to the art of shaved partings, used with Afro-Caribbean hair, to define a parting in short hair. Shaved outlines, used to define the hairline in sculptured designs around the ears and in the nape area, as well as shapes shaved in the hairlines, all require control in the execution to produce the finish required. Facial massage is usually coupled with the shaving process. It is a traditional barbering skill that may be used to relax your client and give him a feeling of well being.

FACIAL SHAVING

Tools and materials

Tools

Razors

The traditional tool for wet shaving is the open razor, a solid blade of metal pivoting from a handle or shield. The blade of the razor can be made of metal of varying hardness and with one of three cross-sectional shapes (or 'grinds'). The grinds are solid or wedge ground (see Figure 13.1), half-hollow ground (see Figure 13.2) and hollow ground.

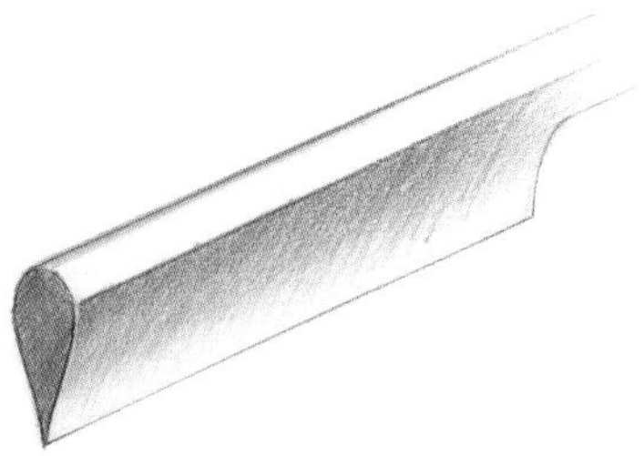

Figure 13.1 Solid ground razor

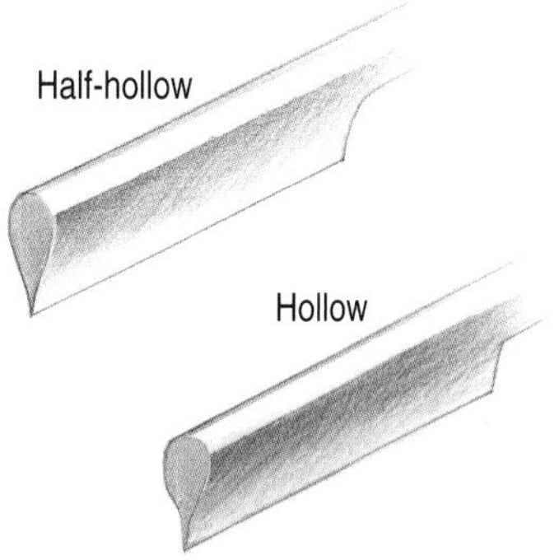

Figure 13.2 Hollow ground razor

The solid grind is the earliest shape and produced a rather heavy razor that could be difficult to manipulate and gave little sensation to the shaver, therefore making it difficult to determine the appropriate shaving pressure to be used. The half-hollow grind (or French) razor gave a little more sensitivity to the shaver. Traditionally made of a soft metal that made it easier to keep sharp but did not retain the edge, this razor was traditionally used for hair cutting and for shaving fine, delicate beards. The hollow ground (or German) razor was most widely used for shaving. Made of a very hard steel, which once sharp retained its edge, the finesse of the blade made it responsive to the shaver and easily manipulated across the face.

These 'fixed blade' open razors require frequent attention to the cutting edge. Immediately following use (to cleanse and dry the cutting edge) and immediately before each use (to polish and smooth the cutting edge) this type of razor requires stropping. Stropping is the process of drawing the cutting edge across a surface, usually leather. There are two types of strop, hanging and solid. The hanging strop is a flexible length of leather attached to a firm hook on the hydraulic chair and held taut at the other end. The leather surface is dressed (to aid its polishing action) with a sweet oil, and the razor is drawn along its length. Some strops also have a canvas surface which is dressed with a hard soap. This surface is used when the razor's edge becomes too dull or blunt for shaving (see Figure 13.3). A hand, Hamon or solid strop is also available. This has a leather surface fixed to a sprung wooden strip. One end is rested on a firm surface and the other held raised by the hand. The surface of the leather is dressed with a specialised stropping paste. Some solid strops also have a surface of balsa wood.

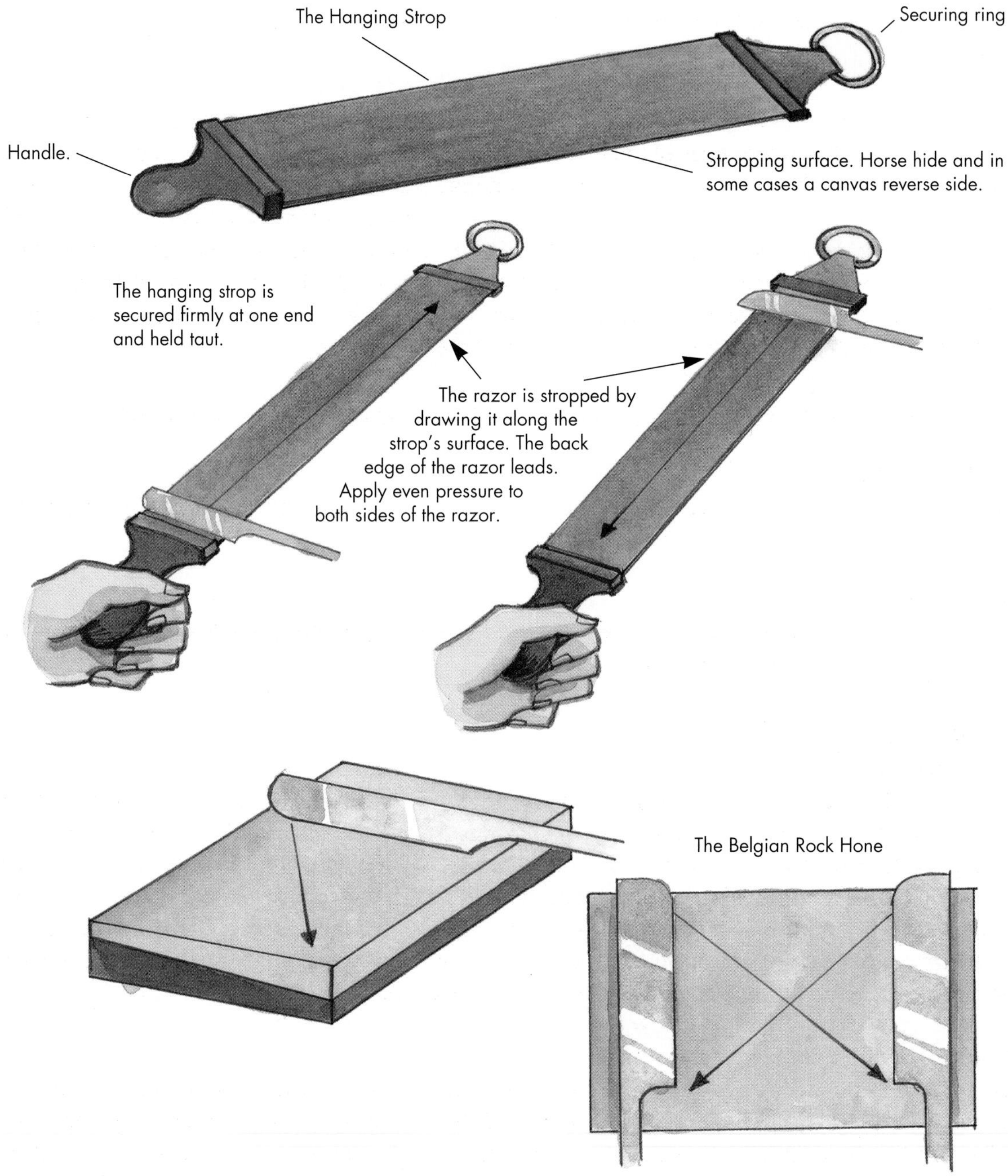
The Hanging Strop
Securing ring
Handle.
Stropping surface. Horse hide and in some cases a canvas reverse side.
The hanging strop is secured firmly at one end and held taut.
The razor is stropped by drawing it along the strop's surface. The back edge of the razor leads. Apply even pressure to both sides of the razor.
The Belgian Rock Hone

Figure 13.3 Stropping

When a razor becomes blunt it requires sharpening. This is accomplished using a hone. This is a slab of stone, either natural or reconstituted, lubricated by water or oil, which improves its bite or ability to sharpen, and the razor's cutting edge is pushed across its surface. Care must be taken to produce an edge which is even both in shape and sharpness (see Figure 13.3).

To test the sharpness of a razor of this type, the cutting edge should be drawn very carefully across the length of the blade over a moistened thumb nail or the moistened end of the thumb. A dragging sensation indicates a sharp edge, a smooth sliding action indicates that the edge is not yet sharp. An uneven edge may appear sharp at some points and blunt at others. The use of a blunt razor will cause considerable client discomfort as well as causing extreme difficulty in hair removal.

To avoid cross infection razors should be washed after every use in hot soapy water, dried and then sterilised.

For commercial shaving these razors are no longer considered hygienically suitable. The difficulty in sterilising the edges of the blades has made them unsuitable for use when there was a risk of puncturing the skin's surface. They are and may still be used safely when used only on one person. For all commercial wet shaving a razor that accepts a disposable blade must be used. There are a number of these commercially available; they consist of a holder for the blade together with a handle/shield. Some styles accept a double edged blade, snapped in half, and others accept specially prepared blades which are fitted from a dispenser. There are also disposable razors available which are made in the style of the open razor.

Your choice of razor may depend on your salon policy or your personal preference.

Lather brushes

The best quality lather brushes are said to have bristles of badger hair. There are brushes available made of both natural and synthetic bristles.

Lather bowls

Clean, sterile bowls are required, one to contain a supply of very hot water in which to warm the lather brush, the second to contain the lather.

Materials

Shaving soap

The solid block form of soap must not be used when shaving commercially as the lather brush is placed on the face, then placed onto the shaving soap and then onto another client's face, facilitating the spread of infection from one client to the next. Powdered shaving soap may be shaken directly onto the bristles of a hot moist lather brush and then applied direct to the face and progressively worked up into a lather, but shaving cream or gel is the more up-to-date product. A small amount is placed into a bowl and then worked into a lather using the lather brush. Aerosol shaving foam is not suitable as working this lather usually decreases its foam.

Astringent

An astringent is a substance that closes the pores and tightens the skin. Cold water may be used as a mild astringent, or after-shave may be used. Take care as the perfume in the lotion may conflict with the cologne used by your client. The stinging effect of after-shave may be reduced by diluting it with water. This is particularly advisable when treating delicate skin. Witch hazel may also be used.

Fine talc

This is used to soothe the skin. The talc should be unperfumed so that it does not clash with your client's cologne.

Coagulant

In case of bleeding, a sterile coagulant such as powdered Alum BP or Ferric Chloride is required.

> ***TIP*** The autoclave sterilises by steaming items, under pressure, at a temperature of 120 °C. Only use an autoclave if you have been trained in its use or by following the manufacturer's directions for safe use.

The shaving process

The shaving process breaks down into a number of steps:

1. preparation of the work area and tools
2. analysis of the beard area
3. preparing the face and softening the beard
4. removing the beard (first time over)
5. re-lathering the beard
6. removing the beard (second time over)
7. removing remaining lather
8. closing the pores
9. cleansing and sterilising tools and materials.

> ***REMEMBER*** Do not use a razor or any other sharp tool near your client without first ensuring that there is adequate clear space around you to prevent other stylists obstructing the process.

Preparation

Prepare all tools prior to undertaking the shave on your client. All tools that will make contact with your client's skin must be clean and sterile. An autoclave may be used to sterilise all metal tools; chemical sterilising fluids should be used to sterilise those tools which have parts that cannot stand high temperatures.

Check that the hydraulic chair is clean and safe for use. Lock the chair in position at its lowest level, with the back upright and head rest in place. Should your client step onto a hydraulic chair footrest when it is not locked in position, the chair may spin away from your client, possibly causing them to fall. This type of chair is at its most stable when the hydraulic lift is at its lowest position, so this is the best position for it to be at when the client sits down. Raise the hydraulic chair to a comfortable working height using the pump, which may be foot-powered or electric. Remember to lock the swivel of the chair in place at all times when adjustment has been completed.

A number of hot steam towels will be required and should be prepared beforehand. Specialist towel steamers are available (see Figure 13.4).

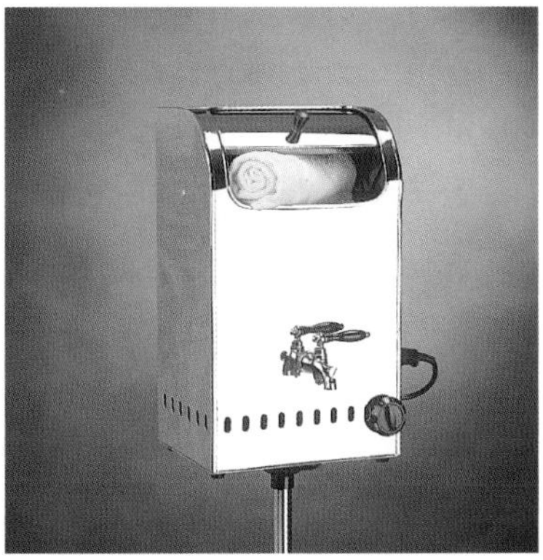

Figure 13.4 Towel steamer

Fold a towel in half, lengthwise, and then in half across the length. Apply a small amount of water to this fold, then roll the towel tightly from the fold towards the loose edges and wring it to spread the moisture through the towel. Place these prepared towels on the shelf in the towel steamer. They will require approximately 20 minutes to heat through. Avoid over-wetting the towel prior to steaming as excessive moisture can scald your client. The case of the towel steamer can become very hot when in use, so inform colleagues and clients to avoid touching this.

HEALTH AND SAFETY Ensure that your hands are clean and that any open sores or cuts on your hands are covered with a waterproof dressing.

Preparing your client

Gown your client, using the cutting cloth – a square sheet with a cut midway along one side. Ensure that your client's clothing is fully protected, draw the cloth up around the client's neck and tuck into the collar (see Figure 13.5).

Always use a clean gown for each client, as this will help to reduce the possible spread of infection from one client to the next. Locate a clean, lightly coloured towel diagonally around the front of your client (see Figure 13.6), tucking the edges into the collar to protect your client's clothing. The use of a lightly coloured towel will reflect light onto the underside of the chin area.

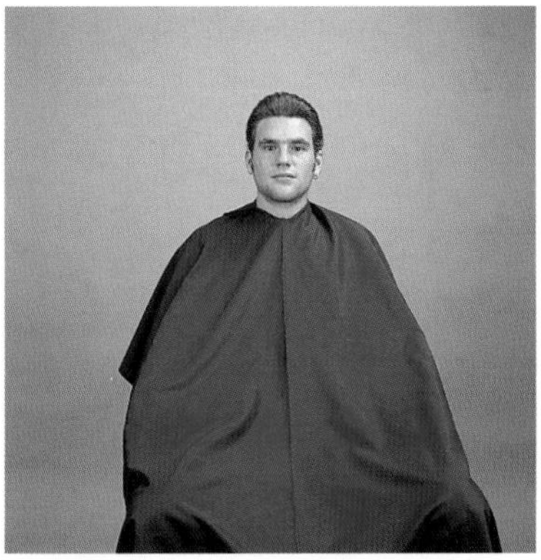

Figure 13.5 Client gowned for a shave

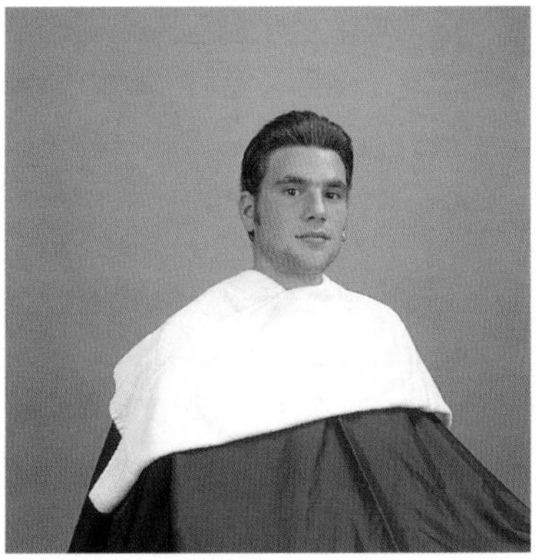

Figure 13.6 White towel round client

Discuss the shaving process with your client, and establish the direction of beard growth by drawing your hands over the beard area. In one direction the beard will feel smooth and in the other the beard will feel at its roughest. The smooth feel will indicate that this is the direction of growth. This is usually in a downward direction on the face. There are, at times, conflicting directions of growth on the client's neck. Check the skin for any conditions that might prevent shaving, including open cuts and abrasions, muscular swelling, contagious skin disorders and pustular eruptions. The location of any unusual features such as moles etc. should be noted, as they will be less apparent once the lather is in place.

Place a clean towel or tissue over the headrest of the chair, ask your client to sit up and then recline the back of the chair to approximately 45 degrees before guiding your client back onto the chair's back, adjusting the headrest to ensure that your client's neck area is not overstretched but exposed and lightly taut. Adjust the height of the chair so that your client's chin is at the level of your elbow. Apply a steam towel to the beard area to help to soften the beard and cleanse the skin. Protecting your hands from the steam using wooden tongs or a dry clean towel, remove a steam towel from the steamer. Wring out any excess moisture, taking care not to allow the hot water to run onto your hands. Unwrap the towel, taking care that the steam given off does not scald your skin. A towel that is too hot may be held without causing you pain by tossing the towel in your hands. This will also help it to cool more rapidly. With the towel still folded in half lengthways, stand at the back of the chair and offer the towel to your client's face (see Figure 13.7).

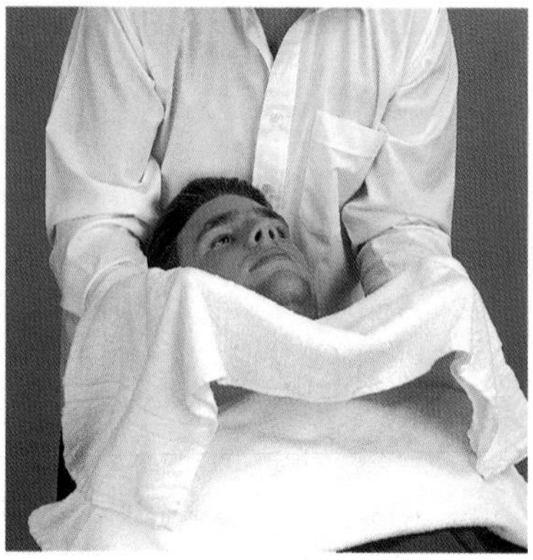

Figure 13.7 Offering hot towel to face

Allow the face to become accustomed to the heat and then wrap the towel loosely around the face, taking care to ensure that all of the beard area is covered, but that the ears do not become covered, as they are sensitive to heat. Gentle pressure onto the towel around the beard area will increase the conduction of heat to the face. Remove the towel before it becomes cool and lather the beard area. The bristles of the lather brush should be pre-heated using hot water. Build up the lather in the lather bowl and then, using a rotary action, apply the lather to the beard area (see Figure 13.8). You can achieve greater control of the lather by gripping the handle and the tops of the bristles. When lathering the top lip, you can achieve a finer spread of the brush through fanning the bristles: press the finger into the base of the bristles (see Figure 13.9).

Lather will soften the beard and help to support the bristles away from the face. Ensure that the face and lather is kept warm throughout the shaving process. To assist in softening the beard, a further steam towel may be applied over the top of the lather. Remove this steam towel before it becomes cold and then re-lather the beard area. Once the lather has built up, the shave

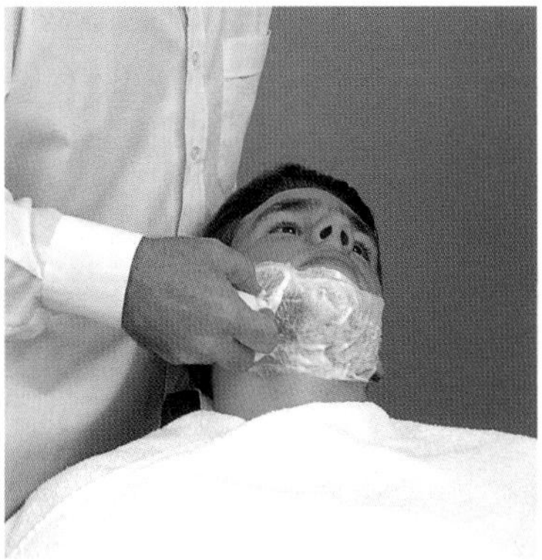

Figure 13.8 Applying lather to beard area

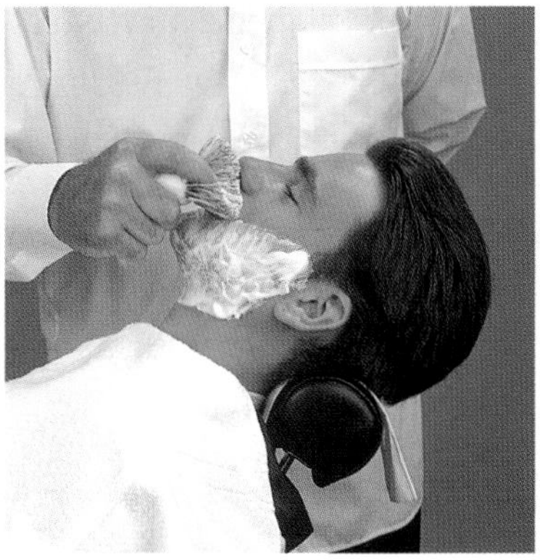

Figure 13.9 Applying lather to top lip

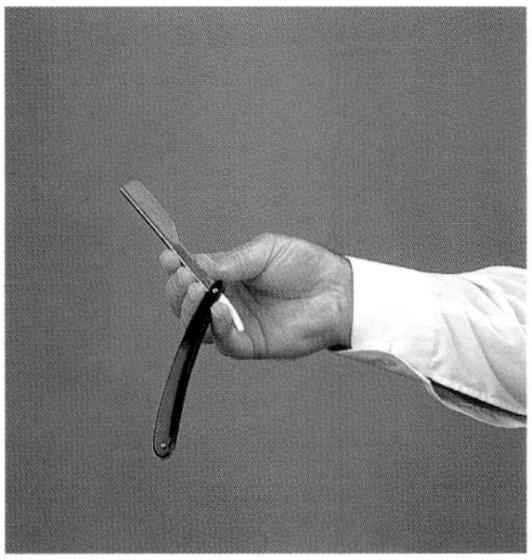

Figure 13.10 Holding the open razor

may be carried out. A clean tissue or towel will be required to wipe the razor on during the shaving process.

The shave

Hold the razor with the first two or three fingers and thumb on the shaft and the remainder on the tang. At all times the razor should be held firmly, with dry hands, so that it may be manipulated from freehand and back hand positions (see Figure 13.10).

> ***NOTE*** Never undertake a shaving stroke without the client's skin being held taut.

The movement of the razor is driven from the wrist. Stretch the skin taut, either behind or in front of the razor: stretching the skin in front of the razor will give a more comfortable, less close shave; stretching behind the razor will give the reverse. If necessary remove lather from areas of the face so that the skin may be stretched more effectively. Lay the razor on the skin, tilting the back of the razor away from the skin at approximately 30 degrees, and firmly but gently draw the razor across the beard. The shaving stroke must move the blade through the beard, avoid using a slicing action that will cut the skin. The shaving stroke is a smooth action extending only as far as the skin is taut. When shaving it is normal to shave standing to the right-hand side of the client and at the back.

Should your client be cut while shaving, apply a small amount of powdered Alum, a powdered styptic, from a sterile dressing. Ferric Chloride may be used as a liquid styptic. Never use an Alum stick, as it may be used on more that one client, and there may be a risk of spreading blood-related disorders.

Careful tensioning of the skin and correct movement of the razor considerably reduces the risk of cutting your client. Take care when shaving over curved surfaces of the face, for example the chin, as it is easy to shave too close and cause short-term bleeding.

> ***HEALTH AND SAFETY*** Do not leave an open razor lying unclosed when not in use as there is a risk of someone accidentally cutting themselves.

First time over shave

The first time over shaving strokes, in the main, follow the direction of beard growth.

1. Standing to the side of your client, with your client's face turned away from you and starting at the lower edge of the sideburn, stretch the skin and shave using a freehand movement, to the corner of the jaw (see Figure 13.12).
2. Follow this with a backhand movement across the cheek. The exact start point for this movement will be determined by the extent of beard growth.
3. Stretching the skin upwards, shave freehand along the jawbone. By stretching up, the jawbone will be free of hair, once released.
4. Stretching both upwards and downwards, shave the under-jaw area using a freehand movement.
5. Turn your client's face towards you, and use a backhand movement to shave from the sideburn down to the corner of the jaw on the other side of the face (see Figure 13.13).
6. This is followed by a freehand movement across the cheek.
7. Stretch the skin upwards and shave, freehand, along the jawbone.
8. Standing slightly forward of your client stretch the under-jaw area, both upwards and downwards and shave the area backhand. This area may require more than one stroke.
9. Move your client's face to a central position. Apply fresh lather, if required.
10. Using a freehand movement and stretching either side of the chin and upwards, shave across the chin area. Take care not to shave too close as this may cause bleeding.
11. Standing slightly to the front of your client, shave freehand down the centre under-jaw area.

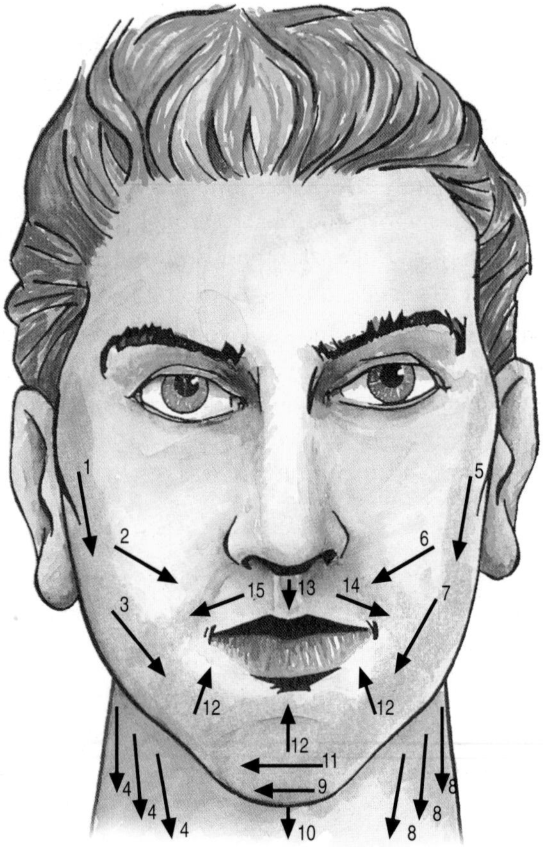

1 = Freehand
2 = Backhand
3 = Freehand
4 = Freehand
5 = Backhand
6 = Freehand
7 = Freehand
8 = Backhand
9 = Freehand
10 = Freehand
11 = Freehand
12 = Freehand reverse
13 = Freehand
14 = Backhand
15 = Freehand

Figure 13.11 First-time over shaving strokes

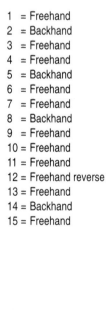

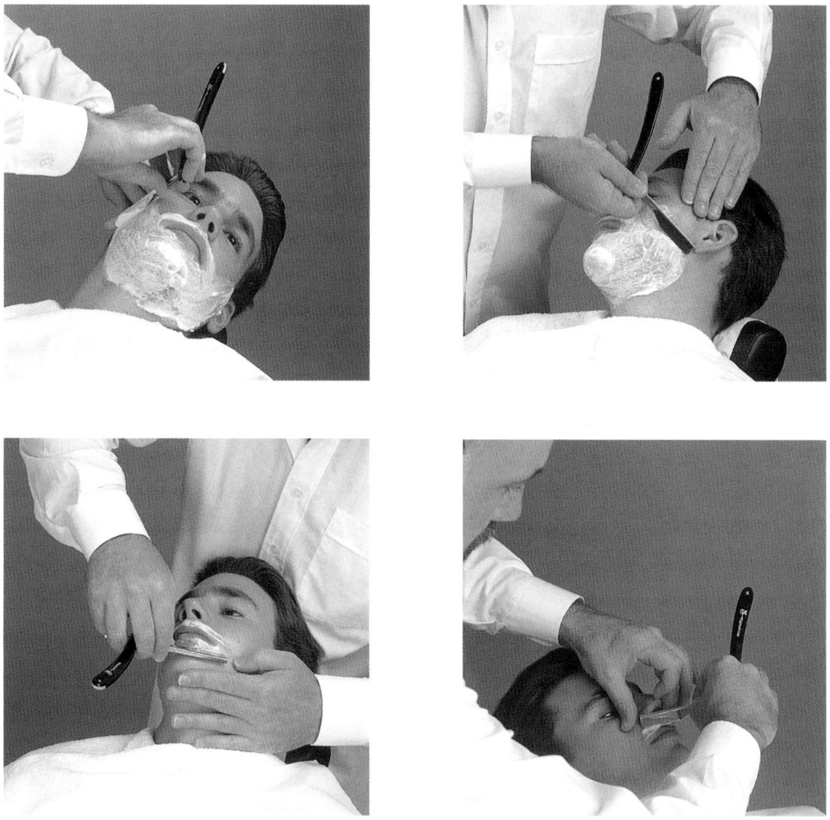

Figures 13.12–15 Basic first time over strokes

12. Return to the side of your client and shave the upper chin area using a freehand movement, taking care not to draw the razor's point along the crease of the chin, below the lip (see Figure 13.14).
13. Shave the area from the lip down to the crease of the skin, using a freehand movement, stretching the skin to either side of the mouth.
14. Shave the top lip freehand down the centre, then shave the near side freehand and the far side backhand in an outward/downward direction (see Figure 13.15).

As the razor's blade becomes clogged or coated with lather and removed beard, wipe the blade by laying it flat on the tissue or towel placed on your client's shoulder for this purpose, and drawing it across the towel with the razor's back leading. Never attempt a shaving movement when the razor's edge cannot be clearly seen.

Second time over shave

> ***TIP*** Do not attempt to shave the skin without a lubricant on the surface.

These movements will remove the remaining beard, giving a closer shave. The shaving stroke will, in the main, go against or across the direction of beard growth. More resistance to the razor will be experienced and firm but gentle movements must be used to overcome this without causing your client discomfort. Re-lather the beard, using fresh supplies of lather and hot water. Once the lather has built up the shave may commence.

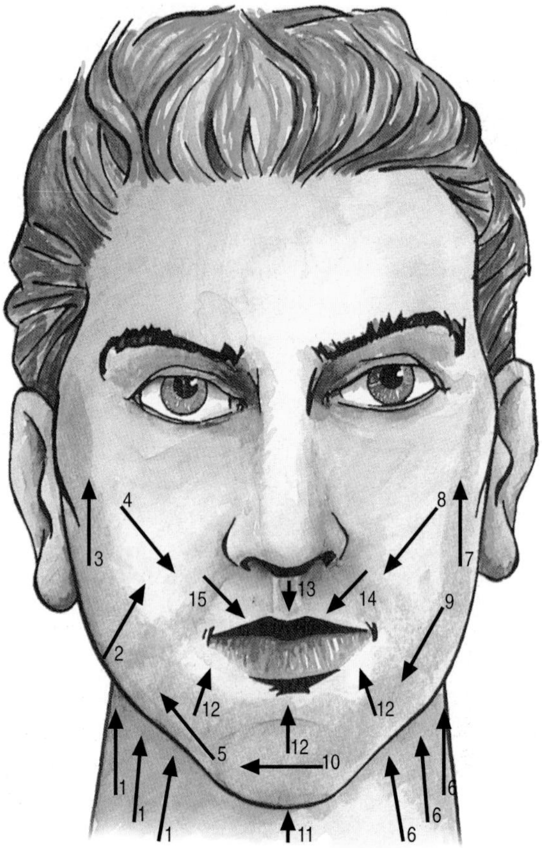

1 = Backhand reverse
2 = Backhand reverse
3 = Backhand reverse
4 = Backhand
5 = Freehand
6 = Freehand
7 = Freehand
8 = Freehand reverse
9 = Freehand reverse
10 = Freehand
11 = Backhand reverse
12 = Freehand reverse
13 = Freehand
14 = Freehand
15 = Backhand diagonal

Figure 13.16 Second time over shaving strokes

1. Direct your client's face away from you, and starting from the hairline on the neck on the left side of your client, stretch down on the neck and shave upwards towards the jawbone using a reverse backhand stroke (see Figure 13.17).
2. The next reverse backhand stroke is used diagonally upwards across the jaw, stretching the skin in front of the razor.
3. This is followed by a reverse backhand movement from the corner of the jawbone upwards towards the sideburn stretching downwards on the skin.
4. A backhand movement follows diagonally across the cheek area, as for the first time over (see Figure 13.18).
5. Finally, on this side of the face, a backhand movement is used towards the chin along the jawbone in the chin area, stretching the skin back towards the corner of the jaw.
6. Move your client's face to face towards you. Standing slightly forward at the side of your client, start at the hairline and use a reverse freehand stroke at the neck, stretching the skin down on the neck (see Figure 13.19).
7. Move behind your client, and reaching over him, using a reverse freehand movement shave from the corner of the jaw towards the sideburn, stretching the skin taut downwards behind the razor.
8. Moving back to the side of the client, shave across the cheek area using a freehand movement, stretching the skin behind (see Figure 13.20). Stretching the skin upwards and back towards the client's ear, use a freehand movement to shave across the area of the jawbone.
9. With your client's face in the central position, and standing forward of the side of your client, use a reverse backhand movement to shave the central area under the chin, stretching downwards and out to each side.

10. Stretch the skin across the chin, pulling this area upwards as well, and shave across the chin using a freehand stroke.

11. Standing at the back of your client and reaching over him, stretch the chin area downwards and using a freehand movement shave the area between the crease of the chin and the bottom lip.

12. Move to the side of your client, shave the centre of the top lip in a downward direction, stretching the skin towards either side.

13. Stretch the nearest side of the top lip outwards and shave with a backhand movement towards the middle. Stretch the furthest side of the top lip outwards and shave towards the centre using a freehand movement. Remove the towel or tissue used to wipe the razor free of lather and beard hair and dispose of it hygienically.

Following the completion of the shave a further hot towel is applied to your client's beard area. This should be removed from the face before cooling and then carefully wrapped around your hand and used to wipe any remaining lather from the face. Pay particular attention to the ear, nose and collar areas.

Having removed the hot towel, apply a cold towel to close the pores, preventing infection and aiding retraction of the facial hair. Allow the cold towel to remain on the face for a few moments, using hand pressure to increase the conductivity of the cooling effect. A cold towel may be prepared in the same manner as a hot towel, using cold water and mild refrigeration to cool. This may be followed by the application of a mild astringent or after-shave which will also close the pores and tighten the skin. When applying astringent, place a small amount on one hand,

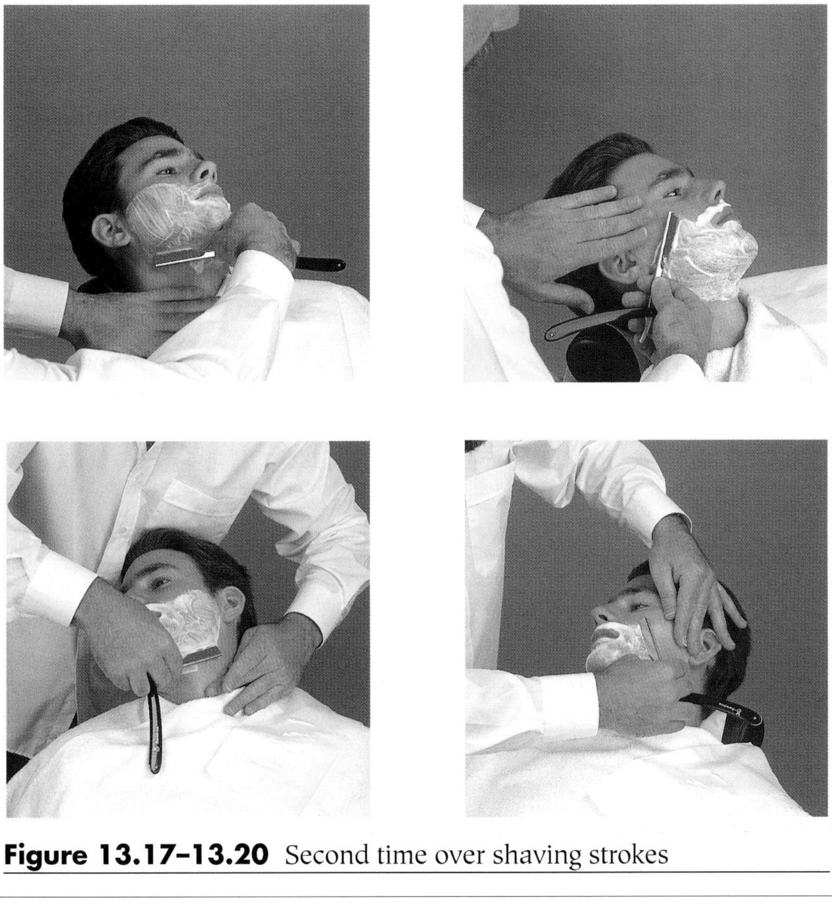

Figure 13.17–13.20 Second time over shaving strokes

work this onto both hands and then using brisk, gentle slapping strokes apply this to the beard area, taking care not to be over-generous or to apply to the areas around the eyes.

Fold a tissue onto your hand and use this to pat the surface of the skin dry before applying unperfumed talc, to soothe and remove shine from the skin. When applying talc to the face, place a small amount onto the hands and apply directly to the beard area or using a talc puffer. Shield your client's eyes and apply directly to the face.

> ***HEALTH AND SAFETY*** Never leave an open razor unclosed.

> ***HEALTH AND SAFETY*** The sharps box, when full, must be hygienically incinerated by a specialised company. Information about such companies may usually be obtained from an environmental health officer.

Remove the towel from your client and place it in the laundry basket, and slowly raise the back of the hydraulic chair. A sudden movement may disorientate your client. Remove the linen gown protecting your client and allow your client to check the surface of his skin using a hand-held mirror.

For safety, before allowing your client to step from the hydraulic chair , ensure that the chair has been lowered and is locked into position.

These shaving movements will provide you with a basic procedure to enable you to complete the shave. Provided that the shave can be completed safely and effectively, without causing your client discomfort, these shaving strokes may be modified and adapted to suit your favoured mode of work and any individual characteristics of the your client's beard area.

When shaving a very dark or heavy beard, an even closer shave may be achieved by sponge shaving. The technique is to shave against and across the direction of beard growth after the first two times over, drawing a warm moist sponge ahead of the razor. This action extends the hair out of the follicle momentarily, allowing the hair to be cut closer before it retracts. Care must be taken as skin irritation may result from shaving too close, particularly on a client unaccustomed to wet shaving.

> ***TIP*** In all forms of shaving, high levels of hygiene are required at all times. All equipment must be thoroughly sterilised both before and after use.

Clean-up

Immediately after the shave, all materials used must either be disposed of or washed and sterilised. Towels and gowns must be laundered, used tissue disposed of in a covered bin, the blade from the open razor must be removed, if you are uncertain of how to remove the blade ask for guidance from your stylist or trainer, the used blade must be placed in a 'sharps box'.

For reasons of hygiene, a razor blade should only be used on one client. The casing of the razor should be washed, dried and placed in a liquid sterilising agent. Lather brushes must be washed and the bristles also placed in liquid sterilising fluid. All bowls and other non-disposable items must be cleaned and sterilised ready for their next use. All work surfaces should be wiped down using a proprietary surface cleaner.

OUTLINE SHAVING

When shaving the outline of facial hair use inverted electrical clippers to define the outline of the beard, moustache or sideburns. Moisten those areas of the beard to be removed using lather, carefully applied so as not to affect the areas which are not to be shaved. Larger areas may have the lather applied using rotary movements with the lather brush, but smaller areas may require a stroking movement. The exact shaving strokes and their direction will be determined by the nature of the shape being outlined. Shaving strokes may have to be adapted to facilitate the clean and close removal of the unwanted beard.

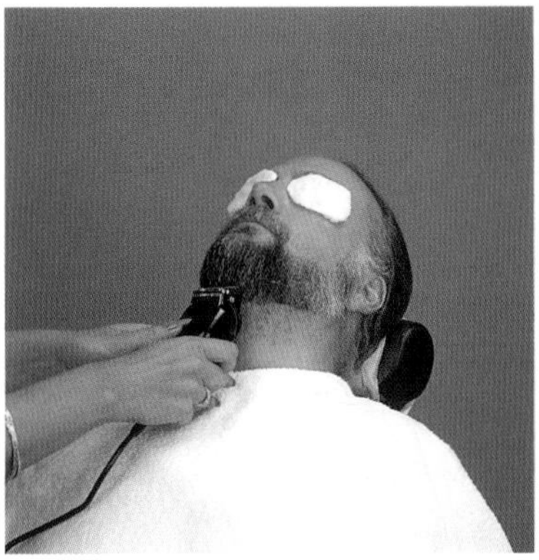

Figure 13.21 Inverted clipper to outline

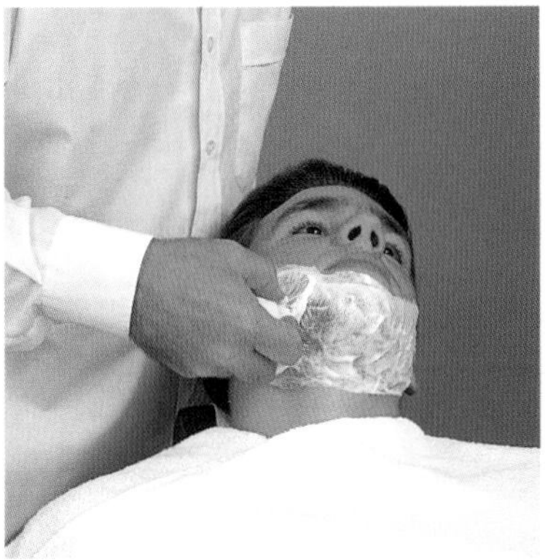

Figure 13.22 Lather beard area

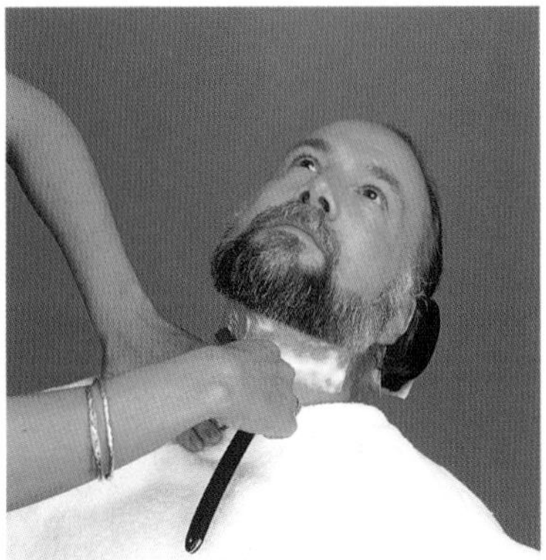

Figure 13.23 Shaving the outline

Shaved hairlines

Some nape hairlines may be shaved using an open razor. These may:

- be clearly defined areas outside of the desired hairline
- have excessively dark or vigorous hair growth
- have very low points of growth.

All of the usual hygiene precautions must be observed. The area to be shaved is normally moistened with water and then, holding the skin taught, the hair is removed by shaving in the direction of hair growth. The skin, once dry, should be soothed by the application of fine talc. Take care not to shave too close or cause soreness or bleeding. Skin unaccustomed to this treatment will be particularly susceptible to soreness and irritation.

In the case of closely graduated sides, very low hairlines around the ears may be shaved, using short shaving strokes, taking care not to cut into the curve where the ear joins the scalp.

In some Afro-Caribbean hair it is necessary to shave areas of the front hairline, when the hairline is particularly low or square. In very short Afro-Caribbean hair types it is necessary to

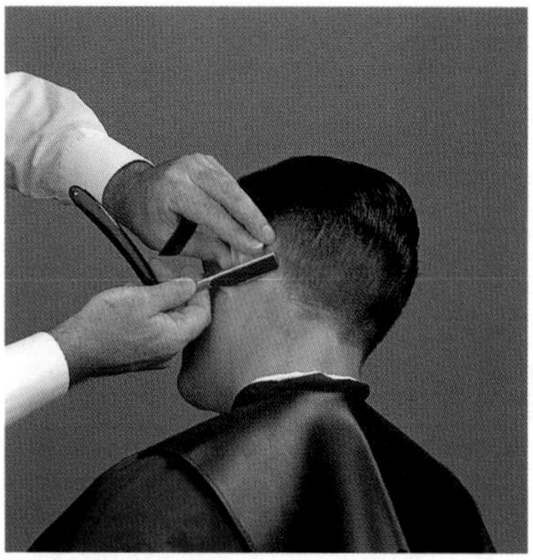

Figure 13.24 Shave side of nape hairline

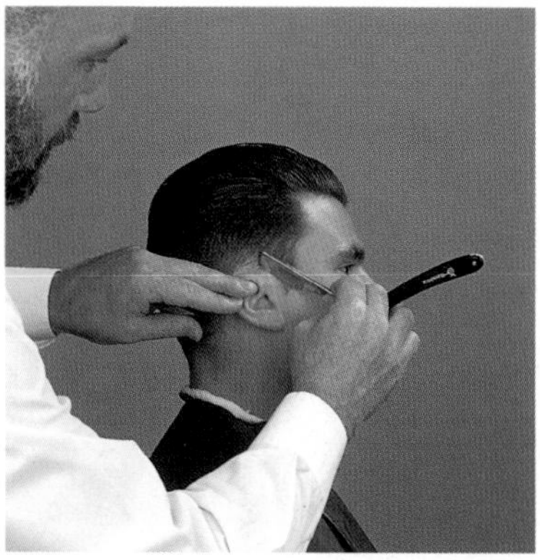

Figure 13.25 Shave above the ear

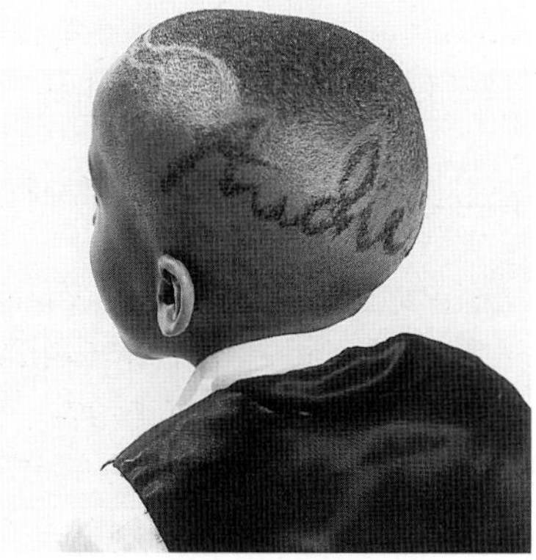

Figure 13.26 Decorative shaving in Afro-Caribbean hair

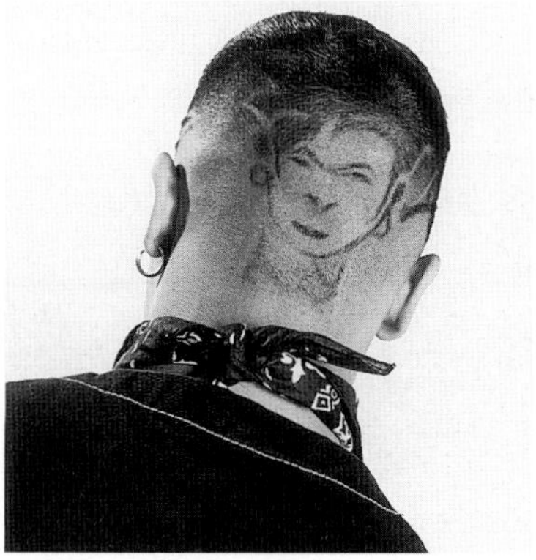

Figure 13.27 Decorative shaving in Afro-Caribbean hair

shave parting areas, to give clear definition. Shave a parting of approximately 3 mm width, having first used electric clippers to mark its position.

FACIAL MASSAGE

This may be used to improve muscle tone and relax your client. This service may be given to the client independently of any other service or following a wet shave.

Tools and materials required

You will require:

- a clean gown or cape
- clean towels
- suitable massage lotions for (a) dry skin – a moisturising cream; (b) greasy skin – a 'roll out' cream; (c) normal skin; a massage cream
- mild astringent lotion
- fine talc

- vibro massager with sponge applicator
- supply of steam towels
- supply of cold towels
- a clean spatula
- tissue.

Client preparation

Ensure that your hands are clean and that any cuts or open sores are covered with a waterproof dressing. When offering this service to your client for the first time, take time to explain the process, giving him an overview of the massage, and the benefits that he will obtain, the time it will take and if the client is unaware, the costs. Seat your client on the hydraulic chair and discuss his skin type with him. Check if his skin is dry, greasy, normal or combination. This will determine the type of massage lotion that you will use. Check for any skin condition which might prevent the massage and gown your client in the same manner as for a wet shave.

Procedure

1. Recline the chair and guide your client into position. Adjust the height of the chair to enable you to reach your client's face while standing behind the chair, and without your body resting on theirs.
2. Locate a clean tissue to cover the headrest of the chair, to prevent the spread of infection from one head to another.
3. Gown your client in the same manner as for a wet shave, if your client's hair falls forward onto the forehead, this should be held back and protected from the massage cream by using a head band or a clean towel wrapped around the head.
4. Apply a hot steam towel to your client's face. This will help to relax your client, open the pores and cleanse the skin. Remove this before it cools and apply massage cream to the face, spotting it over the areas to be massaged.

   The massage cream will lubricate the surface of the skin, allowing the hands and other massage tools to move smoothly, causing no discomfort to your client. These creams contain additives, which will be beneficial to the skin.

HEALTH AND SAFETY Remove massage cream from the tub using a clean spatula, placing the cream onto the back of your hand. This will help to prevent cross-infection caused by passing skin disorders from the client's skin into the product in the tub.

5. Use a clean spatula to remove the massage cream from its container, this will help to prevent cross infection, and place the cream on the back of your hand. Using the fingers from your other hand apply the cream. Gently smooth the cream over the area to be massaged and then apply a further steam towel. This will help in the penetration of the skin's surface by the massage cream as well as relaxing your client.
6. Remove the hot towel before it cools, taking care not to wipe the cream from the face.

TIP Your face will be in very close proximity to that of your client's; always ensure that in these situations, that if you have long hair you do not allow this to fall onto their face, and ensure that your breath is clear of unpleasant odours, including those from cigarettes and strong flavoured food.

If necessary apply additional massage cream to the face and then, standing behind your client, commence the facial massage.

The massage

There are three massage movements that are used during the process of facial massage. These are as follows.

Effleurage

A light continuous stroking movement applied with either the fingers or the palm of the hand in a slow rhythmic manner. No pressure is used. The palms work over large surfaces (see Figure 13.28), while the cushions of the fingertips work over small surfaces (e.g. around the eyes) (see Figure 13.29). This has a soothing, relaxing effect.

> ***TIP*** The process of facial massage should be one that relaxes your client, and all massage movements should follow a smooth, rhythmic uninterrupted pattern. A hand should remain in contact with your client's face at all times during the actual massage process.

Petrissage

A kneading movement. Take the skin and underlying flesh between your fingers and the palm of the hand. As you lift the tissues from their underlying structures, squeeze, roll or pinch with a light, firm pressure (see Figure 13.30). This movement invigorates the part being treated.

Tapotement

Consists of tapping, slapping and hacking movements (see Figure 13.31). This form of massage is most stimulating. It should be applied with care.

The frequency of facial massage depends upon the condition of the skin, the age of your client and the condition to be treated (if applicable). As a general rule, normal skin can be kept in excellent condition with a weekly massage, accompanied by proper home care.

The massage movements

Standing at the back of the hydraulic chair place the fingers of your hands at each of the client's temples. Movements should be rhythmic and soothing, not jerky and sharp.

> ***TIP*** Massage should never be given when there is evidence of muscular swelling, cuts, abrasions or contagious disorders present.

1. Massage across the forehead in small circular movements first with one hand from left to right and then with the other hand from right to left. The hands should always return to the resting point at the temples (see Figure 13.32.1).
2. Massage across the forehead using a zig-zag up and down movement, first from left to right and then from right to left (see Figure 13.32.2).
3. Place the first two fingers of your left hand over to the right-hand side of the tip of the nose and with the pads of the fingers, using only slight pressure, draw this upward to the forehead and across the bridge of the nose to the forehead. As one hand almost

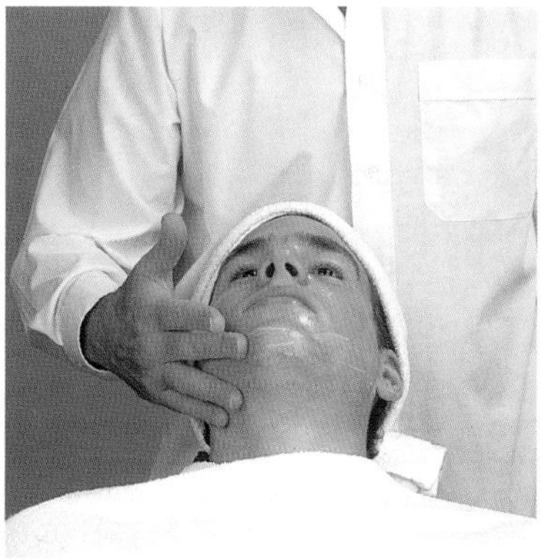

Figure 13.28 Effleurage massage, large areas

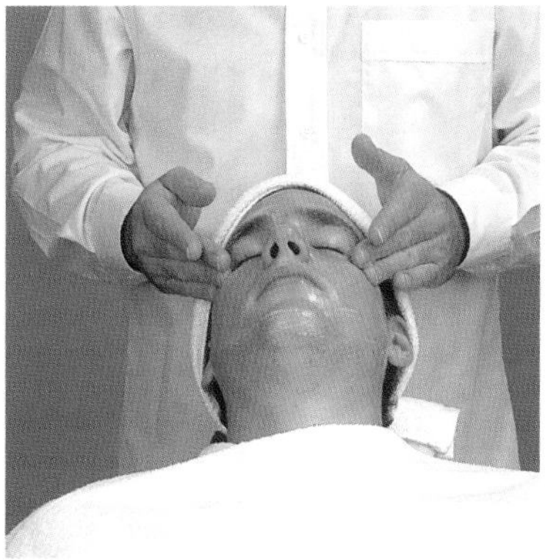

Figure 13.29 Effleurage massage, small areas

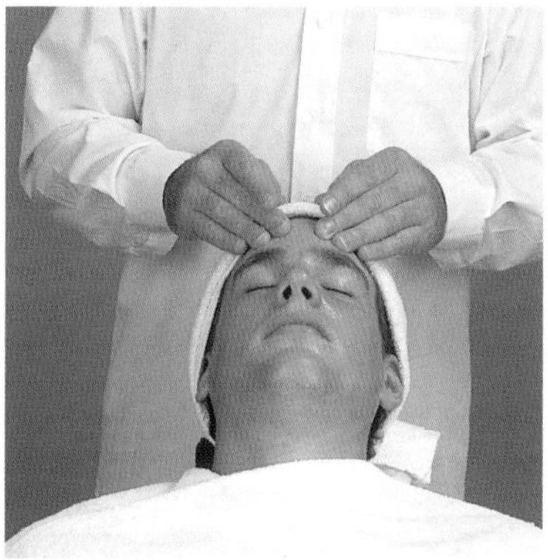

Figure 13.30 Petrissage massage

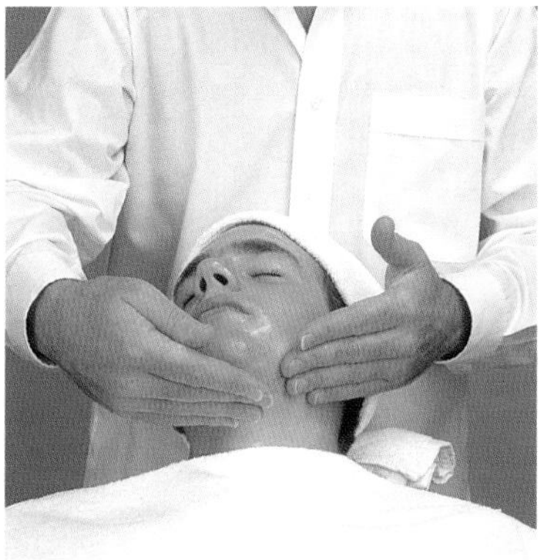

Figure 13.31 Tapotement massage

finishes the movement the other hand should start on the other side. Avoid too much pressure on the tip of the nose as the cartilage can easily be damaged (see Figure 13.32.3).

4. In a co-ordinated manner, simultaneously slide the first two fingers of each hand from the bridge of the nose down the sides of the nose, then in a circular action back up the same side, near the bridge and then around the eye (see Figure 13.32.4).
5. Return your hands to the temples, and simultaneously massage the temples at each side, in small circular movements (see Figure 13.24.8).

TIP Should your client experience discomfort during the massage, you should stop.

6. Simultaneously slide the fingers at both sides down to the corner of the jaw and then, using circular movements, rotate them back up to the temples (see Figure 13.24.6).
7. Slide the fingers to the centre of the chin, and simultaneously using circular movements massage above the jawbone back to the corner of the jaw (see Figure 13.24.7).
8. Cupping the hand either side at a time, draw the palm and fingers, from the corner of the mouth, across the chin to the corner of the jaw, the second finger running in line with the jaw bone and drawing up under the chin. Repeat this on either side (see Figure 13.24.8).

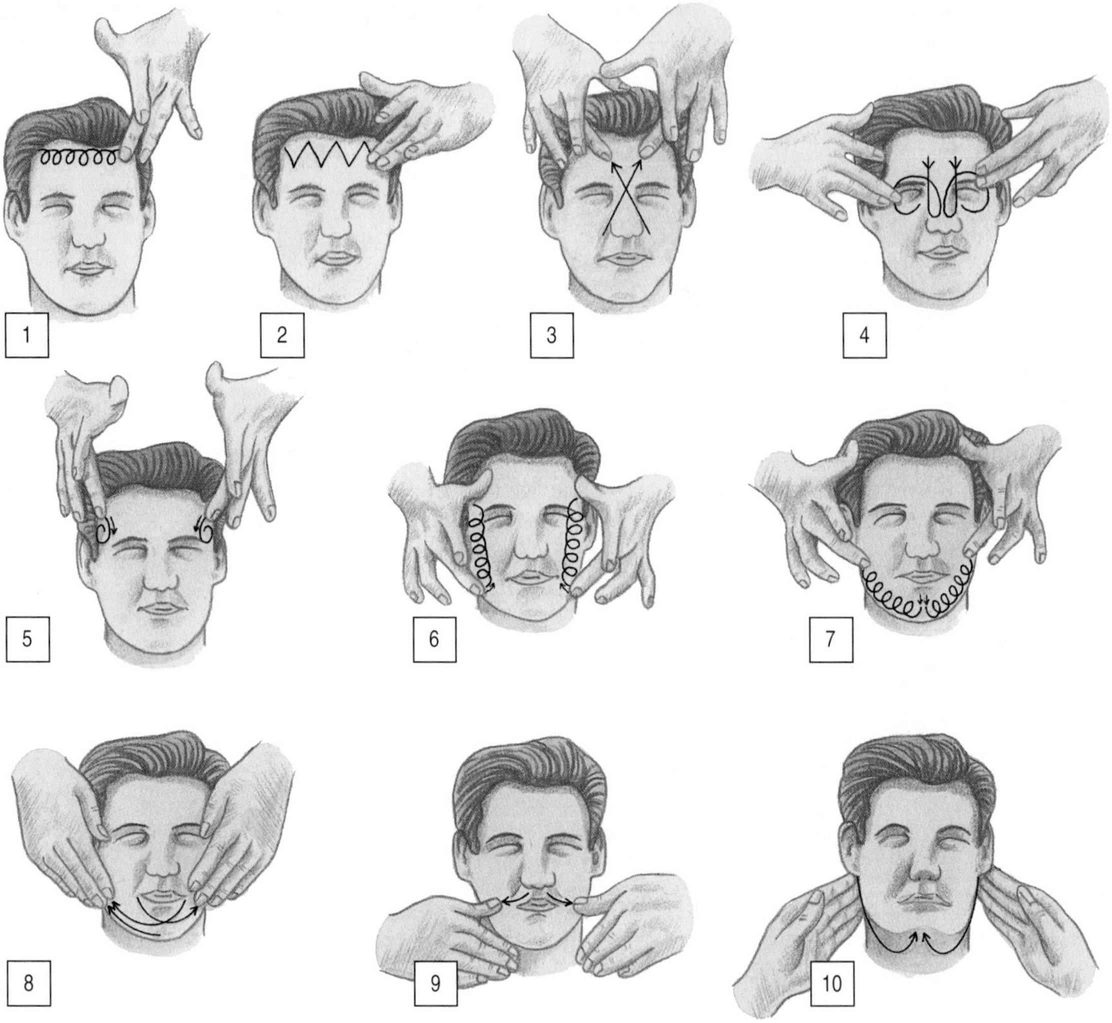

Figure 13.32 Face massage movements

9. Draw the thumbs across the area above the top lip, from the centre outwards to each side (see Figure 13.32.9).
10. Reaching across your client, cup the hand around the neck and draw your hand from just behind the ear, across the front and upwards across the underside of the centre chin (see Figure 13.32.10).

Carry out each movement approximately five times. Avoid too much pressure on the skin. Remember the purpose is to relax, so carry the massage out in a relaxing style.

Once the massage is completed, apply a hot steam towel to the face. This will help in the removal of any excess massage cream or oil. Before it is cool, remove the towel and, having folded it lengthways, use it to wipe the cream from the face. Ensure removal from the areas around the hairline, the nose and ears.

A cold towel may then be applied. This will help to close the pores of the skin, therefore leaving it less exposed to infection. The cold towels may be prepared in a similar method to the hot steam towel, by folding, moistening and rolling the towel, and then placing it in a cool cabinet. Following its removal the application of a mild astringent, for example rose water or witch hazel, may be applied using the palms of your hands. This will serve further to close the pores.

> ***TIP*** Remember, lower the hydraulic chair, to its lowest position, before allowing your client to step off.

Using clean tissue, blot the skin of the face dry and then apply a small quantity of fine talc to soothe and remove shine from the skin. Apply the talc from the palms of your hands or from a talc puffer while you protect the client's nose and eyes with your cupped hand.

Finally check that all excess product is removed from your client's skin. Remove the protective towels from your client and then raise the back of the chair, slowly. Remove the cape and give your client a tissue to wipe his face, should he wish. Give your client the opportunity to assess the effect of the treatment.

Clean up, placing waste in a covered bin and used linen in the laundry basket. Return containers to the storage area and clean all equipment.

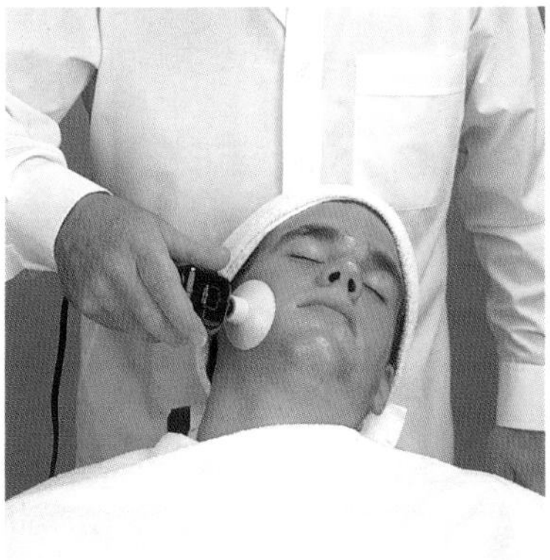

Figure 13.33 Vibro massager in use (1)

Using the vibro massager on the face

The vibro massager may be used, with care, to give facial massage. This should never be given if there are any problems that prevent it, such as muscular swelling, open cuts or sores or the presence of any contagious disorders.

The bell shaped vibro applicator is used for this process (see Figure 13.33.1).

> ***TIP*** Remember to always check the vibro massage and its flex for damage before use. Only use with dry hands.

Prepare the client and his face as for the facial massage already described. Firmly attach the bell-shaped applicator to the massager. Due to the delicate nature of the facial skin, the vibro-massager must be used gently on the skin. Avoid pressure on areas where the jaw bone etc. are prominent. When using the vibro massager on a client for the first time, first allow them to feel the vibratory action in the back of their hand.

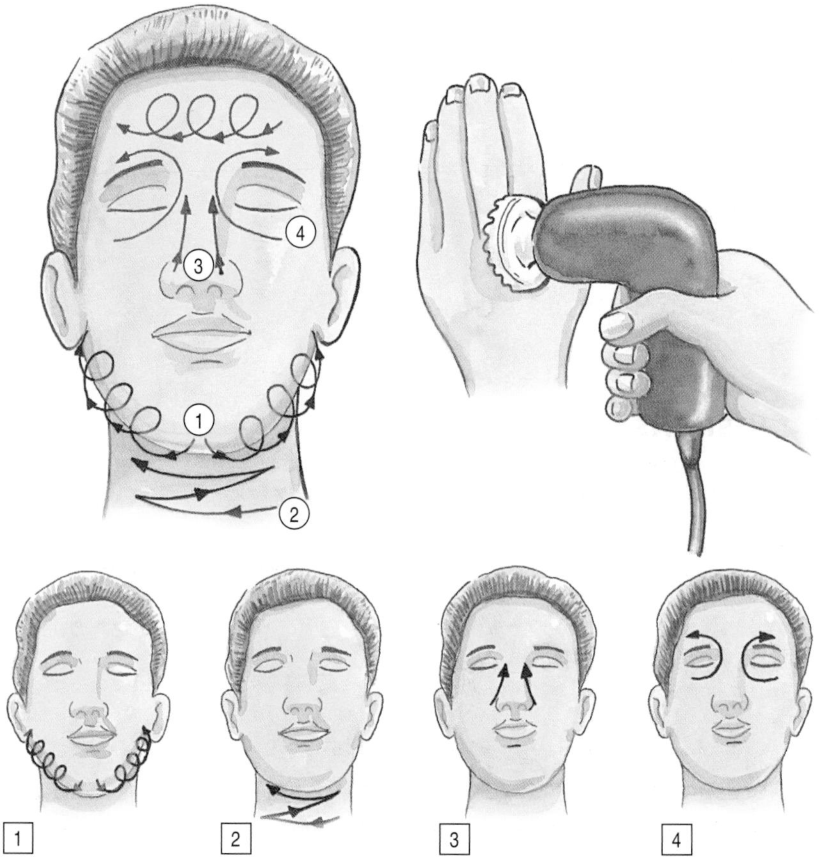

Figure 13.34 Vibro massager movements

1. Use circular movements across the upper jaw area (see Figure 13.34.1).
2. Draw the vibro across the neck in sweeping motions either side of the windpipe (see Figure 13.34.2).
3. Supporting the side of the nose with your free hand, gently draw the vibro along the side of the nose from the tip up towards the forehead. Take care that the applicator does not jar on any prominent bone or cartilage (see Figures 13.34.3 and 13.35).
4. Place the applicator on the back of your free hand and massage the muscle around the eyes using the fingers of this hand (see Figure 13.34.4).

Finish and tidy away material as described previously. Remember to wipe the casing of the vibro massager and to wash, dry and sterilise the applicator.

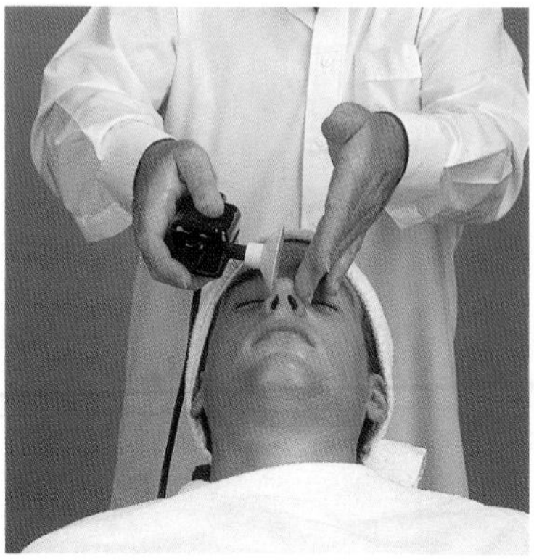

Figure 13.35 Vibro massager in use on side of nose

FURTHER STUDY

- To obtain best results from facial massage, you must have a thorough knowledge of all the structures involved: muscles, nerves and blood vessels. Find out more about them.
- Every muscle and nerve has a motor point. In order to obtain the maximum benefits from a facial massage you must consider the motor nerve points that affect the underlying muscles of the face and neck.
- Local bye-laws may regulate the offering of barbering skills. Find out from your local area what these bye-laws require.

See information about bye-laws in chapter 10 'Health, safety and security in the salon', page 208

REVIEW QUESTIONS

1. State two circumstances which may prevent you from carrying out a wet shave.
2. What steps should be taken should your client's skin be cut while shaving?
3. Suggest two reasons for stretching the skin while shaving.
4. When shaving, what benefit is gained by the use of steam towels?
5. What is the purpose of astringent lotions applied to the skin following a wet shave?
6. What directions should the first time over shaving strokes follow?
7. How should 'sharps' be disposed of?
8. What benefit is obtained by shaving the nape hairline?
9. What benefits, for your client, are achieved by facial massage?
10. What is the purpose of using cold towels following a facial massage?

CHAPTER 14

The hair and scalp

This section will give you the essential knowledge about the structure and properties of the hair, scalp and skin. This section will also help you to identify hair, scalp and skin disorders and to be aware of those that may preclude hairdressing processes and those that do not.

Level 1	
Unit 105	
Element 105.2	Support health and safety at work
Level 2	
Unit 201	
Element 201.1	Consult with and maintain effective working relationships with clients
Unit 202	
Element 202.3	Condition hair and scalp

Contents

INTRODUCTION

As a hair stylist, it is important to have a technical knowledge of the hair and scalp. This knowledge will be an asset to you as a professional hairdresser.

Hair, like people, comes in a variety of colours, shapes and sizes. To keep hair healthy and attractive, proper attention must be given to its care and treatment. Applying a harsh cosmetic, such as one that contains a lot of alcohol, or providing improper hairdressing services can cause the hair structure to become weakened or damaged. Knowledge and analysis of the client's hair, tactful suggestions for its improvement and a sincere interest in maintaining its health and beauty should be primary concerns of every hair stylist.

HAIR

The study of the hair, technically called trichology, is important because stylists deal with hair on a daily basis. The chief purposes of hair are adornment and protection of the head from heat, cold and injury.

Hair is an appendage of the skin, a slender, threadlike outgrowth of the skin and scalp (see Figure 14.1). There is no sense of feeling in hair, due to the absence of nerves.

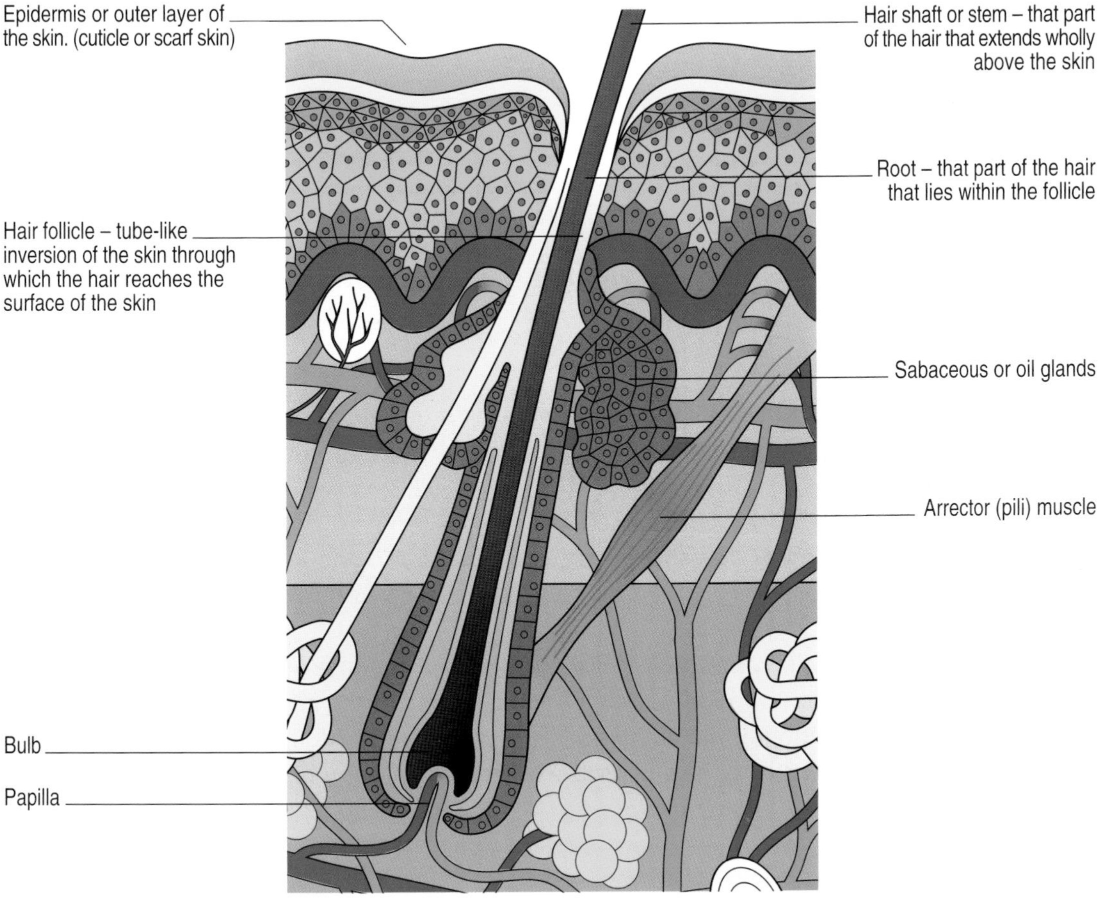

Figure 14.1 Cross-section of skin and hair

Composition of the hair

Hair is composed chiefly of the protein keratin, which is found in all horny growths including the nails and skin. The chemical composition of hair varies with its colour. Darker hair has more carbon and less oxygen; the reverse is true for lighter hair. Average hair is composed of 50.65% carbon, 6.36% hydrogen, 17.14% nitrogen, 5.0% sulphur and 20.85% oxygen.

Divisions of the hair

Full-grown human hair is divided into two principal parts: the root and the shaft.

- *The hair root* is that portion of the hair structure located beneath the skin's surface. This is the portion enclosed within the follicle.
- *The hair shaft* is that portion of the hair structure extending above the skin's surface.

Structures associated with the hair root

The three main structures associated with the hair root are the follicle, bulb and papilla. The follicle is a tube like depression or pocket in the skin or scalp that encases the hair root (see Figure 14.1). Each hair has its own follicle, which varies in depth depending on its thickness and the location of the skin. One or more oil glands (sebaceous glands) are attached to each hair follicle.

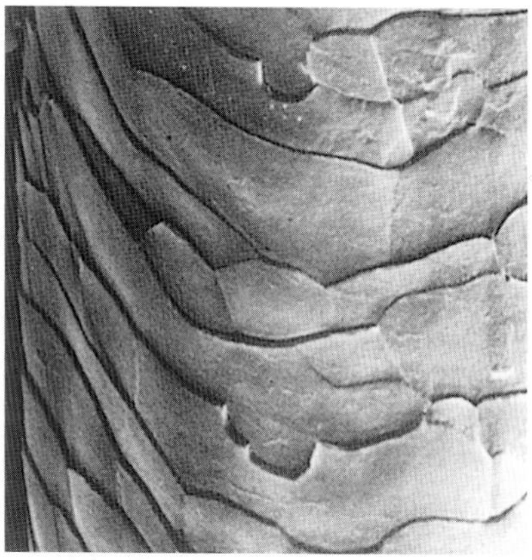

Figure 14.2 Magnified view of hair cuticle, which is composed of keratin

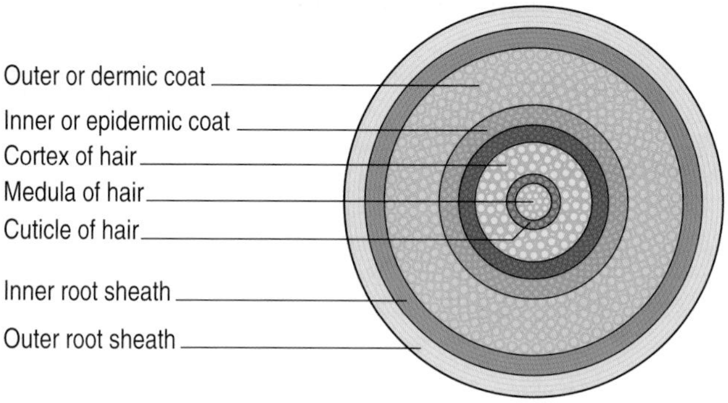

Figure 14.3 Cross-section of the hair and follicle

The follicle does not run straight down into the skin or scalp, but is set at an angle so that the hair above the surface flows naturally to one side. This natural flow is sometimes called the 'hair stream' or 'hair fall'.

The *bulb* is a thickened, club-shaped structure that forms the lower part of the hair root. The lower part of the hair bulb is hollowed out to fit over and cover the hair papilla.

The *papilla* is a small, cone-shaped elevation located at the bottom of the hair follicle. It fits into the hair bulb. There is a rich blood and nerve supply in the hair papilla that contributes to the growth and regeneration of the hair. It is through the papilla that nourishment reaches the hair bulb. As long as the papilla is healthy and well nourished, it produces hair cells that enable new hair to grow.

Structures associated with hair follicles

Arrector pili muscle

The *arrector pili* muscle is a small involuntary muscle attached to the underside of a hair follicle. Fear or cold causes it to contract and the hair stands up straight, giving the skin the appearance of 'gooseflesh'. Eyelash and eyebrow hair do not have arrector pili muscles.

Sebaceous (or oil) glands

These glands consist of little sac-like structures in the dermis. The ducts are connected to and open into the hair follicle. Sebaceous glands frequently become troublesome by over-producing oil and bringing on a common form of oily dandruff. Normal secretion from these glands of an oily substance called sebum gives lustre and pliability to the hair and keeps the skin surface soft and supple. The production of sebum is influenced by diet, blood circulation, emotional disturbances, stimulation of endocrine glands and drugs.

- *Diet* influences the general health of the hair. Eating too much sweet, starchy and fatty food can cause the sebaceous glands to become overactive and to secrete too much sebum.
- *Blood circulation.* The hair obtains its nourishment from the blood supply, which in turn depends on the foods we eat for certain elements. In the absence of necessary foods, the health of the hair can be affected.
- *Emotional disturbances* are linked with the health of the hair through the nervous system. Unhealthy hair can be an indication of an unhealthy emotional state.
- *Endocrine glands.* The secretions of the endocrine glands influence the health of the body. Any disturbance of these glands can affect the health of the body and, ultimately, the health of the hair.
- *Drugs,* such as hormones, can adversely affect the hair's ability to receive permanent waving and other chemical services.

Hair shapes

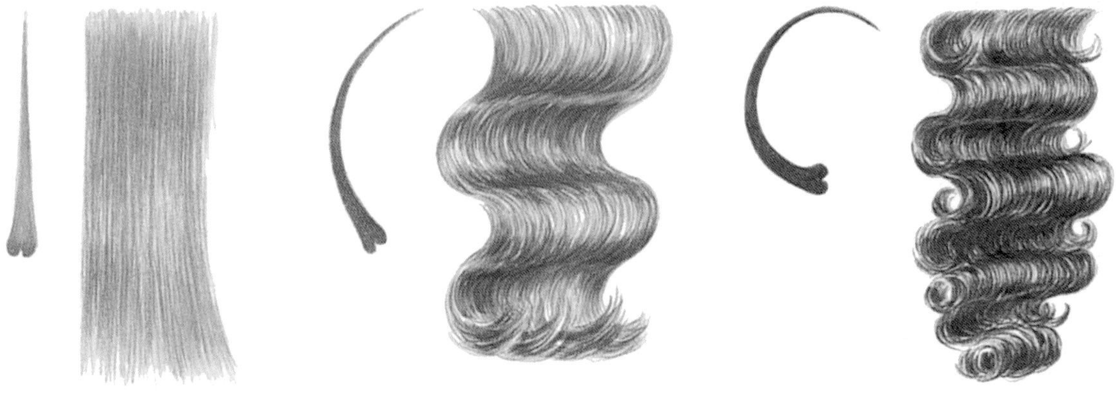

Figure 14.4 a Straight hair; b Wavy hair; c Curly hair

Hair usually has one of three general shapes (see Figure 14.4). As it is pushed out and hardens, hair assumes the shape, size and curve of the follicle. A cross-sectional view of the hair under the microscope reveals that:

- *Straight hair* is usually round in section
- *Wavy hair* is usually oval in section
- *Curly or kinky hair* is almost flat in section.

There is no strict rule regarding the cross-sectional shapes of hair. Oval, straight and curly hair have been found in all shapes.

Direction of hair growth

Hair flowing in the same direction is known as hair stream or hair fall. It is the result of the follicles sloping in the same direction. Two such streams, sloping in opposite directions, form a natural parting of the hair.

- *Crown.* Hair that forms a circular pattern, as at the top, is called a crown. Two whorls at either side of the crown is known as a *double crown* (see Figure 14.5). Whorls are often located at the nape, *nape whorls* requiring special consideration when styling (see Figure 14.6).
- *Cowlick.* A tuft of hair standing up is known as a cowlick. Cowlicks are more noticeable at the front hairline. However, they may be located on other areas of the scalp. When shaping or styling the hair, it is important to consider the direction and lift caused by the cowlick (see Figure 14.7).
- *Widows peek.* A strong pointed shape of the front hairline, forming a bold 'V' shape.

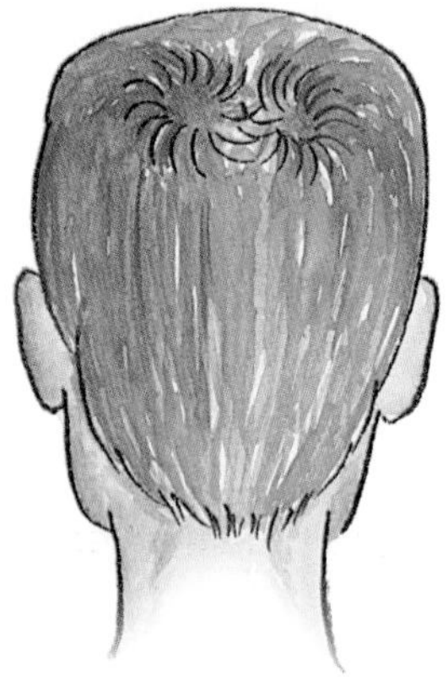

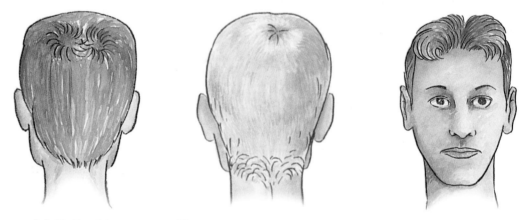

Figure 14.5 Double crown

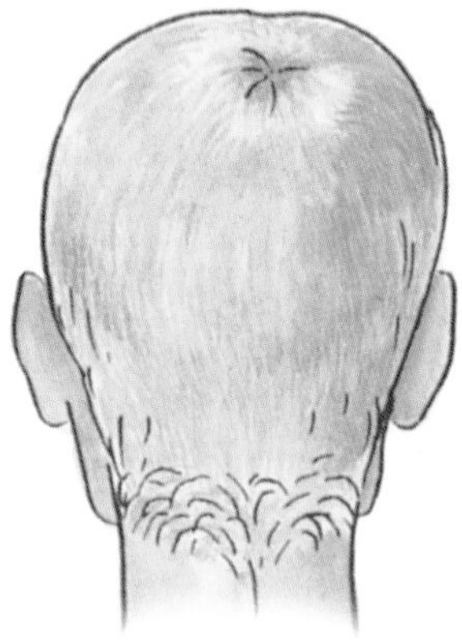

Figure 14.6 Nape whorls

Figure 14.7 Cowlick

Layers of the hair

The structure of the hair is composed of cells arranged in three layers (see Figure 14.3 on page 280):

- *Cuticle.* The outside horny layer is composed of transparent, overlapping, protective scale-like cells, pointing or overlapping away from the scalp towards the hair ends. Chemicals raise these scales so that solutions such as chemical relaxers, permanent hair colour or wave solutions can enter the cortex. The cuticle protects the inner structure of the hair (see Figure 14.2).
- *Cortex.* The middle or inner layer, which gives strength and elasticity to the hair, is made up of a fibrous substance formed by intertwined elongated cells. This layer contains the natural pigment that gives the hair its colour.
- *Medulla.* The innermost layer is referred to as the pith or marrow of the hair shaft and is composed of a honeycomb structure of moisture and air pockets. The medulla may be absent in fine and very fine hair and in other textures of hair may be variable in thickness.

Hair distribution

Hair is distributed all over the body, except on the palms of the hands, soles of the feet, lips, eyelids and the terminal joints of the fingers and toes. There are three types of hair on the body:

- *Terminal hair* protects the scalp against the sun's rays and injury, and adorns the head. This hair also grows in the armpits and pubic areas of both sexes and on the faces of men. Male hormones, however, make a man's facial hair coarser than a woman's.
- *Vellus hair* is fine, soft, downy hair on the cheeks, forehead and nearly all other areas of the body. It helps in the efficient evaporation of perspiration.
- *Lanugo hair* grows on the body of the human foetus, being shed at about one month before birth when vellus hair starts to grow.

Technical terms given to hair on the head and face

The different types of hair on the head and face are referred to by the following terms:

- *Barba* – the face
- *Capilli* – the head
- *Cilia* – the eyelashes
- *Supercilia* – the eyebrows (see Figure 14.8)

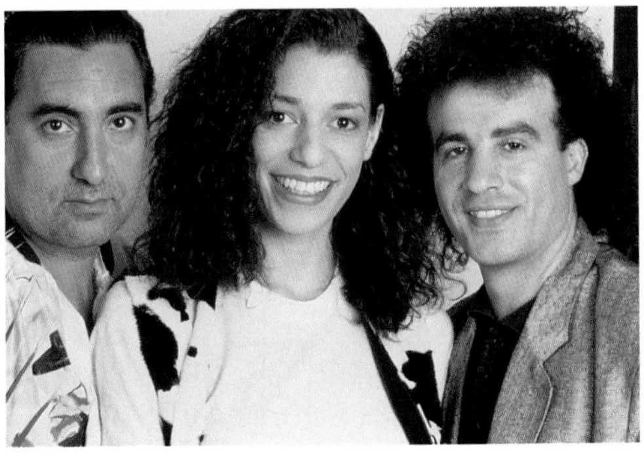

Figure 14.8 Hair on the head and face

Hair growth

If the hair is normal and healthy, each individual hair goes through a steady cycle of events: *growth, fall* and *replacement*. You will notice that the average growth of healthy hair on the scalp is about 1.25 cm per month. The rate of growth of human hair differs on specific parts of the body, between sexes, among ethnic groups and with age. Scalp hair also differs among individuals in strength, elasticity and degree of wave/curl.

The growth of scalp hair occurs rapidly between the ages of 15 and 30, but declines sharply between 50 and 60. Scalp hair grows faster on women than on men. Hair growth is also influenced by seasons of the year, nutrition, health and hormones.

Climatic conditions and seasonal changes affect hair in the following ways:

- Humidity and moisture encourages wavy hair to curl.
- Cold air causes hair to contract.
- Heat causes hair to swell or expand and absorb moisture.

Here are some myths about hair growth:

- Close clipping, shaving, trimming, cutting or singeing have an effect on the rate of hair growth. This is not true.
- The application of ointments and oils increases hair growth. This is not true. Ointments and oils lubricate the hair shaft, but they do not feed the hair.

- Hair grows after death. This is not true. The flesh and skin contract, and there is the *appearance* of hair growth.
- Singeing the hair seals in the natural oil. This is not true.

Normal hair loss

A certain amount of hair is shed daily. This is nature's method of making way for new hair. This average daily shedding is estimated at 50 to 100 hairs. Hair loss beyond this estimated average indicates some scalp or hair abnormality.

Life and density of the hair

The average life of hair ranges from 4 to 7 years, the *Anagen* period of hair growth. Factors such as sex, age, type of hair, heredity and health have a bearing on the duration of hair life.

The area of an average head is about 780 cm^2. There is an average of 1000 hairs to the square inch (645 mm^2). The average number of hairs on the head varies with the colour of the hair: blond, 140,000; brown, 110,000; black, 108,000; red, 90,000.

The growth cycle of hair

Hair depends on the papilla for its growth. As long as the papilla is not destroyed, the hair will grow. If the hair is pulled out from the roots, it will grow again. But should the papilla be destroyed, the hair will never grow again. In humans, new hair replaces old hair in the following manner:

- The bulb loosens and separates from the papilla, *Catagen* (see Figure 14.9).
- The bulb moves upward in the follicle, *Telogen*.
- The hair moves slowly to the surface where it is shed.
- The new hair is formed by cell division, which takes place at the root of the hair around the papilla, *Anagen*, the growth period of hair (see Figure 14.10).

Eyebrows and eyelashes are replaced every four to five months.

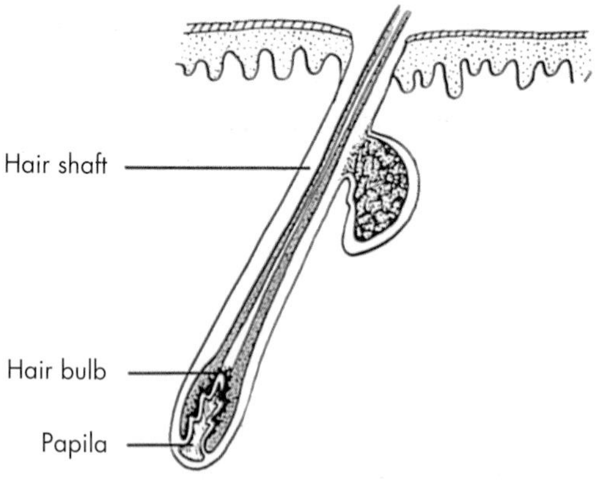

Figure 14.9 At an early stage of shedding, the hair shows its separation from the papilla

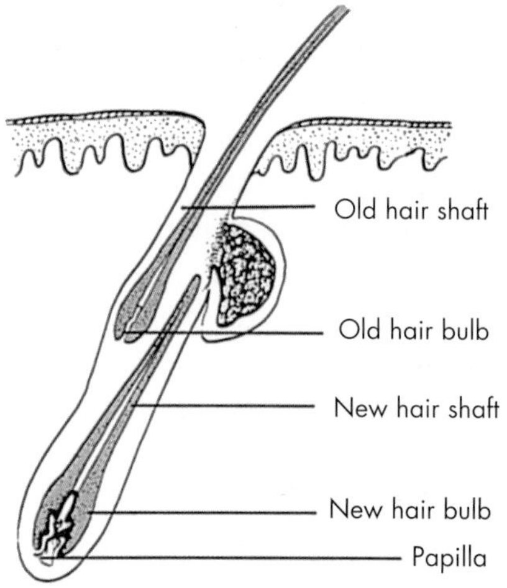

Figure 14.10 At a later stage of the hair shedding, you will note a new hair growing from the same papilla

Colour of hair

The natural colour of hair, its strength and its texture depend mainly on heredity. The cortex contains colouring matter, minute grains of melanin or pigment. Although there is no definite scientific proof, it appears that pigment is derived from the colour forming substances in the blood, as is all pigment of the human body. The colour of a person's hair, how light or dark it is, depends on the number of grains of pigment in each strand.

An albino is a person born with white hair, the result of an absence of colouring matter in the hair shaft, accompanied by no marked pigment colouring in the skin or irises of the eyes.

To give successful hair lightening and tinting services, you need to know about natural hair colour and distribution of hair pigment.

Greying of hair

Grey hair is caused by a mixture of hair without pigment in the cortex (white hair) and naturally coloured hair. The more grey the appearance the greater percentage of white hair in the mix.

In most cases, the greying of hair is a result of the natural ageing process in humans, although greying can also occur as a result of some serious illnesses or nervous shock. An early diminishing of pigment brought on by emotional tensions can also cause the hair to turn grey.

Premature greying of hair in a young person is usually the result of a defect in pigment formation occurring at birth. Often it will be found that several members of a family are affected with premature greyness.

Disorders of the hair

None of the following conditions are contagious.

Canities

Canities is the technical term for grey hair. Its immediate cause is the loss of natural pigment in the hair. There are two types:

- Congenital canities exists at or before birth. It occurs in albinos and occasionally in persons with normal hair. A patchy type of congenital canities may develop either slowly or rapidly depending upon the cause of the condition.
- Acquired canities may be due to old age, or onset may occur prematurely in early adult life. Causes of acquired Canites may be worry, anxiety, nervous strain, prolonged illness or heredity.

Ringed hair

Ringed hair has alternate bands of white and dark hair.

Hypertrichosis

Hypertrichosis or *hirsuties* means superfluous hair, an abnormal development of hair on areas of the body normally bearing only downy hair. Treatment: Tweeze or remove by depilatories, electrolysis, shaving or epilation.

Trichoptilosis

Trichoptilosis is the technical term for *split ends* (see Figure 14.11). Treatment: The hair should be well-oiled to soften and lubricate the dry ends. The splits must be removed by cutting. Split ends may be temporarily treated by proprietary brands of split-end treatments, but these are purely temporary.

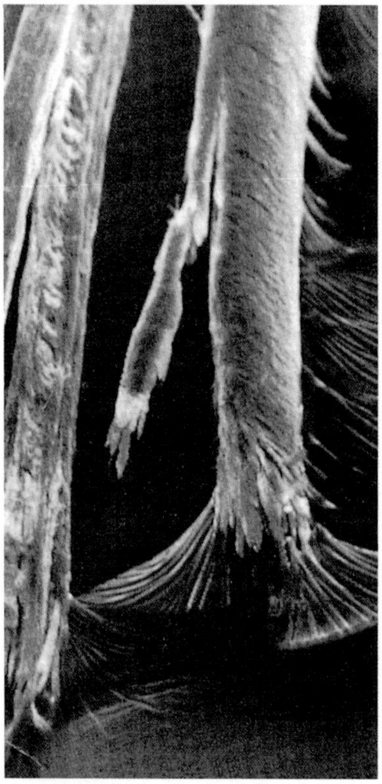

Figure 14.11 Split ends

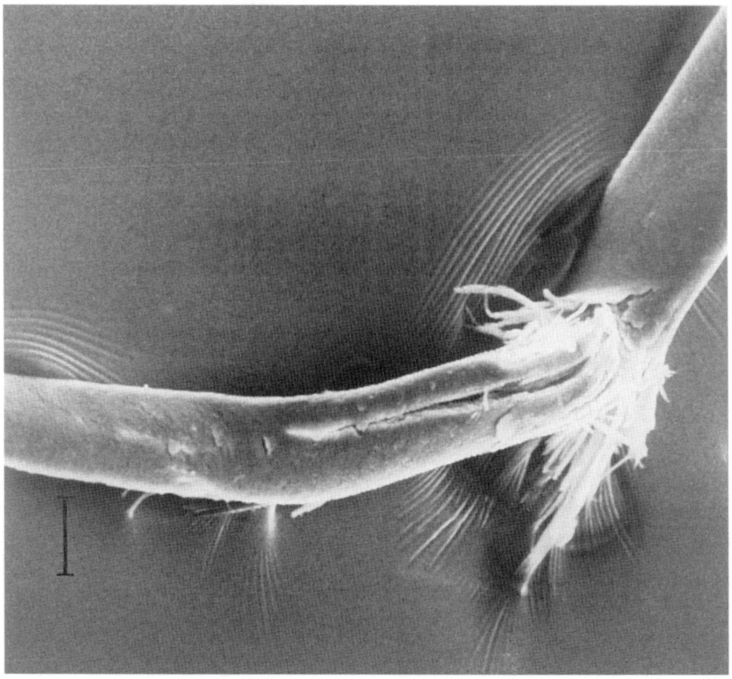

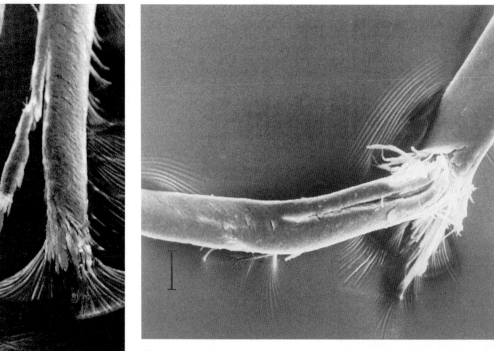

Figure 14.12 Knotted hair

Trichorrexis nodosa

Trichorrexis nodosa or *knotted hair*, is a dry, brittle condition including the formation of nodular swellings along the hair shaft (see Figure 14.12). The hair breaks easily and there is a brush-like spreading out of the fibres of the broken-off hair along the hair shaft. Softening the hair with conditioners may prove beneficial.

Monilethrix

Monilethrix is the technical term for *beaded hair* (see Figure 14.13). The hair breaks between the beads or nodes. Scalp and hair treatments may improve the hair condition.

Fragilitas crinium

Fragilitas crinium is the technical term for *brittle hair* or split ends. The hairs may split at any part of their length. Conditioning hair treatment may be recommended, most effective is to cut and remove the split.

Disorders of the scalp

Just as the skin is continually being shed and replaced, the uppermost layer of the scalp is also being cast off all the time. Ordinarily, these horny scales loosen and fall off freely. The natural shedding of these horny scales should not be mistaken for dandruff.

Dandruff

Dandruff consists of small, white scales that usually appear on the scalp and hair. The medical term for dandruff is *pityriasis*. Long neglected, excessive dandruff can lead to baldness. The nature of dandruff is not clearly defined by medical authorities although it is generally believed to be of infectious origin. Some authorities hold that it is due to a specific microbe.

A direct cause of dandruff is the excessive shedding of the epithelial, or surface cells. Instead of growing to the surface and falling off, these horny scales accumulate on the scalp.

Indirect or associated causes of dandruff are a sluggish condition of the scalp, possibly due to poor circulation, infection, injury, lack of nerve stimulation, improper diet and uncleaniness. Contributing causes are the use of strong shampoos and insufficient rinsing of the hair after shampooing. The two principal types of dandruff are:

- Pityriasis capitis simplex dry type (see Figure 14.14).
- Pityriasis steatoides – a greasy or waxy type (see Figure 15.15).

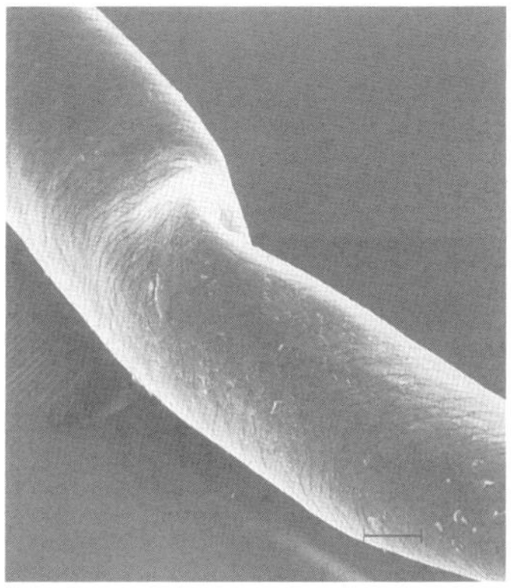

Figure 14.13 Beaded hair

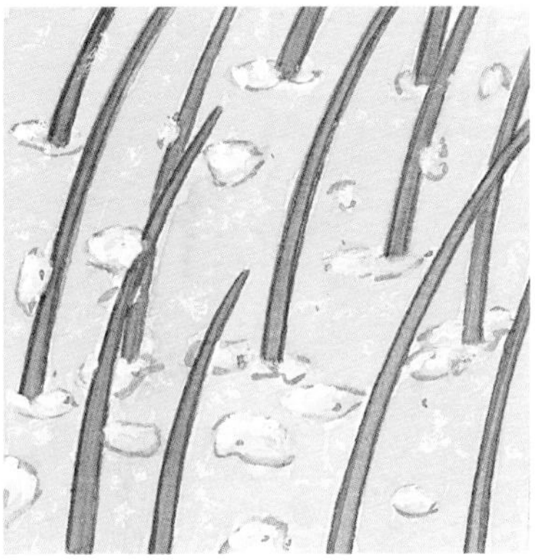

Figure 14.14 Pityriasis capitis simplex

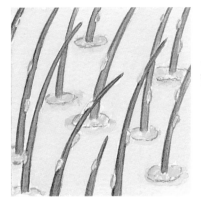

Figure 14.15 Pityriasis steatoides

Pityriasis capitis simplex (dandruff) is characterised by an itchy scalp and small white scales, which are usually attached to the scalp in masses, or scattered loosely in the hair. Occasionally, they are so profuse that they fall to the shoulders. Dry dandruff is often the result of a sluggish scalp caused by poor circulation, lack of nerve stimulation, improper diet, emotional and glandular disturbances, or uncleaniness. Treatment: Frequent scalp treatments, use of mild shampoos, regular scalp massage, daily use of antiseptic scalp lotions, and applications of scalp ointments.

Pityriasis steatoides (greasy or waxy type of dandruff) is a scaly condition of the epidermis (surface skin). The scales become mixed with sebum, causing them to stick to the scalp in patches. There may be itchiness, causing the person to scratch the scalp. If the greasy scales are torn off, bleeding or oozing of sebum may follow. Medical treatment is advisable. Both forms of dandruff are considered to be contagious and can be spread by the common use of brushes, combs and other articles. Therefore, the hairdresser must take the necessary precautions to sterilise everything that comes into contact with the client.

Alopecia

Alopecia is the technical term for any abnormal hair loss. The natural falling out of the hair should not be confused with alopecia. As we learned earlier, when hair has gone through its growing stage (Anagen), it falls out and is replaced by a new hair. The natural shedding of hair occurs most frequently in spring and autumn. Hair loss due to alopecia is not replaced unless special treatments are given to encourage hair growth. Hairstyles such as ponytails and tight braids cause tension on the hair and can contribute to constant hair loss or baldness.

Alopecia senilis is the form of baldness that occurs in old age. This loss of hair is permanent. It is not contagious.

Alopecia prematura is the form of baldness that begins any time before middle age with a slow, thinning process. This condition is caused when hairs fall out and are replaced by weaker ones. It is not contagious.

Alopecia areata is the sudden falling out of hair in round patches, or baldness in spots, sometimes caused by anaemia, scarlet fever, typhoid fever or syphilis. Patches are round or irregular in shape and can vary in size from 1.25 to 5 or 7.5 cm (½" to 2" or 3") in diameter. Affected areas are slightly depressed, smooth and very pale due to a decreased blood supply. In most conditions of alopecia areata, the nervous system has been subjected to some injury. Since the flow of blood is influenced by the nervous system, the affected area also is poorly nourished (see Figure 14.16).

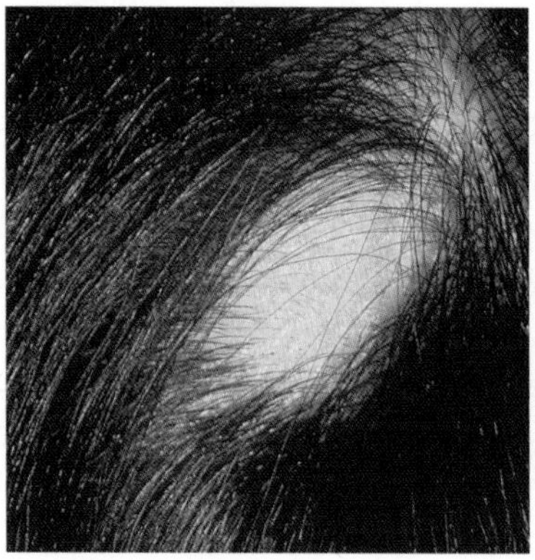

Figure 14.16 Alopecia areata

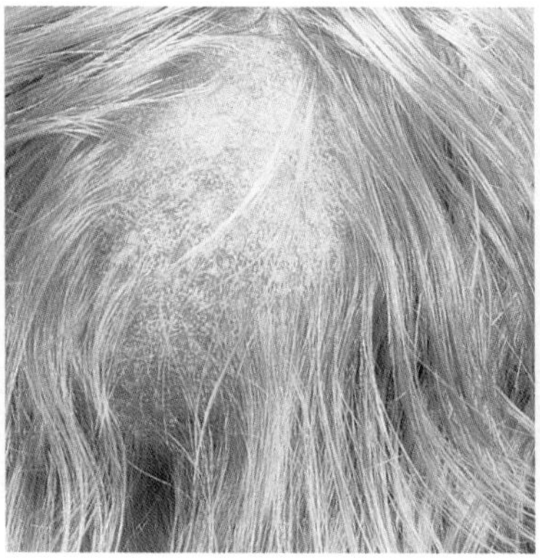

Figure 14.17 Tinea capitis

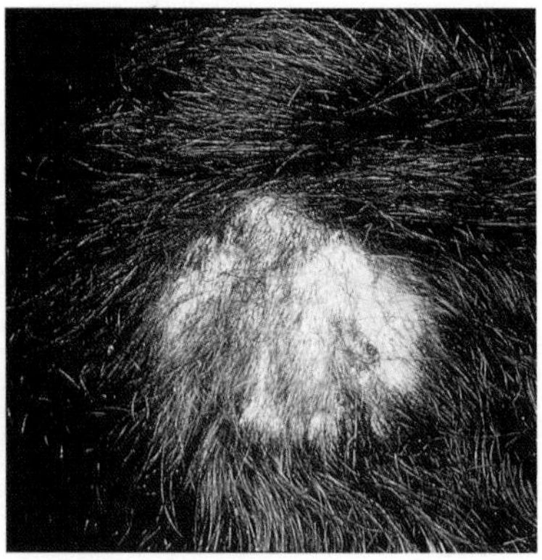

Figure 14.18 Tinea favosa (honeycomb ringworm)

Treatment for alopecia

Alopecia appears in a variety of different forms, caused by many abnormal conditions. Sometimes an alopecia condition can be improved by proper scalp treatments.

Infections

All the infections covered below are contagious.

Fungal infections

Tinea is the medical term for ringworm. Ringworm is caused by a fungus. All forms are contagious and can be transmitted from one person to another. The disease is commonly carried by scales or hairs containing fungi. Bathtubs, swimming pools and unsterilised articles are also sources of transmissions.

Ringworm starts with a small, reddened patch of little blisters. Several such patches may be present. Any ringworm condition should be referred to a medical practitioner.

Tinea capitis, ringworm of the scalp, is characterised by red papules, or spots, at the opening of the hair follicles (see Figure 14.17). The patches spread and the hair becomes brittle and lifeless. It breaks off, leaving a stump, or falls from the enlarged open follicles.

Tinea favosa, also *favus* or *honeycomb ringworm* is characterised by dry sulphur yellow cuplike crusts on the scalp, called **scutula**, which have a peculiar odour (see Figure 14.18). Scars from favus are bald patches that may be pink or white and shiny. It is very contagious and should be referred to a medical practitioner.

Animal parasitic infections

Scabies 'itch' is a highly contagious, animal parasitic skin disease, caused by the itch mite. Vesicles and pustules can form from the irritation of the parasites or from scratching the affected areas.

Pediculosis capitis is a contagious condition caused by the *head louse* (animal parasite) infesting the hair of the scalp (see Figure 14.19). The adult female is 3–4 mm long, the male slightly smaller. The female adult, during their life span of approximately one month, lays 7–10 eggs per day. The eggs hatch in about 8 days and the louse becomes sexually mature within a further 8 days.

As the parasites feed on blood at the scalp, itching occurs and the resultant scratching can cause infection. The head louse may be transmitted from one person to another by contact with infested hats, combs, brushes or other personal articles. To kill head lice advise the client to apply a proprietary brand of treatment, following the manufacturer's instructions. Proprietary brands of treatment shampoo may be used to remove the infestation. However, to prevent re-infestation usually the application of a treatment lotion is required. The duration of an infestation may be calculated by the position of the egg along the hair's length. The female adult lays its egg on the hair next to the scalp, therefore eggs located 1 cm from the scalp will have been produced one month previous. The unsightly husks of the 'nit' or egg may be removed using a fine toothed comb.

Staphylococci infections

A *furuncle* or boil is an acute staphylococci infection of a hair follicle that produces constant pain (see Figure 14.20). It is limited to a specific area and produces a pustule perforated by hair.

A *carbuncle* is the result of an acute staphylococci infection and is larger than a furuncle. Refer the client to a medical practitioner.

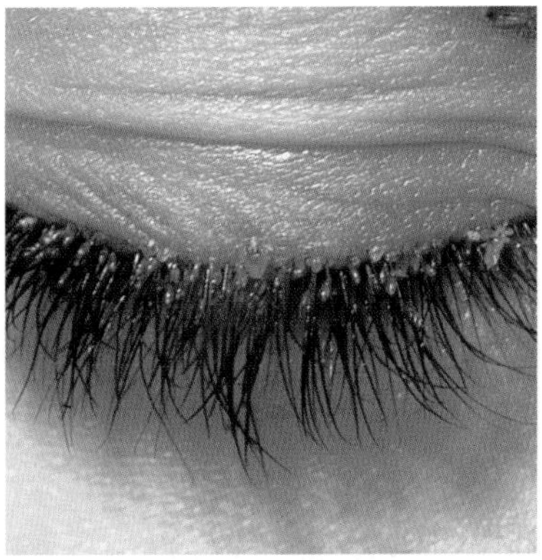

Figure 14.19 Pediculosis capitis

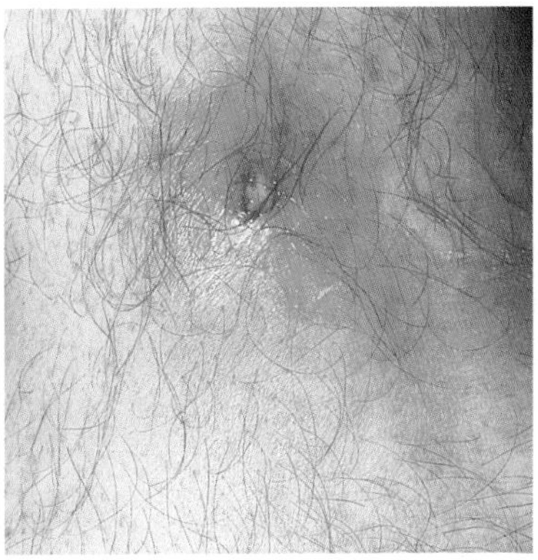

Figure 14.20 Furuncle, or boil

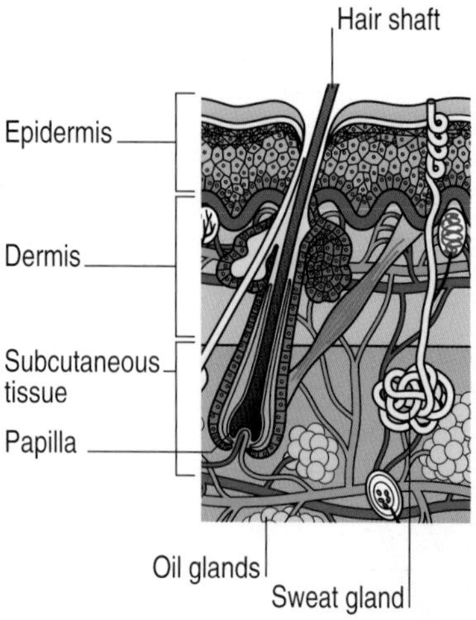

Figure 14.21 Microscopic section of skin

SKIN

The skin is the largest and one of the most important organs of the body. The scientific study of the skin and scalp is important to the hairdresser and beautician because it forms the basis for an effective programme of skin care, beauty services and scalp treatments. A hairdresser who has a thorough under-standing of skin, its structure and functions is in a better position to give clients professional advice on scalp, facial and hand care (see Figure 14.21).

A healthy skin is slightly moist, soft and flexible; posses a slightly acid reaction; and is free from any disease or disorder. The skin also has immunity responses to organisms that touch or try to enter it. Its texture (feel and appearance) ideally is smooth and fine grained. A person with a good complexion has fine skin texture and healthy skin colour. Appendages of the skin are hair, nails and sweat and oil glands.

Skin varies in thickness. It is thinnest on the eyelids and thickest on the palms and soles. Continued pressure on any part of the skin can cause it to thicken and develop a callus.

The skin of the scalp is constructed similarly to the skin elsewhere on the human body. However, the scalp has larger and deeper hair follicles to accommodate the longer hair of the head (see Figure 14.22).

Histology of the skin

The skin contains two main divisions: the epidermis and the dermis.

The *epidermis* is the outermost layer of the skin. It is the thinnest layer of skin and forms a protective covering for the body. It contains no blood vessels, but it has many small nerve endings. The epidermis is made up of the following layers:

- The *stratum corneum*, or horny layer, is the outer layer of the skin. Its scale-like cells are continually being shed and replaced by underneath cells coming to the surface. These cells contain the protein keratin, and combined with a thin covering layer of oil help make the stratum corneum almost waterproof.
- The *stratum lucidum*, or clear layer, consists of small, transparent cells through which light can pass.
- The *stratum granulosum*, or granular layer, consists of cells that look like distinct gran-

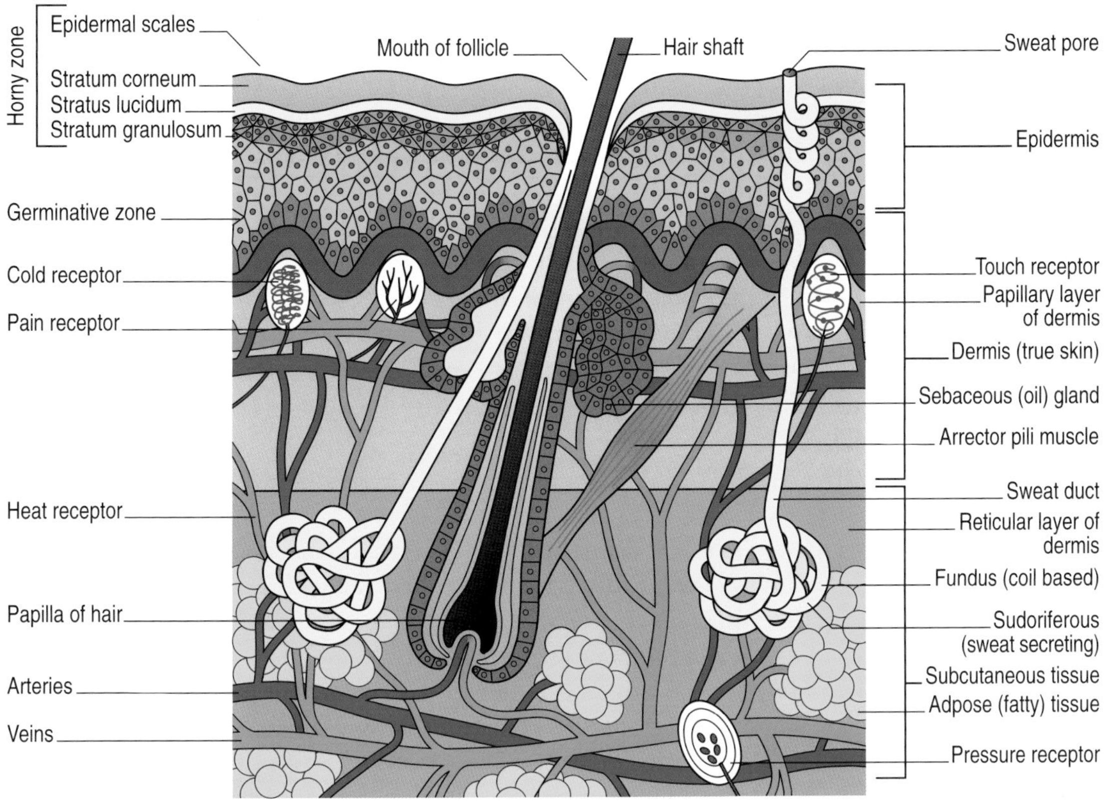

Figure 14.22 A cross section of the scalp

ules. These cells are almost dead and are pushed to the surface to replace cells that are shed from the stratum corneum.

- The *stratum germinativum*, formerly known as the *stratum mucosum* and also referred to as the basal or Malpighian layer, is composed of several layers of different-shaped cells. The deepest layer is responsible for the growth of the epidermis. It also contains a dark skin pigment, called melanin, which protects the sensitive cells below from the destructive effects of excessive ultraviolet rays of the sun or of an ultraviolet lamp. These special cells are called *melanocytes*. They produce melanin, which determines skin colour.

The *dermis* is the underlying, or inner, layer of the skin. It is also called the *derma, corium, cutis* or *true skin*. It is about 25 times thicker than the epidermis. It is a highly sensitive and vascular layer of connective tissue. Within its structure there are numerous blood vessels, lymph vessels, nerves, sweat glands, oil glands, hair follicles, arrector pili muscles and papillae. The dermis is made up of two layers: the papillary, or superficial layer and the reticular or deeper layer.

- The *papillary layer* lies directly beneath the epidermis. It contains small cone-shaped projections of elastic tissue that point upward into the epidermis. These projections are called *papillae*. Some of these papillae contain looped *capillaries*; others contain nerve fibre endings, called *tactile corpuscles*, which are nerve endings for the sense of touch. This layer also contains some of the melanin skin pigment.
- The *reticular layer* contains the following structures within its network: fat cells, blood vessels, lymph vessels, oils glands, sweat glands, hair follicles, arrector pili muscles. This layer also supplies the skin with oxygen and nutrients.

Subcutaneous tissue is a fatty layer found below the dermis. Some histologists consider this tissue as a continuation of the dermis. This tissue is also called *adipose*, or *subcutis* tissue and varies in thickness according to the age, sex and general health of the individual. It gives smoothness and contour to the body, contains fats for use as energy and also acts as a protective cushion for the outer skin. Circulation is maintained by a network of *arteries* and *lymphatics*.

How the skin is nourished

Blood and lymph supply nourishment to the skin. As they circulate through the skin, the blood and lymph contribute essential materials for growth, nourishment and repair of the skin, hair and nails (note hair and nails are not able to repair themselves as they are dead materials). In the subcutaneous tissue are found networks of arteries and lymphatics that send their smaller branches to hair papillae, hair follicles and skin glands.

Nerves of the skin

The skin contains the surface endings of many nerve fibres. They are:

- *Motor nerve fibres*, which are distributed to the arrector pili muscles attached to the hair follicles. This muscle can cause gooseflesh when you are frightened or cold.
- *Sensory nerve fibres*, which react to heat, cold, touch, pressure and pain. These sensory receptors send messages to the brain (see Figure 14.23).
- *Secretory nerve fibres*, which are distributed to the sweat and oil glands of the skin. These nerves regulate the excretion of perspiration from the sweat glands and control the flow of sebum to the surface of the skin.

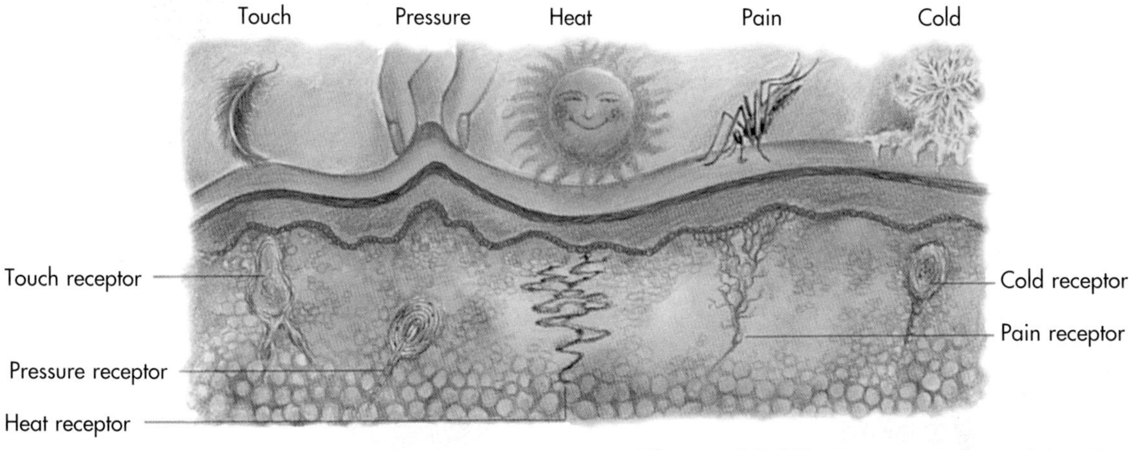

Figure 14.23 Sensory nerves of the skin

Sense of touch

The papillary layer of the dermis houses the nerve endings that provide the body with the sense of touch. These nerve endings register basic sensations; touch, pain, heat, cold, pressure or deep touch. Nerve endings are most abundant in the fingertips. Complex sensations, such as vibrations, seem to depend on the sensitivity of a combination of these nerve endings.

Skin elasticity

The pliability of the skin depends on the elasticity of the dermis. For example, healthy skin regains its former shape almost immediately after being expanded.

Ageing skin

The ageing process of the skin is a subject of vital importance to many people. Perhaps the most outstanding characteristic of the aged skin is its loss of elasticity. One factor that contributes to the loss of elasticity is that as we age subcutaneous tissue shrinks and is not as effective a support system in preventing the skin from wrinkling.

Skin colour

The colour of the skin, whether fair, medium or dark, depends, in part, on the blood supply to the skin and primarily on melanin, the colouring matter that is deposited in the stratum germinativum and the papillary layers of the dermis. The colour of pigment varies from person to person. The distinctive colour of the skin is a hereditary trait and varies among ethnic origins and races. Melanin protects sensitive cells from sunburn and tanning beds with ultra violet rays. A sun protection factor (SPF) should be used to help the melanin in the skin and protect it from burning.

Glands of the skin

The skin contains two types of duct glands that extract materials from the blood to form new substances: the *sudoriferous*, or *sweat glands* and the *sebaceous* or *oil glands*.

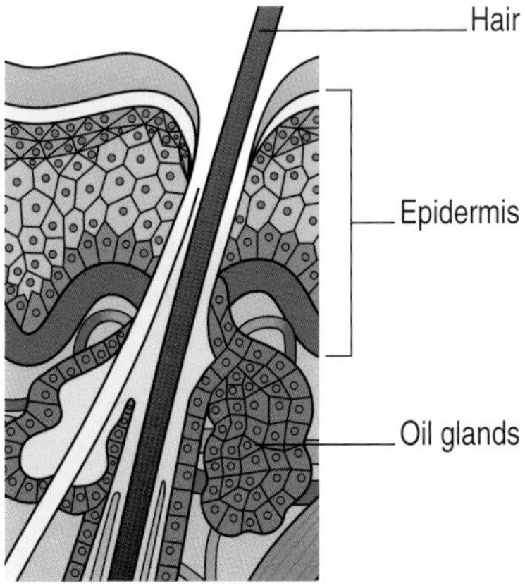

Figure 14.24 Body hair and follicle

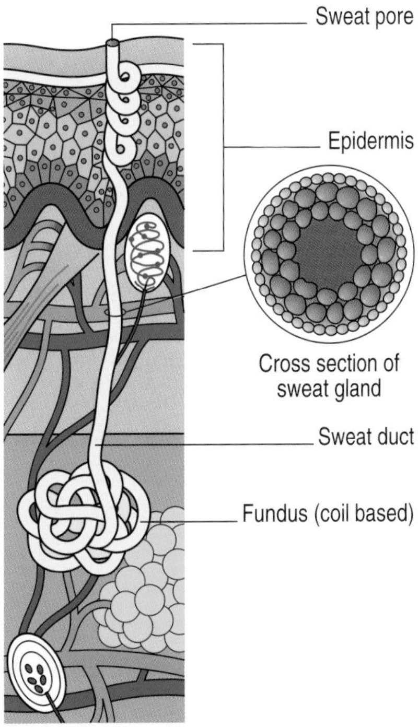

Figure 14.25 Sweat gland

Sweat glands

The sweat glands (tubular type), which excrete sweat, consist of a coiled base, or *fundus*, and a tube-like duct that terminates at the skin surface to form the sweat pore. Practically all parts of the body are supplied with sweat glands, which are more numerous on the palms, soles, forehead and in the armpits.

The sweat glands regulate body temperature and help to eliminate waste products from the body. Their activity is greatly increased by heat, exercise, emotions and certain drugs.

The excretion of sweat is controlled by the nervous system, Normally, 1 to 2 pints of liquids containing salts are eliminated daily through sweat pores in the skin.

Oil glands

The oil glands (saccular type) consist of little sacs whose ducts open into the hair follicles. They secrete sebum, which lubricates the skin and preserves the softness of the hair. With the exception of the palms and soles, these glands are found in all parts of the body, particularly in the face and scalp where they are larger

Sebum is an oily substance produced by the oil glands. Ordinarily, it flows through the oil ducts leading to the mouths of the hair follicles. However, when the sebum becomes hardened and the duct becomes clogged, a blackhead is formed.

Functions of the skin

The principal functions of the skin are protection, sensation, heat regulation, excretion, secretion and absorption.

- *Protection.* The skin protects the body from injury and bacterial invasion. The outermost layer of the epidermis is covered with a thin layer of sebum, thus rendering it waterproof. It is resistant to wide variations in temperature, minor injuries, chemically active substances and many forms of bacteria.
- *Sensation.* By stimulating sensory nerve endings, the skin responds to heat, cold, touch, pressure and pain. When the nerve endings are stimulated, a message is sent to the brain. You respond by saying 'ouch' if you feel pain, by scratching an itch, or pulling away when you touch something hot. Sensory nerve endings, responsive to touch and pressure, are located near hair follicles.
- *Heat regulation* means that the skin protects the body from the environment. A healthy body maintains a constant internal temperature of about 98.6 Fahrenheit (37 Celsius). As changes occur in the outside temperature, the blood and sweat glands of the skin make necessary adjustments and the body is cooled by the evaporation of sweat.
- *Excretion.* Perspiration from the sweat glands is excreted through the skin. Water lost through perspiration takes salt and other chemicals with it.
- *Secretion.* Sebum, or oil, is secreted by the sebaceous glands. This oil lubricates the skin, keeping it soft and pliable. Oil also keeps hair soft. Emotional stress can increase the flow of sebum.
- *Absorption* is limited, but it does occur. Female hormones, when an ingredient of a face cream, can enter the body through the skin and influence it to a minor degree. Fatty materials, such as lanolin creams, are absorbed largely through hair follicles and sebaceous gland openings.

Disorders of the skin

In your work as a hairdresser in a salon you will come in contact with skin and scalp disorders. You must be prepared to recognise certain common skin conditions and must know what you can and cannot do with them. If a client has a skin condition that the hairdresser/beautician does not recognise as a simple disorder, the person should be referred to a medical practitioner.

Most important is that a client who has an inflamed skin disorder, infectious or not, should not be treated in the salon. The hairdresser/ beautician should be able to recognise these conditions and suggest that appropriate measures be taken to prevent more serious consequences. Therefore the health of the hairdresser/beautician as well as the health of the public are safeguarded.

Definitions about skin disorders

Listed below are a number of important terms that should be familiar to the hairdresser for an understanding of the subject of skin, scalp and hair disorders.

- *Dermatology*. The study of the skin, its nature, structure, functions, diseases and treatment.
- *Dermatologist*. A medical skin specialist.
- *Pathology*. The study of disease.
- *Trichology*. The study of the hair and scalp and its disorders and diseases.
- *Etiology*. The study of the causes of disease.
- *Diagnosis*. The recognition of a disease by its symptoms.
- *Prognosis*. The foretelling of the probable course of a disease.

Lesions of the skin

A lesion is a structural change in the tissues caused by injury or disease. There are three types: primary, secondary and tertiary. The beautician is concerned with primary and secondary lesions only. If you are familiar with the principal skin lesions you will be able to distinguish between conditions that may or may not be treated in a salon (see Figure 14.26).

The symptoms or signs of diseases of the skin are divided into two groups:

- *Subjective symptoms* are those that can be felt, such as itching, burning or pain.
- *Objective symptoms* are those that are visible, such as pimples, pustules or inflammation.

Definitions about primary lesions

The following is a list of important terms and definitions that should be familiar to the beautician.

- *Macule*. A small, discoloured spot or patch on the surface of the skin, such as freckles. These are neither raised nor sunken.
- *Papule*. A small, elevated pimple on the skin, containing no fluid, but which might develop pus.
- *Wheal*. An itchy, swollen lesion that lasts only a few hours. Examples include hives, or the bite of an insect, such a mosquito.
- *Tubercle*. A solid lump larger than a papule. It projects above the surface or lies within or under the skin. It varies in size from a pea to a walnut.
- *Tumour*. An abnormal cell mass, varying in size, shape and colour. Nodules are also referred to as tumours, but they are smaller.

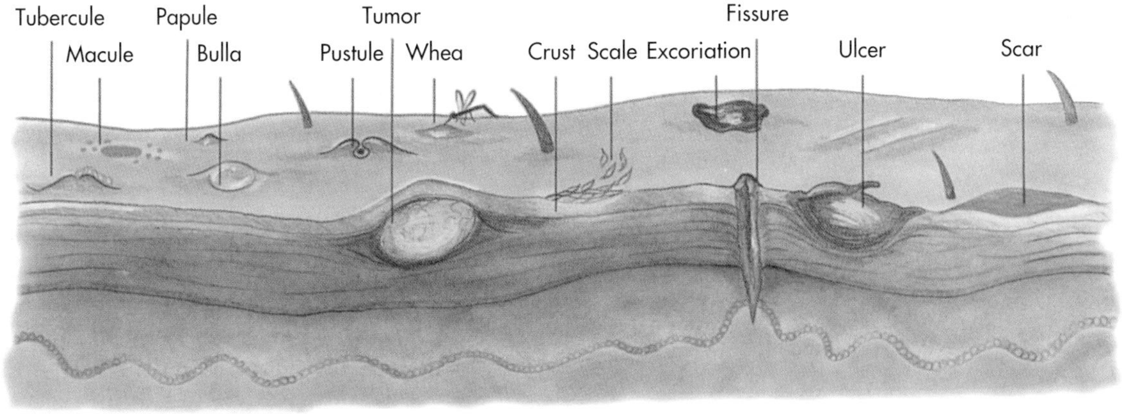

Figure 14.26 Lesions of the skin

- *Vesicle.* A blister with clear fluid in it. Vesicles lie within or just beneath the epidermis; for example, poison ivy produces small vesicles.
- *Bulla.* A blister containing a watery fluid, similar to a vesicle, but larger.
- *Pustule.* An elevation of the skin having an inflamed base, containing pus.
- *Cyst.* A semi-solid or fluid lump above and below the skin.

Definitions about secondary lesions

Secondary skin lesions are those that develop in the later stages of disease. These are:

- *Scale.* An accumulation of epidermal flakes, dry or greasy. Example: abnormal or excessive dandruff.
- *Crust.* An accumulation of sebum and pus, mixed perhaps with epidermal material. Example: the scab on a sore.
- *Excoriation.* A skin sore or abrasion produced by scratching or scraping. Example: a raw surface due to the loss of the superficial skin after injury.
- *Fissure.* A crack in the skin penetrating into the dermis, as in the case of chapped hands or lips.
- *Ulcer.* An open lesion on the skin or mucous membrane of the body, accompanied by pus and loss of skin depth.
- *Scar.* Likely to form after the healing of an injury or skin condition that has penetrated the dermal layer.
- *Stain.* An abnormal discoloration remaining after the disappearance of moles, freckles or liver spots, sometimes apparent after certain diseases.

NOTE The terms 'infectious disease', 'communicable disease' and 'contagious disease' are often used interchangeably.

Definitions about disease

Before describing the disease of the skin and scalp so that they will be recognisable to the hairdresser/beautician, it is necessary to understand what is meant by disease.

- *Contagious disease.* One that is communicable by contact.
- *Disease.* Any departure from a normal state of health.
- *Skin disease.* Any infection of the skin characterised by an objective lesion (one that can be seen), which may consist of scales, pimples or pustules.
- *Acute disease.* One with symptoms of a more or less violent character such as fever and usually of short duration.
- *Chronic disease.* One of long duration, usually mild but recurring.
- *Infectious disease.* One due to germs (bacterial or viral) taken into the body as a result of contact with a contaminated object or lesion.
- *Congenital disease.* One that is present in the infant at birth.
- *Seasonal disease.* One that is influenced by the weather, as prickly heat in the summer, and forms of eczema, which is more prevalent in cold weather.
- *Occupational disease* (such as dermatitis). One that is due to certain kinds of employment, such as coming in contact with cosmetics, chemicals or metals (nickel).
- *Parasitic disease.* One that is caused by vegetable or animal parasites, such as pediculosis and ringworm.
- *Pathogenic disease.* One produced by disease-causing bacteria, such as staphylococcus and streptococcus (pus-forming bacteria), or viruses.

- *Systemic disease.* Due to under- or over-functioning of internal glands. It can be caused by faulty diet.
- *Venereal disease.* A contagious disease commonly acquired by contact with an infected person during sexual intercourse.
- *Epidemic.* The appearance of a disease that simultaneously attacks a large number of persons living in a particular locality. Infantile paralysis, influenza or smallpox are examples of epidemic-causing diseases.
- *Allergy.* A sensitivity that some people develop to normally harmless substances. Skin allergies are quite common. Contact with certain types of cosmetics, medicines and tints or eating certain foods all can cause an itching eruption, accompanied by redness, swelling, blisters, oozing and scaling.
- *Inflammation.* A skin disorder characterised by redness, pain, swelling and heat.

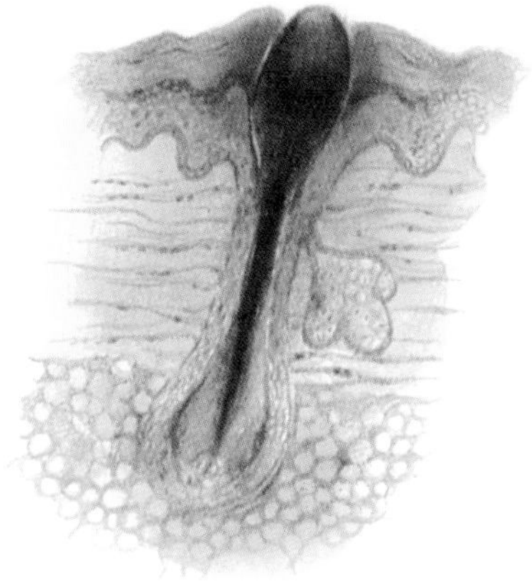

Figure 14.27 Blackheads

Disorders of the sebaceous (oil) glands

There are several common disorders of the sebaceous (oil) glands that the hairdresser/beautician should be able to identify and understand.

Comedones, or blackheads, are wormlike masses of hardened sebum, appearing most frequently on the face, especially the forehead and nose.

Blackheads accompanied by pimples often occur in youths between the ages of 13 and 20. During this adolescent period, the activity of the sebaceous glands is stimulated, thereby contributing to the formation of blackheads and pimples (see Figure 14.27).

When the hair follicle is filled with an excess of oil from the sebaceous gland, a blackhead forms and creates a blockage at the moth of the follicle. Should this condition become severe, medical attention is necessary.

To treat blackheads, the skin's oiliness must be reduced by local applications of cleansers and the blackheads removed under sterile conditions. Thorough skin cleansing each night is a very important factor. Cleansing creams and lotions often achieve better results than common soap and water.

Milia, or whiteheads, is a disorder of the sebaceous (oil) glands caused by the accumulation of sebaceous matter beneath the skin. This can occur on any part of the face, neck and, occasionally, on the chest and shoulders. Whiteheads are associated with fine-textured, dry types of skin.

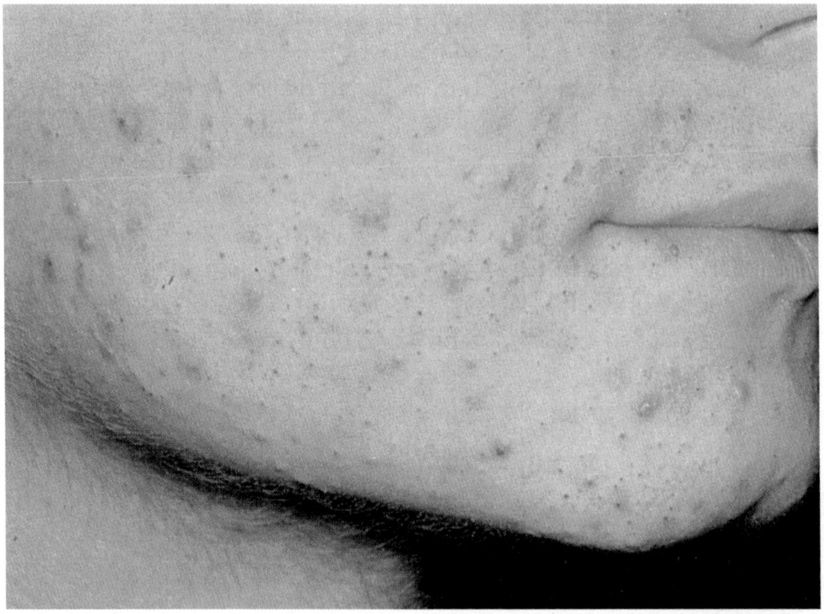

Figure 14.28 *Acne simplex*, or *acne vulgaris*

Acne is a chronic inflammatory disorder of the sebaceous glands, occurring most frequently on the face, back and chest. The cause of acne is generally believed to be microbic, but predisposing factors are adolescence and perhaps certain foods in the diet. Acne, or common pimples, is also known as *acne simplex* or *acne vulgaris* (see Figure 14.28).

Acne appears in a variety of different types, ranging from the simple (non contagious) pimple, to serious, deep-seated skin conditions. It is always advisable to have the condition examined and diagnosed by a medical practitioner before any service is given in a salon.

Seborrhea is a skin condition caused by an excessive secretion of the sebaceous glands. An oily or shiny condition of the nose, forehead or scalp indicates the presence of seborrhea. On the scalp, it is readily detected by an unusual amount of oil on the hair.

Asteatosis is a condition of dry, scaly skin, characterised by absolute or partial deficiency of sebum, due to senile changes (old age) or some bodily disorders. It can be caused by alkalis, such as those found in soaps and washing powders.

Rosacea, formerly called acne rosacea, is a chronic inflammatory congestion of the cheeks and nose. It is characterised by redness, dilation of the blood vessels and the formation of papules and pustules. The cause of rosacea is unknown. Certain things are known to aggravate rosacea in some individuals. These include consumption of hot liquids, spicy food or alcohol, being exposed to extremes of heat and cold, exposure to sunlight and stress.

Steatoma, or sebaceous cyst, is a subcutaneous tumour of the sebaceous gland. It is filled with sebum and ranges in size from a pea to an orange. It usually appears on the scalp, neck and back. A steatoma is sometimes called a wen.

Definitions about disorders of the sudoriferous (sweat) glands

Bromidrosis or *osmidrosis*. Foul-smelling perspiration, usually noticeable in the armpits or on the feet.

Anhidrosis, or lack of perspiration. Often a result of fever or certain skin diseases. It requires medical treatment.

Hyperhidrosis, or excessive perspiration. Caused by excessive heat or general body weakness. The most commonly affected parts are the armpits, joints and feet. Medical treatment is required.

Miliaria rubra, or *prickly heat*. An acute inflammatory disorder of the sweat glands, characterised by an eruption of small red vesicles and accompanied by burning and itching of the skin. It is caused by exposure to excessive heat.

Definitions about inflammations

Dermatitis. A term used to indicate an inflammatory condition of the skin. The lesions come in various forms, such as vesicles or papules.

Eczema. An inflammation of the skin, of acute or chronic nature, presenting many forms of dry or moist lesions. It is frequently accompanied by itching or a burning sensation. All cases of eczema should be referred to a medical practitioner for treatment. Its cause is unknown.

Psoriasis. A common, chronic, inflammatory skin disease whose cause is unknown. It is usually found on the scalp, elbows, knees, chest and lower back, rarely on the face. The lesions are round, dry patches covered with coarse, silvery scales. If irritated, bleeding points occur. It is not contagious.

Herpes simplex. A recurring virus infection, commonly called fever blisters. It is characterised by the eruption of a single vesicle or group of vesicles on a red swollen base. The blisters usually appear on the lips, nostrils or other parts of the face and rarely last more than a week. It is contagious (see Figure 14.29).

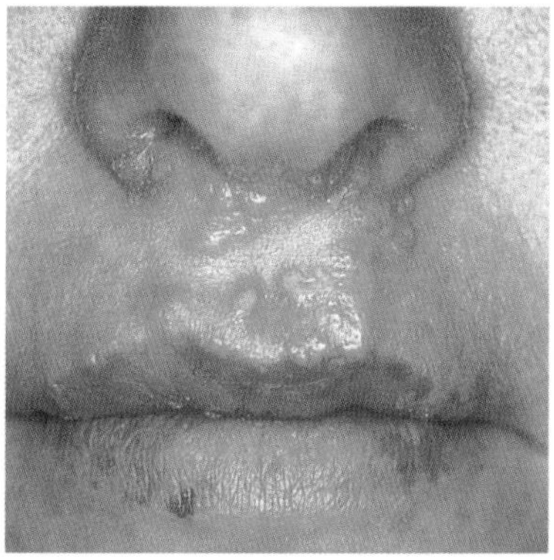

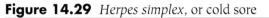

Figure 14.29 *Herpes simplex*, or cold sore

Occupational disorders in hairdressing

Abnormal conditions resulting from contact with chemicals or tints can occur in the course of performing services in the salon. Some individuals may develop allergies to ingredients in cosmetics, antiseptics, cold waving lotions and aniline derivative tints. These can cause eruptive skin infections known as *dermatitis venenata*. It is important that hairdressers employ protective measures, such as the use of rubber gloves or protective creams whenever possible.

> ***TIP*** Your employer may have set in place procedures to follow when using certain chemicals. These procedures should reduce risk to an acceptable level.

Research in many countries has shown that between 10 – 50% of hairdressers (male and female) suffer from eczema. Hairdressers' eczema is caused when the skin comes in contact with:

- water
- chemicals including shampoo, hair bleaches and liquids used with permanent colouring
- nickel (in scissors, combs, blow dryers and money)
- air flows (blow dryers and wind).

Respiratory disorders may be produced by the inhalation of products such as bleach powder, hair sprays and permanent waves.

FURTHER STUDY

1 - Find out your salon's procedures for advising clients who may have a contagious scalp disorder.
- Find out who you should inform, within your salon, when encountering a contagious scalp disorder.
- Investigate which shampoos and lotions are available, and their methods of use, to recommend to clients in the treatment of *Pediculosis capitis*.
- Find out if your salon has guidelines in the safe use of chemicals such as perm lotion, powder bleach.

REVIEW QUESTIONS

1 **1.** What are infectious conditions?
2. How should you protect yourself from the effects of chemicals when working on clients?
3. What term is used for abnormal hair loss?
4. For how long does the female head louse live?
5. What is the most effective treatment for split ends in hair?
6. What is the period of hair growth known as?
7. Name the three areas of the hair root.
8. Name the three layers found in hair.
9. Name a fungal parasitic scalp disorder?
10. Name the term given to excessive production of sebum.

CHAPTER 15

Model answers

CHAPTER 1

1. Client's name (including initial), client's address, client's telephone number, the name of any products used on the hair, the costs.
2. To the manager/manageress.
3. Confused look on their face, lack of response, fidgeting.
4. By their surname (if known), introduce self and ask them their name, or sir or madam.
5. Contagious conditions including Pediculosis capititis (head lice), Tinea capititis (ringworm of the scalp). Recommend that they consult a medical practitioner.
6. Texture.
7. Porosity.
8. When wet.
9. Cowlick – strong upward movement at front hairline.
   Nape whorls – strong circular growth patterns at the nape area.
   Double crown – two strong circular conflicting growth pattern at the crown.

CHAPTER 2

1. A range of commercial or proprietary brand names and their related hair/scalp types.
2. Lime scale can form, blocking the jets.
3. When the client's hair cannot be made wet or when drying would be difficult.
4. On the back of the hand.
5. Circular movements using the pads of the fingers.
6. Zinc Pyrethione and Selenium Sulphide.
7. 4.5 to 5.5.
8. Coats the cuticle of the hair, making it feel smoother and less likely to tangle.
9. To even out the hair's porosity before perming
   To protect hair from the effect of chemicals.
10. Increased blood flow.
    Stimulation of the sebaceous gland.
    Client relaxation.
11. Deep kneading and gripping movement using the pads of the fingers.
12. Open cuts or sores on the scalp.
    Muscular swelling.
    Client experiencing discomfort.
13. Moist heat swells the hair shaft allowing the conditioner to penetrate more effectively.
14. Distilled or de-ionised water.

CHAPTER 3

1. Hydrogen bonds.
2. Golf ball size.
3. From a distance of at least 30 cm, avoid wet patches or spraying onto the client's face or neck.
4. Speed up elastic recoil, the set/blow dry will drop.
5. The required style, the hair type and the client's preference.
6. By blow drying into the root area of upheld meshes of hair. By drying the root area against the direction of the style.
7. By directing the air flow in the direction of the style.
8. The diffuser.
9. Styling wax.
10. Heavy, greasy appearance.

CHAPTER 4

1. Hair type, direction of hair growth, the length of the hair, client's personal preference.
2. To protect the client and their clothing from hair clippings.
3. With the thumb and third finger.
4. Club cutting.
5. Taper cutting and thinning.
6. Graduation.
7. An area where additional bulk is created by the volume of hair.
8. Drawing the fingers through meshes of hair from either side of the head and comparing, using the dressing point mirror or by drawing strands of hair from even points on each side, whose hair ends should meet in the middle.
9. The hair may be cut closer to the head than can be done with the hair held in the fingers.
10. Wet hair.

CHAPTER 5A

1. It provides the client with hairstyle options which otherwise would not be available.
2. The ability of hair to absorb moisture.
3. How thick or thin an individual hair is.
4. The ability of hair to be stretched and then return to its original length.
5. The number of hairs, on the scalp, per square centimetre.
6. Winding the hair spirally along the rod, usually from root to point.
7. Winding the hair around itself on the rod, from point to root.
8. a) Introduces hydrogen to the hair, which breaks down the disulphide bonds in the hair.

   b) Introduces oxygen to the hair, which removes the hydrogen, allowing the sulphur bonds to reform into disulphide bonds.
9. The degree or strength of curl required.
10. A pre-processed curl used to determine correct lotion choice.
11. Strength of lotion used.

    Hair type.
12. Slow down the processing or extend the processing time.

13. Hair lacking in elasticity, hair breakage.
14. Rapid drop of curl, uneven curl.
15. To remove the perm lotion from the hair.
16. Hydrogen peroxide.

CHAPTER 5B

1. Two chemicals often used in chemical hair relaxing products are sodium hydroxide and ammonium thioglycolate.
2. The term 'base' means, in relation to hair relaxation processes, a petroleum cream designed to protect the scalp during the straightening process.
3. The client's hairline and face should be protected during relaxing chemical processes, by the application to the complete hairline of barrier cream and moist cotton wool.
4. The three main stages of the chemical hair relaxation process are processing, neutralising and conditioning.
5. The strand test is used to determine the hair's porosity and elasticity.
6. The hairdresser should wear protective gloves when working with relaxing/straightening substances.
7. Straightener products should be applied no closer than 5 cm from the scalp.
8. The main stages of a two-step perm are rearrange the curl (straighten the hair), wind and curl the hair, neutralise the hair, condition the hair.
9. 'Over-directing' when curler winding, means to comb the hair upwards and away from the direction of the wind.
10. Little or no tension should be used when winding the hair during a two-step perm.

CHAPTER 6

1. To cover grey hair, to boost their image, to correct unwanted colour, for fashion purposes.
2. Skin and eye colouring, their job, their personal preference, their natural hair colour.
3. A combination of spot lights (incandescent) and fluorescent.
4. Strand test.
5. Behind the client's ear or in the fold of their elbow.
6. Before every application.
7. Melanin.
8. Porosity.
9. Depth of colour, how light or dark. A level 7 is *medium blonde*.
10. Matt or drab.
11. Temporary, semi-permanent and permanent.
12. Mousse coats the cuticle.
13. The dye penetrates to the cortex layer where it combines with the oxygen, from the hydrogen peroxide to form a molecule too large to escape.
14. Scalp heat will speed up and increase the lightening effect of the product at the root area therefore the product should be applied to the middle lengths and ends of the hair first (to within 1.5 cm of the scalp), and then applied to the root area after lightening has begun.
15. By the use of moist tint.
16. Oxidation continuing after the product has been removed from the hair, the colour changes.

CHAPTER 7

1. No, not without permission of salon management.
2. With a smile, courteously and if possible by name.
3. To greet clients, phase appointments, receive client payments, undertake retail sales, answer the telephone.
4. The client's name, contact telephone number and the service required.
5. By repeating the details back to the client for confirmation.
6. A reminder to the client of the date and time of their next appointment and an advertisement for the salon.
7. Phasing appointments is to schedule appointments so that work is carried out in an efficient manner, particularly when more than one client may be treated at the same time.
8. Pass the message to that person as soon as it is practical to do so.
9. The client's signature matches that of the card, the start and expiry dates are valid and the amount does not exceed the guarantee limit.
10. To enable change to be given to clients with a minimum of delay.
11. The level above which authorisation must be obtained, from the card company, to guarantee payment.

CHAPTER 8

1. A Professional Development Plan is a personal plan for your career and how you will achieve it.
2. Exposed cuts must be covered with a waterproof dressing while working with clients.
3. The style of heels best suited to be worn by the hairdresser while at work are flat and broad.
4. To reduce fatigue, the hairdresser's spine should be straight while working on the client.
5. Phasing customer appointments enables the hairstylist to carry out work on more than one client at a time, therefore increasing personal efficiency.
6. Two topics of conversation that should be avoided with the client are politics and religion.
7. The hairdresser should be aware of the features, benefits and costs of products which are retailed to their clients.
8. Clients' concerns must be dealt with as soon as they become apparent.
9. The ideal occasion to raise issues that are relevant to a working team is within a team or staff meeting.
10. One focus that an appraisal interview may follow is: plan future work, review performance.

CHAPTER 9

1. Resource items that will require monitoring before each working day include: shampoo, conditioner, retail products, professional use products, towels and gowns, perm curlers.
2. Stock rotation is the principle of using the older stock before the new.
3. You should protect yourself when topping up potentially hazardous materials by seeking guidance if uncertain of correct use, and by wearing protective gloves and overalls.
4. Spillages of liquids should be mopped up as soon as possible.

5. Ideal storage conditions for stock are cool, dark, and dry.
6. Heavy products should be lifted by bending the knees and lifting with your back straight.

CHAPTER 10

1. The person responsible for undertaking COSHH risk assessment for a business is the employer.
2. The method of sterilising in the salon using moist heat at high pressure is the autoclave.
3. The hairdresser should cover any exposed cuts, when working on a client, using a waterproof dressing.
4. Floor surfaces should be swept at least once a day.
5. Tools are prepared by washing and drying before being placed in an ultra-violet sterilising cabinet.
6. Protective gloves should be used when handling perm lotion.
7. Employees must inform their employer of any loss or damage to personal protective equipment which has been supplied.
8. The possible consequences in not following accident, emergency and evacuation procedures, are injury to self or client and the possible neutralising of compensation rights.
9. Damaged equipment should be reported to the responsible person in the salon.
10. Failure to sweep up hair clippings from the floor may result in someone slipping and being injured.

CHAPTER 11

1. A set is retained in the hair until affected by moisture from the atmosphere or by shampooing.
2. The type of hair roller most likely to mark bleached or very porous hair is the spiked roller.
3. When roller setting, the curler diameter determines the strength of curl achieved.
4. The section taken should be the same as the size of roller to be used.
5. Hair in its unstretched state is known as alpha keratin.
6. The term 'over directing', when setting hair, means to direct the roots of the mesh of hair away from the direction of the set.
7. The hair should be brushed in the direction of the intended style prior to dressing.
8. Back combing should normally follow the direction of the hair style.
9. Always protect the client's face and neck when applying hair fixing spray.
10. Fine pins should be positioned in a downwards direction so that they do not fall out of the dressing.

CHAPTER 12

1. The electric clipper should be inverted to outline a beard.
2. The hydraulic chair should be locked in its lowest position when the client is invited to sit.
3. Light coloured towels are used when beard trimming to reflect light under the beard area and to give a contrast with the beard.

4. The largest size clipper grader available is 'number 8'.
5. A clean tissue placed on the chair's head rest while trimming the beard to reduce the risk of the spread of infection from one client to the next.
6. When beard trimming, the area beneath the chin will appear longer when the head is upright.
7. Scissor-over-comb techniques are used when a very short haired result is required.
8. Hair should be dry when using electric hair clippers.
9. The essential feature of a graduated neckline is that there is no clear definition where the hairline ends and the neck begins.
10. The razor used on wet hair.

CHAPTER 13

1. Contraindications to the provision of a wet shave are: open cuts or sores on the face, muscular swellings, contagious skin conditions.
2. Should the client's skin be cut while shaving, powdered alum of ferric chloride should be applied to a clean sterile dressing and then held against the cut.
3. Two reasons for tensioning the skin while shaving are to provide a closer shave and to prevent cutting the client.
4. Steam towels provide moist heat that relaxes the client, improves the softening action of the lather, cleanses the skin's surface.
5. Astringent lotions are applied to the skin following a wet shave to close the skin's pores and help prevent infection.
6. First time over shaving strokes usually go with the direction of beard growth.
7. Sharps should be placed in an appropriate container which is then incinerated by a specialist company.
8. The benefit obtained by shaving the nape hairline is a cleaner defined outline, which will last longer.
9. The benefits from facial massage are improved muscle tone and relaxation.
10. Use of cold towels following a facial massage will close the pores, preventing the spread of infection and reducing any discomfort that may be experience if an astringent lotion is applied.

CHAPTER 14

1. Infectious conditions are those diseases passed on by contact with a contaminated object.
2. You should protect yourself from the effects of chemicals when working on clients by wearing protective gloves and overalls.
3. The term used for abnormal hair loss is Alopecia.
4. The female head louse lives for approximately one month.
5. The most effective treatment for split ends in hair is to cut them off.
6. The period of hair growth is known as Anagen.
7. The three areas of the hair root are the follicle, the bulb and the papilla.
8. The three layers found in hair are the cuticle, the cortex and the medulla.
9. A fungal parasitic scalp disorder is Tinea Capitis (ringworm).
10. The term given to excessive production of sebum is Seborrhea.

CHAPTER 16

Your personal skill check

The section may be photocopied for your own personal ongoing use, to enable you to evaluate your own development towards competence and to help you identify existing competence.

HOW TO USE

Within the table you will find questions about your job or hairdressing experience, in the adjacent columns you will tick as appropriate. If you never carry out a particular task tick the first column, if you carry the task out but need considerable guidance from your trainer in doing this tick the second column, if you can carry out the task without guidance from others then tick the third column and if the task forms your normal job role that you carry out on a regular basis you should tick the fourth column. If you intend to claim existing competence or wish to plan how your competence will be assessed, use the evidence identification section to help identify where and how you will collect this. This table may help you identify which award is most appropriate to your competence/needs and expectations.

LEVEL 1 AND 2 HAIRDRESSING

Task	Never done	With assistance	Little assistance	Regularly done	What evidence to support range
Consult with clients on technical services and products Level 2					
Advise clients on after care procedures and future salon services Level 2					
Maintain effective working relationships with clients Levels 1 & 2					
Shampoo and surface condition hair Level 1					
Shampoo and condition hair and scalp Levels 1 & 2					
Dry below shoulder length hair Level 1					
Dry hair into shape: include detail of the range of hair and drying techniques Level 2					

Task	Never done	With assistance	Little assistance	Regularly done	What evidence to support range
Create a finished look on dry hair Level 2					
Cut hair to produce a variety of one length looks Level 2					
Cut hair to achieve a variety of layered looks Level 2					
Cut hair to achieve a variety of fashion looks Level 2					
Carry out basic perms on virgin hair and chemically treated hair Level 2					
Neutralise perms and relaxers Levels 1 & 2					
Relax hair using a range or straighteners Level 2					
Add temporary colour to hair Level 1 & 2					

Task	Never done	With assistance	Little assistance	Regularly done	What evidence to support range
Add semi-permanent colour to hair Level 2					
Permanently change hair colour Level 2					
Create highlight and lowlight effects in hair Level 2					
Remove colouring and lightening products from hair Levels 1 & 2					
Attend to visitors and enquiries Levels 1 & 2					
Schedule appointments for salon services Levels 1 & 2					
Handle payments from clients for the purchase of services and retail products Level 2					
Organise your own work role Level 2					

Task	Never done	With assistance	Little assistance	Regularly done	What evidence to support range
Work with others as part of a team *Levels 1 & 2*					
Improve your personal effectiveness within your job-role *Level 1*					
Maintain personal health, hygiene and appearance *Levels 1 & 2*					
Operate safely in the salon *Levels 1 & 2*					
Set hair to achieve a variety of looks *Level 2*					
Dress out set hair *Level 2*					
Dress long hair into style *Level 2*					
Cut facial hair into shape *Level 2*					
Cut hair to achieve a variety of one length looks *Level 2*					

Task	Never done	With assistance	Little assistance	Regularly done	What evidence to support range
Cut hair to achieve a variety of layered looks Level 2					
Remove hair by shaving Level 2					
Provide face massage Level 2					
Cut hair using barbering techniques Level 2					

Index